Public Health and the American State

PUBLIC HEALTH AND
THE AMERICAN STATE

Edited by Gaetano Di Tommaso, Dario Fazzi and
Giles Scott-Smith

EDINBURGH
University Press

Edinburgh University Press is one of the leading university presses in the UK. We publish academic books and journals in our selected subject areas across the humanities and social sciences, combining cutting-edge scholarship with high editorial and production values to produce academic works of lasting importance. For more information visit our website: edinburghuniversitypress.com

Edinburgh University Press Ltd
The Tun – Holyrood Road
12(2f) Jackson's Entry
Edinburgh EH8 8PJ

Typeset in 11/13 Sabon by
IDSUK (DataConnection) Ltd, and
printed and bound in Great Britain

A CIP record for this book is available from the British Library

ISBN 978 1 3995 1933 5 (hardback)
ISBN 978 1 3995 1935 9 (webready PDF)
ISBN 978 1 3995 1936 6 (epub)

Contents

Illustrations

Notes on Contributors

Nancy K. Bristow is Professor of History at the University of Puget Sound, Tacoma, WA. She pursues research and teaching in the area of twentieth-century American history, with an emphasis on race and social change. She is currently researching state-sanctioned violence against African Americans in the Black Power era of the late 1960s and early 1970s.

Jonathan Chilcote is Assistant Professor of History at Florida College, where he teaches courses in American history and Western Civilization. He earned his PhD at the University of Kentucky, specialising in US foreign relations, transnational history and pandemics.

Kerri Culhane is an architectural historian whose experience spans twenty years of professional historic preservation and planning practice, ranging from restoration of individual buildings to landscape-scale planning and sustainable development projects.

Emma Day is Research Associate at the Rothermere American Institute at University of Oxford. An historian of the twentieth-century United States, she has a particular focus on the histories of sexuality, gender, race and activism.

Gaetano Di Tommaso is a Postdoctoral Researcher at the Roosevelt Institute for American Studies, Middelburg, The Netherlands. His research focuses on the role of natural resources in US history. He is interested in how US extraction and use of specific raw materials, especially fossil fuels, have impacted life and politics on different scales, from local environments and communities to global ecosystems.

Dario Fazzi is Professor in Transatlantic and Environmental History at Leiden University and the Roosevelt Institute for American Studies, Middelburg, The Netherlands. His research focuses on the interplay between US social and foreign policy history. In particular, he is interested in the impact of public intellectuals and social movements on US Cold War relations.

Yifei Li is a doctoral candidate at University College London. Her research project explores the processes of policy feedback through a case study of Medicare, a major public health insurance programme for the elderly in the United States.

Richard M Mizelle, Jr. is Associate Professor of History at the University of Houston, Texas. His research, writing and lecturing focuses on the history of race and healthcare politics, chronic disease, environmental health, and the historical connections between gender, identity and ethnicity in medicine.

Stefano Morello is a doctoral candidate in English at the Graduate Center and a Teaching Fellow at Queens College, City University of New York. His academic interests include American Studies, poetics, popular culture, modern and contemporary American literature, queer theory and transnational screen cultures.

Bob H. Reinhardt is Assistant Professor in the History Department of Boise State University, Idaho. Prior to coming to Boise State, he served as Executive Director of the Willamette Heritage Center, a 5-acre museum in Salem, Oregon. He also coordinates the department's internship programme and is the director of Boise State's Working History Center.

Naomi Rogers is Professor of the History of Medicine in the Section of the History of Medicine at the Yale Medical School and in Yale University's Program in the History of Science and Medicine, with courtesy appointments in the History Department and the Women's, Gender and Sexuality Studies Program. Her historical interests include gender and health; disease and public health; disability; medicine and film; and alternative medicine/CAM.

Giles Scott-Smith is Professor of Transnational Relations and New Diplomatic History at Leiden University, The Netherlands, and is Dean of Leiden University College. Research interests involve a broad exploration of the multiple forms of diplomacy in international history, with specific attention given to investigating the 'Transnational Transatlantic' – tracking and explaining the governmental and non-governmental linkages that have bound North America and Europe since the Second World War.

Sarah B. Snyder is a Professor at the American University School of International Service, Washington, DC, specialising in Cold War history and human rights activism. Her award-winning work explores the influences of the 1960s social movements on US human rights policy and the impact of human rights advocacy on the end of the Cold War.

Olga Thierbach-McLean is an independent scholar, journalist, musician and literary translator. After studying North American literature, Russian literature and musicology at the University of California Berkeley and the University of Hamburg, she earned her doctorate in American Studies at the latter. She is the author of various articles on US political culture, as well as the book *Emersonian Nation* which traces the resonance of Emersonian individualism in current US discourses on personal rights and social reform.

Introduction

Gaetano Di Tommaso, Dario Fazzi and
Giles Scott-Smith

Providing affordable, accessible and effective healthcare services to the highest number of people has been one of the main challenges of modern societies. Countries across the globe have tried to address the issue in various ways, often by adopting policies and frameworks very different from each other, mirroring the discrepancies in the structure and ideology of their political regimes. The result has been a patchwork of approaches to healthcare research, delivery and reform. Particularly for democracies, improving and ensuring access to quality healthcare – a key dimension of the UN Human Development Index – has been a defining struggle that governments have not always won.[1]

This is also true for the United States, where debates about access to public health have been fierce and highly consequential for social change, and where life expectancy has recently seen the biggest drop in a century amid a deep economic and institutional crisis.[2] The difficulties in managing the COVID-19 pandemic, which caused over 1 million deaths in the United States, are the main reasons for this dramatic fall, but not the only ones. Drug overdoses – driven mainly by the opioid epidemic that has engulfed the country – are the second leading cause of decreased life expectancy and are evidence of another recent, major public health failure.[3] Meanwhile, diseases long considered eradicated, such as polio, have made a dire comeback in states like New York.[4]

These developments demonstrate how complex and multifaceted health governance is and how difficult it remains, even today, to address public health challenges effectively, even for a state like the United States, whose resources, reach and ambitions have grown immensely during the last century. The chapters presented in this volume explore Washington's attempts to take up the daunting task of ensuring people's well-being from a historical perspective. They explain how US public health policy has been deeply intertwined with the evolution of the American state, its federal structure, its domestic and international politics, and its socio-cultural and economic relations.

Through a series of topical and chronologically ordered essays, the book discusses the relationship between the changing nature of public health and the evolution of American power over the past century. More specifically, it addresses how the emergence and proliferation of concerns over the health and safety of the US population since the early twentieth century have transformed American governance and interacted with the ever-expanding role and action of the federal government – at home and abroad. Two pandemics, the Spanish 'flu in 1918–1920 and the outbreak of COVID-19 in 2019–2021, vividly provide the temporal boundaries for analysing the choices made by the US government – the responsibilities, policies and opportunities taken, along with those evaded, rejected or missed by Washington – in its attempt to face health threats within the country and in the rest of the world. The concept of public health and the implementation of public health measures are therefore critically examined here in connection with the growth of American power during a period in which the latter went through a series of profound transformations involving its institutional framework as well as its foreign entanglements.

In 1941, Henry Luce pointed to the advent of an era of US ascendancy that he famously labelled the 'American Century'. At the time, Luce saw the world as already profoundly influenced, if not dominated, by US economic weight, industrial capacity and cultural production. The expression, therefore, was meant to encapsulate a reality already favourable to American interests as much as to inspire a vision for the future, where the United States would further project its power on a global scale. Luce aimed to rally domestic support for US intervention in the Second World War and advocate for Washington's global leadership; behind his effort was the conviction that American hegemony – the quintessential element of the American Century – would result in a democratic and open world order organised around liberal-capitalist principles.[5]

Such an international system did materialise in the second half of the twentieth century, although it tragically failed to live up to its original promises in many respects. In the last couple of decades, scholars, commentators and politicians have debated whether the era of US supremacy has reached an end. Instead of providing a definitive answer to that question, this volume investigates what a century of US power has meant for the understanding, development, and implementation of public health policies within and outside the nation. In other words, the chapters use the 'American Century' as a theme to critically examine the changing importance of state power and state–market relations for the provision of social welfare in the United States. This means that the 'century' is approached in two ways. First, it designates a broad hundred years bracketed by the Spanish 'flu and the COVID-19 pandemics. Secondly, and more conceptually, it is used to track the policies and political will of the US federal government to secure a 'safe society' through the eradication of threats to public health. This is treating the idea of the 'American Century' more in the guise of its original usage by Henry Luce – a call for the United States to assert leadership as a superpower of 'humanitarian capitalism'. The 1918–2021 spread between global pandemics, therefore, provides a neat century-long frame for the second use of the 'American Century' as a metaphor for exploring US political ambitions and civilian expectations.

The historical analysis revolves around two issues that the authors address through different case studies. On the one hand, the contributors try to understand to what extent public health has represented a challenge in the projection of American power and, simultaneously, an opportunity for its growth. Safeguarding people's health and safety determined a net expansion of the breadth and scope of the US federal government as well as a profound rethinking of its relationship with citizens, state legislatures and other nations. On the other hand, the chapters in this collection expound how the ideals, values and principles that characterised the American experiment in the last century – individualism, progressivism, militarism, free enterprise, consumerism and racial hierarchy – have shaped the quest for common and effective responses to public health threats and diseases.[6] By following the path of American public health policy and discourse during the American Century, the book shows how issues of epidemiology, sanitation and toxic contamination, among others, became deeply interwoven with the work of defining and redefining US citizenship and democracy.

Traditional narratives tend to depict the progression of federal healthcare regulations as steady and extensive.[7] As many contributors of this volume acknowledge, public health concerns precipitated the creation of new federal offices and agencies, whose actions enabled the US government to face recurrent threats to the people's health and safety. The strengthening of the federal apparatus has proved to be crucial to overcoming the inefficiencies of or, most simply, the lack of resources in the local systems of prevention and caring.[8] The federal national Public Health Service (PHS) and the many following agencies, like the National Institute of Health (NIH) and the Department of Health and Human Services, have played the fundamental role of mediating between different levels of governance and establishing a shared, all-American approach to healthcare. Such a result stemmed from the transformation of the early sanitary system of late colonial times and the early republic years, when public health issues were managed by local boards or left to the initiative of individual trail-blazers, into a modern and much more complex field of public policy.[9]

However, the chapters in this volume indicate that public health development and reform did not follow a linear path and represented a highly contested process. The approach helps to problematise the growth of the federal state – its structural changes at home and its interactions with the rest of the world – and provides an original way of looking at the connection between public health, citizens' rights and American power. The current structure of public health management, while centring on the federal government, represents a multifaceted institutional arrangement combining various levels of public governance and powerful private actors. Such a system is the result of complex historical processes shaped by the interactions between competing political, social and economic interests – and needs. The continuous negotiations between these colliding parties inevitably led to the acceptance of suboptimal compromises and unbalanced outcomes on multiple occasions during the last century. Most contributors to this collection have highlighted those trade-offs, arguing that the expansion of federal competencies in matters relating to public health has naturally replicated the shortcomings – and thus contributed to perpetuating the flaws – of a markedly unequal, individualist and fragmented social system. The contradictions that accompanied the institutionalisation of public health in the Unted States have hindered, at times, the country's ability to deal with health crises efficiently. Furthermore, the tensions and contradictions that characterised the engineering of a national – and possibly global – American approach to people's well-being are what the authors of this volume found most interesting when analysing the connection between the growth of US power and the development of public health in the United States.

The existing literature concerning the evolution of public health in the United States mainly follows the development of the field, focusing on scientific and medical advances, the proliferation and expansion of healthcare institutions, and the consequences of improved healthcare access and services.[10] This volume, instead, takes a different approach, shedding new light on four interconnected themes or patterns. These issues emerge as elements of continuity in the analysis that the chapters provide on the dynamics that determined federally coordinated responses to public health challenges in the last century.

The first is the ever-present and, at times, overwhelming influence of economic and military interests. Since the late nineteenth century, the growth of American power went hand in hand with that of commercial and defence industries. Their perceived importance, which is to say, the high value attached to attaining specific industrial and security goals, deeply affected how the country identified and addressed public health threats. Business and security interests acted as powerful elements in formulating and implementing federal policies, factoring in, if not determining, how the federal government allocated funds, what resources were available, and what incentives were used.[11] As happened in many other fields, the presence of these actors led to the establishment of an inextricable and interdependent relationship between the public and the private sector. Over time, private investments and initiatives have become an inherent and inescapable component of the US public health system.

The second point, closely related to the first, is the interchange of functions and resources between public and private operators that has marked the very functioning of the American public health system. Private entities, like foundations, civil society organisations and commercial enterprises, have been crucial in the very administering of public health in the United States. On the one hand, such a partnership has guaranteed an inflow of funds for research and development; it has pushed the country to the forefront of pharmaceutical science and ensured that the public health machinery did not run short of human capital and material infrastructure. On the other hand, however, it has also led to the commodification and privatisation of public health, according to a quintessentially American model, infused with capitalist, individualist (and predominantly masculine, as Olga Thierbach-McLean (Chapter 12) and Emma Day (Chapter 10) demonstrate in their chapters) values and norms, which the country has tried to frame as a universal standard of efficiency.[12]

The third common theme or element emerging from the following chapters is the relevance of public health crises as political and social battlegrounds. More specifically, one of the main arguments in this volume is that federal public health policies and programmes, and how these have been enacted, have played a role in the constant mediation and renegotiation of American citizenship. The lack of universality is a defining feature of the American public health system. Indeed, its formulation and institutionalisation has mirrored the racial divisions at the very basis of US society. In some cases, the expansion of public health services has followed patterns of (violent) assimilation or segregation meant to assuage the fears of the White American population while leaving other citizens outside the light cone.[13] The analyses presented here help to contextualise such dynamics in the twentieth century and amid the long civil rights struggles that characterised it. The chapters show how public health has become contested ground, an arena where the process of progressive expansion of legal rights and civil liberties has been tested. Therefore, they show how public health programmes and practices became not only a tool for the expansion of federal power, but also another manifestation of its limits and innermost contradictions.[14]

The fourth theme, which further problematises the expansion of US power vis-à-vis the emergence of public health concerns and demands, is politicisation. Public health programmes and policies were also caught in the ideological crossfire as partisanship grew in the United States. They became a target of political opportunism and fuel for the fire of internal divisiveness. The rising level of polarisation in the country effectively turned disagreement over public health issues, typical of democratic countries, into hostility and conflict, as evidenced by the highly contentious management of the COVID-19 pandemic. The result has been the dissolution of a shared idea – or ideal – of the common good and a higher degree of disengagement by the federal government from the management of public health in the United States. The weaponisation of public health has worked against the expansion of public healthcare and has forced a constant renegotiation of its principles and application. In this regard, this volume helps to understand how deep are the historical roots of this process.[15]

While addressing these four broad themes, the chapters in this volume also help to place a fresh emphasis on the connection between public health and the projection of American power abroad, furthering the understanding of public health as a vector of the expansion of American hegemony worldwide.[16] Indeed, public health science and practices remained vital components of American ascendancy throughout the twentieth century. In the interwar years, the initiative was left mainly in the hands of private entrepreneurs, who worked to distribute the benefits of American scientific and technological advancements and, by doing so, ended up promoting the primacy of American medicine. During the Cold War, healthcare became part of the international fight against Communism; yet, as Sarah Snyder shows (Chapter 9), it was also instrumental in strengthening and disseminating the precepts of American liberalism. The investment in creating a global 'Great Society' was as much an outward projection of domestic transformations as a function of the consolidation of American ascendancy.[17]

The volume maintains an interdisciplinary and polycentric approach that aims to connect political history with the history of medicine, diplomatic history, environmental history and socio-economic history. Such a perspective allows us to see how, through crisis after crisis, the US healthcare institutions have renegotiated their shape and purpose, adapting and responding to the simultaneous modifications taking place in US politics and society. To highlight this tortuous trajectory, the chapters are arranged according to a broadly chronological framework, charting the rising importance of public health as a responsibility of the US government and, ultimately, as a litmus test for the functioning of American democracy.

Jonathan Chilcote (Chapter 1), shows how the Spanish influenza epidemic reshuffled the relationship between public health and the federal government in the United States. While federal supervision over public health had been growing prior to the influenza epidemic, this chapter argues that the congressional appropriation to combat it marked a critical turning point in the evolution of public health and its acceptance as a necessary and vital function of the federal government. In Chapter 2, Nancy Bristow enters into a conversation with Chilcote's argument, highlighting Washington's shortcomings in moments of national emergency instead. In doing that, Bristow draws an interesting parallel between the experience of the COVID-19 pandemic and that of 1918, calling attention, among other things, to the inequitable distribution of psychological trauma and loss that constituted one of the central features of both public health crises.

In Chapter 3, Naomi Rogers follows the story of polio and its eradication to discuss critical issues in US public health crises, such as the role of political leadership, the importance of scientific expertise, the emergence of social divisions and scepticism towards public authorities. Rogers identifies the presence of socio-economic and regional inequalities in access to healthcare in her case study, confirming the existence of a recurring problem in US health governance. Indeed, discrimination and disease politicisation are also visible in Chapter 4 in which Stefano Morello and Kerri Culhane demonstrate that the dynamics at play during the COVID-19 pandemic echoed long-standing patterns of racial exclusion and migrants' stigmatisation.

The framework of the long Progressive Era is also the backdrop against which Gaetano Di Tommaso (Chapter 5) explores the intersection of oil, modernity and public health in the United States. Di Tommaso analyses the early struggles to balance progress and people's safety. His chapter explores the role of the federal government in managing the evolving and often conflicting needs of economic prowess and public health by focusing on two separate but connected issues: the controversy surrounding the introduction of leaded gasoline in the early 1920s and the public reaction to the mounting evidence of oil contamination of US water bodies and coastal regions. Richard Mizelle (Chapter 6) continues the exploration of the legacies of the long Progressive Era by looking at the tragic history of medical racism and segregation in the United States. Mizelle illustrates how the colour line affected – slowed down, in fact – the democratisation of public health in the United States. He links the struggle to expand civil rights with that to guarantee access to healthcare for American minorities. The chapter discusses the clashes, confrontations and, not coincidentally, crucial litigations that characterised both paths to equality.

Dario Fazzi (Chapter 7) shifts the volume's focus and brings in the national security dimension. Fazzi's chapter analyses the early Cold War's impact on medical research by looking at the early 1950s nuclear fallout debate. Despite people's growing anxiety over nuclear radioactivity and the concerns of several American medical professionals, the federal Atomic Energy Commission greenlighted the expansion of the US nuclear programme, ending up heralding the subordination of public health to national security. The following two chapters by Bob Reinhardt (Chapter 8) and Sarah Snyder (Chapter 9) continue to explore the domestic–foreign policy linkage in public health during the second half of the twentieth century. Their work shows how healthcare became a field of soft power confrontation as the Cold War developed. In the 1960s, in particular, the United States engaged in efforts to globalise public health through either federal action or private initiatives – or a combination of the two – as part of a broader humanitarian and development effort.

In Chapter 10, Emma Day further problematises the picture of the US government's involvement in public health by focusing on the AIDS epidemic of the 1980s. Day shows how HIV testing in the 1980s became interwoven with structural inequalities beyond homophobia, including the struggle over abortion and reproductive rights in an era of conservative backlash. The chapter argues that the official response to the epidemic used AIDS as a wedge to expand power over women's bodies and contributed to the devaluation of women's right to motherhood. According to Day, the HIV-AIDS epidemic drew a line between those who, for the US government, deserved support and those who did not. The redefinition of the idea of the 'public', and the process of healthcare commodification that accompanied it are also central in Yifei Li's chapter (Chapter 11), which describes how the US healthcare system became largely dominated by private interests and market-oriented strategies in the last part of the twentieth century. In Chapter 12, Olga Thierbach-McLean also looks into the socio-cultural components that came to define US healthcare policy. She explains that the ideological tensions over the national response to the COVID-19 pandemic, usually attributed to the polarising and inconsistent messaging of the Trump administration, are better understood as the result of a much broader and more profound intellectual tradition of individualism and masculinity.

The book's Conclusion assesses the historical legacies of public health policies in the United States. As an autonomous field of public policy, as a political objective and as a catalyst of socio-economic inequality, healthcare has tested the core principles of the American Century, that is, the cooperation between the market and the state and the construction of a democratic society despite deep fractures along the lines of race, gender and class. Overall, the historical trajectory of public health in the United States reveals that the federal government has been primarily reactive and exclusionary in providing access to effective and affordable health services. However, the chapters presented in this volume also provide several examples of comprehensive, expansive reforms and struggles for global inclusivity. How the US government will manage these two opposing tendencies, and overcome the system's long-standing limits and contradictions, will represent one of the main litmus tests for the functioning and continuous appeal of US democracy worldwide.

Notes

1. Niels Lind, 'A Development of the Human Development Index', *Social Indicator Research* 46 (2019), 409–23.
2. 'Life Expectancy at Birth, Total for the United States', *FRED*, 3 May 2022, available at: https://fred.stlouisfed.org/series/SPDYNLE00INUSA, accessed on November 17, 2022. Robert H. Shmerling, "Why life expectancy in the US is falling," *Harvard Health Publishing*, October 20, 2022, online at https://www.health.harvard.edu/blog/why-life-expectancy-in-the-us-is-falling-202210202835, last accessed 17 November 2022.
3. 'Drug Overdose Deaths Remain High', US Center for Disease Control and Prevention, available at: https://www.cdc.gov/drugoverdose/deaths/index.html, last accessed 17 November 2022.
4. 'Why Polio, Once Eliminated, is Testing NY Health Officials', *New York Times*, 3 October 2022, available at: https://www.nytimes.com/2022/10/03/nyregion/polio-new-york-eradication.html, last accessed 17 November 2022.
5. Andrew J. Bacevich, 'Life at the Dawn of the American Century', in Andrew J. Bacevich (ed.), *The Short American Century: A Postmortem* (Cambridge, MA: Harvard University Press, 2012), 1–14.
6. Natalia Molina, *Fit to Be Citizens? Public Health and Race in Los Angeles, 1879–1939* (Berkeley: University of California Press, 2006).

7. J. Kim, 'Development of Public Health in America: "Guaranteed Issue" Mandates', *Journal of Public Health* 39:3 (2017), 433–39; Christopher Hamlin, 'The History and Development of Public Health in Developed Countries', in Roger Detels et al. (eds), *Oxford Textbook of Global Public Health*, 7th edn (New York: Oxford University Press, 2021).
8. Fitzhugh Mullan, *Plagues and Politics: The Story of the United States Public Health Service* (New York: Basic Books, 1989).
9. Bernard Turnock, *Public Health What It Is and How It Works*, 6th edn (Burlington, MA: Jones & Bartlett Learning, 2015).
10. John Duffy, *The Sanitarians: A History of American Public Health* (Champaign: University of Illinois Press, 1992); George Rosen, *A History of Public Health* (Baltimore, MD: Johns Hopkins University Press, 2015).
11. Bill Frist, 'Public Health and National Security: The Critical Role of Increased Federal Support', *Health Affairs* 21:6 (2002), 117–30; Jennifer Brower and Peter Chalk, *The Global Threat of New and Reemerging Infectious Diseases: Reconciling US National Security and Public Health Policy* (Santa Monica, CA: RAND, 2003); Colin McInnes and Kelley Lee, 'Health, Security and Foreign Policy', *Review of International Studies* 32:1 (2006), 5–23.
12. Daniel S. Goldberg, 'Social Justice, Health Inequalities and Methodological Individualism in US Health Promotion', *Public Health Ethics* 5:2 (2012), 104–15.
13. For example, several studies on the expansion of public health services to Native American communities during the long process of nation – or empire – building of the United States have shown the many reverberations and heavy toll of such a process. See, among others, Tara Watson, 'Public Health Investments and the Infant Mortality Gap: Evidence from Federal Sanitation Interventions on US Indian Reservations', *Journal of Public Economics* 90:8/9 (2006), 1537–60.
14. Nayan Shah, *Contagious Divides: Epidemics and Race in San Francisco's Chinatown* (Berkeley: University of California Press, 2001); Molina, *Fit to Be Citizens?*
15. Lawrence O. Gostin, 'Language, Science, and Politics: The Politicization of Public Health', *Journal of the American Medical Association* 319:6 (2018), 541–2.
16. Matthew Connelly, 'The Cold War in the Longue Durée: Global Migration, Public Health, and Population Control', in Melvyn P. Leffler and Odd Arne Westad (eds), *The Cambridge History of the Cold War, vol. 3: Endings* (New York: Cambridge University Press, 2010), 466–87.
17. Erez Manela, 'A Pox on Your Narrative: Writing Disease Control into Cold War History', *Diplomatic History* 34:2 (2010), 299–323; Daniel Tarantola, 'A Perspective on the History of Health and Human Rights: From the Cold War to the Gold War', *Journal of Public Health Policy* 29 (2008), 42–53.

1

Beyond Control of Local Authorities: The Spanish Influenza Epidemic and Federal Supervision of Public Health

Jonathan Chilcote

'We have gone to the rescue frequently in the case of floods and other visitations which were local . . . but I think in this case the work is national and affects the welfare of the war work as well as the welfare of the part of the country where the scourge is raging most severely.'[1] This statement from Senator Henry Cabot Lodge of Massachusetts came in September 1918 as Congress discussed the rapidly spreading Spanish influenza epidemic. The epidemic presented a crisis for the United States. Beyond its effects on the lives of millions of Americans, the virus threatened the federal government's power. Because the epidemic's effects were too expansive for the existing public health structure to handle, the epidemic had the potential to severely disrupt the war effort in Europe and hamper the ability of industry to supply needed war materials. Not only was influenza devastating to human life, but also its enhanced destructive power during wartime was alarming to Cabot Lodge and other elected officials.

As Congress surveyed the US response to Spanish influenza in late September, it recognised how quickly the epidemic had overwhelmed the ability of state and local governments to cope. Tens of thousands of cases were reported in major cities, but while local authorities closed schools, businesses and attempted other methods of slowing the spread of the disease, nothing worked. The number of those sick, hospitalised and dying spiralled upward. State and local government health boards were similarly helpless in their efforts to stop the epidemic or to treat those already sick, and even when they pooled their resources, the government entities were unable to combat an epidemic of the magnitude of Spanish influenza.

The epidemic also wreaked havoc in the military. Thousands of soldiers at camps inside the United States lay suffering or dead, with similar situations on Atlantic transport ships and among the American

Expeditionary Force (AEF) in France.[2] On 26 September, just as the AEF began the Meuse-Argonne offensive, the AEF Provost Marshal General cancelled draft calls for new recruits.[3] The outbreaks in camps and facilities were so devastating that the US military could not risk exposing more personnel to influenza, and they temporarily halted new soldier training. Not only did influenza threaten those already in the military, but also the ability of the US government to supply and transport healthy reinforcements as it began its largest offensive since the Civil War.

Industrial war work was similarly threatened. Labour shortages because of sickness were reported across the country, including thousands of workers at key production facilities and munitions' factories. While many were unable to work, others stayed home for fear of catching influenza. This virus significantly hindered production in the United States just as the country displayed its industrial and military capacity to the world. The presence and pervasiveness of Spanish influenza threatened both the military and industrial power of the United States and drove Congress to action.

The epidemic pushes Congress

These forces – the inability of state and local institutions to counter the disease, and the threat to military and industrial efforts – pushed Congress to action on 28 September 1918. Citing the devastating capabilities of Spanish influenza on the military and industry, and the reality that influenza was beyond the ability of state and local health authorities to control, Congress hastily passed a unanimous resolution appropriating $1 million to suppress the disease by coordinating public health efforts among the three levels of American government.[4] Under the plan, Congress called on the federal government and its primary public health arm, the US Public Health Service (PHS), to provide leadership and administration for the effort. Until that point the PHS cared for seamen, enforced quarantines, inspected immigrants, conducted research, led sanitation drives and, beginning in 1917, protected public health around domestic military installations. But this was a new role for Congress and the PHS; while Congress annually appropriated money to an 'epidemic fund' on which the PHS could draw to target various outbreaks in various locations, this resolution ordered a national campaign against a specific disease.[5]

While, in hindsight, Spanish influenza did not catastrophically disrupt the US military effort or its industrial capacity during the First World War, the epidemic nonetheless forever transformed American public health. The congressional resolution gave the PHS new statutory authority and resources and presented an opportunity for federal oversight to grow. In its suppression efforts, the PHS assumed leadership over state and local public health efforts and entrenched federal supervision of public health.[6] Health officials, across all levels, established trust between each other and in the efficacy of federal leadership. The epidemic established the credibility of the federal government to oversee coordinated responses of public health matters.

The federal government, as well as state and local governments and many private citizens, believed that public health coordination was vital to national interests and was clearly a federal responsibility. The cooperative model created during the epidemic characterised governmental public health work during the American Century. The federal government became the more dominant partner in the federal–state–local public health structure because of the epidemic, but federalism and the needed cooperation of state, local and private health agencies constrained its overall authority. The success of federal intervention in the suppression of the Spanish influenza epidemic, then, marks a critical turning point in the centralisation and expansion of federal power through the PHS, but the PHS remained limited by its need to work with other public health actors.

Growing, but disorganised: public health work to 1918

In the early twentieth century, American public health efforts were largely split between the federal government and those of states and local areas. The PHS originated with the Marine Health Service (MHS) in 1798 and operated under the Treasury Department, tasked with the care of American seamen. The MHS spent much of the nineteenth century in those efforts, but after the Civil War, the service expanded as the United States did, establishing hospitals and facilities for seamen along waterways and ports. As such, the MHS became the only health organisation with a national reach, even though the service was disorganised and primarily concentrated along the Atlantic and Pacific coasts.[7] Because federal police power over public health matters is not enumerated in the Constitution, under the Tenth Amendment almost all other public health concerns were left to states. State and local governments were the source of most health actions, including safety measures and quarantines.[8]

Beginning in the 1870s the duties of the MHS expanded. The agency provided doctors and federal assistance to states when epidemics of select diseases struck, such as yellow fever and the plague.[9] States lacked the health infrastructure to deal with such outbreaks and, when asked by the states, the MHS provided coordination and resources. As the MHS became more involved in the inspection of immigrants arriving in the United States, and with increasing scrutiny on the introduction of disease from abroad, the Quarantine Act was passed in 1893. The Act placed authority for operating quarantines with the federal officials, taking away responsibility from individual states. In 1902, the Marine Health Service was renamed by Congress as the Public Health and Marine Hospital Service and its head, the surgeon general, was granted the ability to call conferences with state and territorial health officers to promote public health. This ensured the existence of at least a small level of cooperation between the federal and state levels of health officials at the beginning the twentieth century.[10]

At the end of the nineteenth century the federal government confined its health activities to caring for specific groups, conducting international health relations and scientific research, overseeing interstate and intragovernmental relations, and providing health information to the public. These duties, however, were often more potential than actual, especially in dealing with interstate and intragovernmental issues.[11] Even as the difficulties of urbanisation, industrialisation and the bacteriological revolution stimulated health work across all levels of government, the PHS could not overawe other public health agencies. Although the PHS had the power to request that state officials meet in conferences, state officials could not be compelled to attend or cooperate.[12] State public health agencies were still entrusted with most health work based on the American system of federalism, which divides power between states and the federal government. In that division the police power over health and sanitation issues fell to states, and only in matters of interstate concern could the federal government exercise jurisdiction. In most instances, only when states failed noticeably did the federal government perform such oversight.[13] Most aspects of public health work practiced in the late nineteenth and early twentieth centuries were deemed as the proper jurisdiction of states and local governments, rather than a federal responsibility.

The Progressive Era increased the level of federal control over the nation's health in many areas yet left state and local boards of health with wide independence. By 1902, forty-five states had established state boards of health. As the medical industry became more institutionalised and professional, advances in bacteriology changed research, leading state legislatures to appropriate funds to deal with endemic issues within their borders.[14] Local governments similarly created health departments – often at the behest of state governments – to cope with local issues, such as rural sanitation in less-populated areas or outbreaks of typhoid fever in major cities.[15] These boards, both state and local, were frequently weak and ineffective. Some states, because of a lack of respect for the value of public health (and therefore a lack of allocated funding), prevented their health boards from doing anything beyond encouraging local officials to inform the public of medical advancements. Other state boards found that local counterparts ignored their orders or refused even to form boards or register vital statistics. When outbreaks of disease did occur, at times state legislatures refused to allocate extra money to state health boards for suppression. While some states made progress in public health, many others were wholly unprepared for health crises.[16]

The quest for efficiency

Public health workers, across all levels, shared the same goal of promoting and protecting health. Although jurisdictional lines made complete cooperation difficult, by the early twentieth century state boards of health and the PHS were coordinating in select initiatives, such as rural sanitation and educational campaigns. Because they had more resources and expertise, the PHS often took the lead.[17] But the goodwill between federal, state and local health officials was not a firm foundation on which to build. While all health officials might have the same goals, their methods of attaining them could be very different. State and local officials might hamper federal initiatives if they objected to federal oversight, and state legislatures could refuse to appropriate funds to their own health boards if state health authorities could not persuade their legislatures to provide extra financial support. While the federal government had the ability to accomplish some health work on its own, without the trust and willing cooperation of state and local health officials, there was little chance of successfully integrating all public health officials into one empowered organisation.[18]

The necessity for federal–state–local coordination led to calls for centralised public health efforts, and, perhaps, a new federal agency to oversee health concerns for federal government and the entire nation.[19] While the PHS was the most prominent of the federal health agencies, it was just one of several health groups operating under different cabinet departments, creating an overlap of duties and questions of ultimate authority.[20] In 1906, Progressive reformers organised a committee to pressure the federal government to consolidate its health functions into one body, arguing that healthcare was a national concern and resource, and needed to be under the jurisdiction of one department run by experts so as to increase efficiency.[21] In 1908, both major political parties incorporated calls for a unified health bureau into their election-year platforms, although both parties recognised that even a national health agency should not interfere with the jurisdictions of state health authorities.[22]

Within four years at least thirteen bills calling for a national health department were introduced into Congress, but such a department was never created. In 1910, a bill providing for the creation of a department of public health was introduced, which would control all the federal agencies involved in any public health work.[23] While reformers backed the changes, critics came out strongly against them. Critics included those opposed to vaccinations, vivisections and purveyors of patent medicine who rejected government oversight of healthcare. They were joined in opposition by members of Congress concerned about federalism and threats to individual liberties and privacy. Oddly enough, one of the most determined opponents was the surgeon general of the PHS at the time, Walter Wyman. Wyman feared that such a national organisation would absorb the PHS and decrease its prominence, and he worked to scuttle the bill. He died a short time later, and Congress, hesitant to approve controversial legislation, instead passed a watered-down public health bill in 1912. The new bill increased the authority of the PHS yet stopped short of creating a national health agency.[24] Many viewed this new bill as a compromise between those who advocated for the creation of a new federal department of health, and those who opposed the bill as a violation of individual rights.[25]

The 1912 legislation changed the nature of the PHS, but not its overall priorities. The PHS was granted authority to investigate diseases without state and local cooperation, if necessary, and to fund increased research. As new Surgeon General Rupert Blue noted, the law recognised 'the Public Health Service as the central health agency of the Nation'.[26] The legislation did not, though, completely reorganise federal health activities and Blue, with an accomplished background working with state and local health officials in campaigns against yellow fever and plague, chose to increase the level of cooperation with boards of health, rather than attempt to push the limits of PHS and federal authority to control state and local work.[27] Without federal coercion, state and local boards of health continued to operate with a great deal of autonomy and focused on local issues, working with the PHS only when such efforts suited them. While many public health officials desired a more coordinated approach, the PHS could only hope for voluntary cooperation and mainly devoted its efforts to laboratory research, health and hygiene campaigns, and investigating endemic diseases in the American South, particularly hookworm, trachoma and pellagra.[28]

The inadequate response

The semi-autonomous relationships among governmental public health agencies were challenged when the United States officially entered the First World War in April 1917. The PHS was quickly tasked with constructing public health systems around military posts. The agency enjoyed robust appropriations throughout the summer of 1918, but nearly all the money and PHS doctors and nurses were focused in the areas immediately surrounding military installations.[29] With patriotic spirit running high, state and local boards of health saw many of their trained medical personnel volunteer for military assignments, leaving a dearth of doctors and nurses throughout much of the country. This deficiency left state and local boards unprepared for even normal wartime work and helpless in the face of an epidemic.

When the Spanish 'flu wreaked its wrath on the United States in autumn 1918, the response of state and local boards of health was woefully inadequate. In Massachusetts alone an estimated 85,000 people contracted influenza in September, far outstripping the capacity of medical personnel and hospitals to treat the sick, let alone protect others.[30] State and local health agencies lacked coordination in their responses, and with few doctors and nurses available, confusion and desperation reigned. Many states, too, had exhausted their annual health funds and their legislatures were not in session to appropriate more.[31] The health boards were without many of the tools needed to fight the disease. Governors, state health commissioners and others frantically pleaded with their federal delegations, the PHS and President Woodrow Wilson to secure resources and assistance.[32] State and local health boards simply could not deal with an epidemic like Spanish influenza. As the *Washington Post* summarised, '[Spanish influenza is] . . . apparently beyond control of local authorities.'[33]

With states and local health efforts floundering, the PHS was similarly unprepared to combat Spanish influenza. The epidemic struck with the PHS staff focused on the health of the armed forces, and the PHS lacked the personnel, plans or administrative organisation to counter a disease that affected so many civilians.[34] The PHS, too, prior to Spanish influenza had been without the authority and resources necessary to coordinate a vigorous and multi-government suppression effort, such as Congress demanded in its September 1918 resolution. But now, because of influenza, Congress expanded the power of the PHS granting it new funding so that it could assume control over and direct the public health responses of states and localities. As Representative Joseph Sherley of Kentucky put it, 'If the physicians in localities are left alone to deal with this situation they will not be able to cope with [the epidemic], and it is believed that the Public Health Service . . . can . . . control it.'[35] One representative stated that 'this disease, like other diseases, knows no State boundaries', and another replied that because the disease was a danger to several states, he would support an expansion of PHS power and resources.[36] The severity and crisis of the influenza epidemic convinced members of Congress that a growth of federal authority, increased financial resources, and the centralisation of public health was justified and necessary.[37] It was not the fear of redundancy in health work that spurred this action, but rather the complete inadequacy of the public health response that ultimately overcame traditional objections to increasing federal supervision.

The PHS takes control

The threat and devastation of Spanish influenza pushed state and local boards of health, despite their prior independence, to willingly embrace federal control. In desperate need of funding and resources, state and local boards actively sought PHS money when it became available on 1 October, and enthusiastically accepted federal direction of their influenza suppression programmes.[38] With calls for help coming in from all over the country, the PHS had installed health directors in each state by 15 October. Since the PHS had a relatively small number of commissioned medical officers, it could not directly care for all the sick and instead created a decentralised system where the PHS integrated state and local health officials into its organisation. To coordinate this effort and to encourage cooperation, many state and local health officials were hired as PHS employees, serving in overlapping roles as federal, state and local directors.[39]

Over the next several months, these new PHS officials allocated aid and oversaw the build-up of PHS personnel and resources in their jurisdictions. In this way the PHS greatly expanded its reach into states and avoided redundancy in its work, while simultaneously securing relationships with grateful boards of health and other medical groups.[40] To locate needed physicians for state work, the PHS in October made appeals to the American Medical Association and the Volunteer Medical Service Corps for the names of physicians in their organisations that could be available for emergency duty. The Red Cross, who already had responsibility for recruiting nurses for the military, aided in the recruitment. With the assistance of the Red Cross and private groups, the PHS effectively staffed severely stricken areas with doctors and nurses during the early weeks of the influenza epidemic. The PHS secured over one thousand physicians and over seven hundred nurses and nurses' aides to meet the needs of states and municipalities.[41]

Through the final months of 1918 state boards of health, flush with PHS resources and assistance, directed medical personnel and supplies to needy districts. To overcome legal issues, physicians who volunteered for emergency influenza duty were appointed by the PHS to state boards of health and were then hired as state employees with legal authority to practice medicine anywhere in the state. These physicians and nurses were paid jointly with state and PHS funds.[42] By the end of the epidemic many public health officials, doctors and nurses were at least partially operating as federal employees.[43] Together, federal and state officials established temporary hospitals funded by the federal government and discussed comprehensive plans for coordinating their efforts and combining resources so they could efficiently educate the public, improve sanitation, care for the sick, and, hopefully, slow the spread of influenza.[44] While all states cooperated in these efforts, those with heavily rural populations – especially in the southern and central parts of the country – enthusiastically worked with the PHS and began, almost immediately, lobbying for a long-term connection between state and federal public health work.[45] These state and local health officials did not resist federal encroachment into their traditional jurisdictions; rather, they freely and eagerly cooperated with the PHS, even as it and the federal government established authority over them.

The PHS also worked closely with the American Red Cross to administer care and guidance when the PHS itself lacked the personnel to oversee certain areas. Just three days after the passage of the congressional resolution, the PHS secured the help of the Red Cross in creating an organised response with a multifaceted plan for combating the epidemic. To aid in oversight and efficiency, a PHS officer was detailed to Red Cross headquarters.[46] The Red Cross agreed to recruit, assemble and pay nurses, rent temporary hospital space for emergency care centres, provide resources for both temporary and permanent hospitals, and create a travelling medical team that could be quickly sent to areas of need.[47] The Red Cross also agreed that the PHS would lead the joint effort and allocate doctors, nurses, Red Cross supplies, and coordinate with all state and local boards of health. Red Cross requests for supplies or money were channelled through the PHS for approval.[48] The Red Cross submitted to PHS leadership, as one official phrased it, 'in order to centralize the efforts in combating the disease'.[49]

The connections between the PHS, state and local health boards, and the Red Cross were necessary because each group was unable to suppress the epidemic on its own. Each relied on the others for something each lacked, whether medical personnel, funding, legal jurisdiction or the infrastructure to administer care and spread information across the country. These working relationships were not created by influenza, but rather enlarged, and all parties recognised that they needed the others to carry on their work and overcome their unique obstacles to combat Spanish 'flu.

Pressures from below

By late October the epidemic had waned. Almost immediately, though, states and municipalities pushed Congress to strengthen the PHS so that future epidemics might be avoided. State legislatures, city councils and private groups sent petitions and resolutions to Congress calling for the federal government and the PHS to investigate diseases and protect the nation from future health crises. In these petitions the interested parties made clear the acceptance of federal control over national public health matters and the expectation that Congress should take the lead in building and supporting the PHS, which, as petitioners noted, had proved its credibility and worth during the influenza epidemic.[50]

The American Public Health Association, made up of public health advocates and workers from all levels of government, met for their annual meeting in December 1918. The group advertised, in advance of the gathering, a special symposium regarding the influenza epidemic and published a list of questions for consideration and discussion. One question demonstrated how the minds of public health officials were already turning towards the future, asking, 'How can we take advantage of the epidemic for the benefit of more adequate health appropriations and better community and personal hygiene?'[51] Across all levels of government for public health workers the question was simple: how could the epidemic lay the foundation for the evolution of, and a long-term national investment in, public health?

The actions of both the state boards and the Red Cross demonstrate how tightly intertwined they were with the PHS. While state board personnel flooded Congress with appeals to build up the PHS, in their private correspondence local officials also pledged their allegiance to the PHS and acknowledged their need for oversight. State board officials also begged for a return of the joint appointments as PHS–state–local health officers as were common during the influenza epidemic.[52] The Red Cross prepared for a re-emergence of influenza in 1919 by copying the cooperative framework it had established with the PHS the year before. Red Cross officials assembled lists of potential nurses, allocated money to pay them, stockpiled medical supplies to give to hospitals and appointed liaison officers with state boards of health to coordinate decisions.[53]

The PHS certainly knew they had an opportunity to push their prominence and campaign for more funding and authority. In August 1919, a Republican senator wrote to Surgeon General Rupert Blue, fearful of a recurrence of influenza during the autumn, wanting to know what steps Blue and the PHS were taking to prepare for another epidemic.[54] Blue responded by touting his agency's organisation and coordination with other public health groups, noting joint preparation for future health crises.[55] The reach of the PHS extended further, though, with Blue stating that local health officers were issued statements covering proper procedures to control influenza. The PHS had, in effect, coordinated public health work across government levels with both state and local officials receiving requests and information from the federal government. While also asking for more funding, Blue attempted to use this integration as evidence that the nation's public health forces were ready to confront another influenza epidemic if it emerged.[56]

Inherent in these interactions were trust, and a recognition that all levels of public health workers needed each other. Those working in each level of government saw the opportunity of working with others – through increased authority and control, or by access to federal grants and appropriations – trusting that they all wanted the same result: a robust national public health infrastructure. Each health entity recognised that their constraints made it impossible for any one group to combat a national epidemic. A common goal and need for cooperation – as evidenced during the influenza epidemic – allowed for an expansion of public health after the influenza epidemic's conclusion.

An expanding role: the PHS after the Spanish 'flu

Even as the 1918 epidemic receded in the nation's consciousness, its seeming end was held up as an example of effective federal coordination of the nation's public health resources and agencies. The PHS had, in many minds, accomplished the goals of protecting the nation's health and limiting the destructive power of disease through its organisational and suppression expertise.[57] The perceived success of the PHS in combatting influenza among the public meant that many now came to see the group as a necessity for the nation's health, and one that needed to be reinforced and properly financed to protect Americans from future epidemics. The public accepted the PHS as a credible and capable federal agency that needed to continue directing the nation's public health efforts. States, local governments and private citizens vigorously petitioned Congress and encouraged the US government to maintain the PHS and give the money and support it required.

Congress agreed with the sentiments and quickly created a reserve corps for the PHS, something it had refused to pass before the epidemic. Congress also entrusted the PHS with the care of returning veterans, a massive expansion of PHS responsibilities.[58] As the size of the PHS grew, many other federal agencies and boards created during the war were abolished. But even as Warren G. Harding was elected president in 1920 on a 'return to normalcy' platform and advocated for economy in government and tax reductions, he made sure to include in that platform a call for a maternity bill that would further increase federal responsibilities, such as funding and supervision, for public health.[59] In 1921, Congress approved such a bill – the Sheppard–Towner Act – and during its debate congressmen justified the growth of federal leadership by citing the effective work done by federal health officials during the influenza epidemic.[60] Once the appropriated money became available, forty states requested grants from the federal government, even though by doing so they explicitly accepted PHS oversight of their maternal health programmes.[61]

The Parker Act also demonstrates how quickly attitudes shifted. First proposed in 1926, the Parker Act called for granting the president the power to transfer almost any executive agency involved in public health to the oversight of the PHS, including all personnel, records and unused appropriations. The Parker Act aimed to reduce the duplication of federal health activities and still maintain the constitutionally defined role of aiding, not controlling, state and local health boards.[62] This Act was remarkably like the failed public health bill introduced in 1910, except that instead of creating a new department of public health which consolidated health work, the PHS effectively now served as the coordinator of all federal health activity with the ability to detail its officers to other health agencies.[63]

During the debate over the proposed Parker Act, health officials and politicians argued that an enlargement of power for the PHS was necessary given the changes that had occurred in society since the turn of the twentieth century. PHS Surgeon General Hugh Cumming testified that as commerce and communication increased there was an increased need for uniformity and coordination in the suppression of epidemics, a duty the federal government had gradually assumed over previous decades. The transportation of people and goods across state lines brought the spread of germs, and the federal government was already involved in scientific research into both the diseases and methods of suppressing them. But the increases in trade and inter-action between people brought a danger; epidemics could spread quicker and be more harmful to the nation's economy and society than ever before.[64] In Cumming's view, as the recognition of danger increased among governmental bodies, each entity attempted to deal with public health issues in its own way, creating confusion and over-lap.[65] Only a singular federal agency, then, was fit to oversee public health work and counter threats which spanned state borders and affected the nation's well-being.

Such problems, especially potential epidemics, allowed for pas-sage of the far-reaching Parker Act. Cumming based his testimony on the belief that new public health issues could be handled only by a unified federal response structure, led by a stronger and more expan-sive PHS. If such an empowered organisation were not available to meet new challenges, the nation's welfare was imperilled.[66] The belief that the federal government was capable of and could handle threats to health – as evidenced by the influenza epidemic – made it clear to lawmakers that they needed to strengthen the PHS to protect the nation's future. The Parker Act represented a massive increase in the power of the PHS, and Cumming and the congressmen he testified to knew it. During questioning, one representative asked of Cum-ming: 'Under the provisions of this bill . . . you would have practi-cally unlimited authority to go ahead – unlimited authorization . . . Is not that true?' Cumming did not avoid the question, answering, 'Pretty nearly, Mr. Chairman.'[67] Cumming's arguments based on the fear of another epidemic were successful; the Parker Act passed both chambers of Congress but was vetoed by Calvin Coolidge in May 1928. Members of both political parties, though, still believed in the bill and in the growth of the PHS and the federal government's role in coordinating public health. The Parker Act was resubmitted dur-ing Herbert Hoover's presidency and signed into law in April 1930.[68]

The new foundation for public health work

The federal government considered itself to be a fundamental part of the citizen–health dynamic, an idea shared by most policymak-ers stretching from the president and Congress to state and local governments. But a unified federal public health response, while important, could not fully protect the nation's health; to be truly effective, health work needed to involve the states and their health boards. Congress addressed this need in the 1935 Social Security Act. While the Parker Act allowed the PHS to coordinate federal public health work, the Social Security Act gave the PHS the authority to construct a firm network of state and local health board cooperation and provided grants to states (if matched by the states) for the development of comprehensive health services. These services operated locally but were aided by the federal government, which also paid for the training of public health employees and funded scientific research. Federal authorities took the lead in the investigation of interstate diseases, provided data and information, and issued advice and administrative guidance. States, in turn, carried out their health work but with the support, information and financial backing of the federal government. This cooperative agreement was necessary because of federalism, and incentivised, rather than forced, states to allocate money for public health because adequate funding was a widespread deficiency during the Great Depression. With this structure the PHS officially served as the senior partner in the federal–state–local health relationship, as state and local boards were permanently placed under the oversight of the PHS and were reliant on its funding for public health programmes.[69]

While the relationship was formally ensconced in 1935, the origin of the federal–state–local health cooperation was the result of the Spanish influenza epidemic. The crisis the epidemic created, coupled with the demands of the war, overcame issues of federalism and congressional objections to an empowered federal public health agency. Congress passed the influenza resolution in September 1918 which forever transformed the structure of US public health. The federal government adapted to its new role as supervisor of public health across state and local boundaries, and both health work, and the nation, were changed. After the epidemic and with the credibility of the PHS entrenched, the federal government put greater emphasis on oversight, funding and coordination of efforts. This new role did not happen immediately or without the support and cooperation of state and local officials. Officials from all levels of government and private citizens eagerly lobbied for the evolution of public health. Previous attempts to achieve such public health centralisation had failed; they were successful after 1918, though, because of the influenza epidemic.

As the United States developed its global role, it recognised that health and national interests overlapped, and that the nation needed healthy citizens at home. Citizen health was threatened by epidemics, which, if left unchecked, could seriously disrupt the power that the

United States wished to project. As the US Congress acted in 1918 to cope with such a threat – the Spanish influenza epidemic – it unknowingly created the conditions which allowed for a more national, cooperative and centralised public health structure to emerge. That power and structure – supervised by the PHS and federal government yet constrained by the continual need for state and local assistance – laid the foundation for public health work during the American Century.

Notes

1. *Prevention of Spanish Influenza*, H. J. Res. 333, 65th Congress, 2nd session, *Congressional Record 56* (28 September 1918): S10896.
2. Carol R. Byerly, *Fever of War: The Influenza Epidemic in the US Army during World War I* (New York: New York University Press, 2005), 105, 113–14.
3. 'Influenza Stops Flow to the Camps of Drafted Men', *New York Times*, 27 September 1918.
4. *Prevention of Spanish Influenza*, H10905–10906.
5. Ralph C. Williams, *The United States Public Health Service, 1798–1950* (Washington, DC: Commissioned Officers Association, 1951), 134. The PHS generally engaged in disease research and targeted specific diseases in specific areas, not national campaigns. Much of the funding from these local campaigns came from private donors, such as the Rockefeller Foundation.
6. Jonathan Chilcote, '"This Disease . . . Knows no State Boundaries": The 1918 Spanish Influenza Epidemic and Federal Public Health', *Federal History* 13 (2021), 37–57.
7. Williams, *United States Public Health Service*, 45–7.
8. John Fabian Witt, *American Contagions: Epidemics and the Law from Smallpox to Covid-19* (New Haven, CT: Yale University Press, 2020), 4–5.
9. Williams, *United States Public Health Service*, 114–24.
10. Fitzhugh Mullan, *Plagues and Politics: The Story of the United States Public Health Service* (New York: Basic Books, 1989), 40, 48.
11. Williams, *United States Public Health Service*, 158–9. Examples of groups that were cared for by the federal government included merchant seamen, the military, Native Americans and those with leprosy.
12. Bess Furman, *A Profile of the United States Public Health Service, 1798–1948* (Washington, DC; GPO, 1973), 249.
13. Williams, *United States Public Health Service*, 158–9.
14. Mullan, *Plagues and Politics*, 48.
15. Williams, *United States Public Health Service*, 139–40.
16. John Duffy, *The Sanitarians: A History of American Public Health* (Urbana: University of Illinois Press, 1990), 152–4.
17. Ibid., 48, 55.
18. Furman, *A Profile of the United States Public Health Service*, 286.

19. Laurence F. Schmeckebier, *The Public Health Service: Its History, Activities and Organization* (Baltimore, MD: Johns Hopkins University Press, 1923), 34–5.
20. Ibid., 32.
21. Mullan, *Plagues and Politics*, 55–6.
22. Schmeckebier, *Profile of the United States Public Health Service*, 33–5.
23. Ibid., 35.
24. Duffy, *The Sanitarians*, 241–2.
25. *Public Health and Marine-Hospital Service*, 62nd Congress, 2nd session, *Congressional Record* 48 (13 August 1912): S10790.
26. Furman, *A Profile of the United States Public Health Service*, 286.
27. Williams, *United States Public Health Service*, 480-1.
28. Mullan, *Plagues and Politics*, 63–8.
29. Ibid., 72.
30. Alfred Crosby, *America's Forgotten Pandemic: The Influenza of 1918* (New York: Cambridge University Press, 2003), 53; 'Boston Joins State in Fighting Grippe', *Boston Globe* (morning edition), 26 September 1918.
31. Williams, *United States Public Health Service*, 602.
32. Crosby, *America's Forgotten Pandemic*, 48.
33. 'Death Rate Shows Large Increase in Army Camps Owing to Spanish Grippe', *Washington Post*, 28 September 1918.
34. Mullan, *Plagues and Politics*, 72.
35. *Prevention of Spanish Influenza*, H10905.
36. Ibid., H10906.
37. Ibid., H10905; Chilcote, '1918 Spanish Influenza Epidemic', 42–4.
38. 'Brief Outline of Activities of the Public Health Service in Combating the Influenza Epidemic: 1918–1919', in 'Influenza Epidemic' Box 145, File 1622, Records of the Public Health Service Central File, 1897–1923, RG 90, NARA College Park.
39. Schmeckebier, *Profile of the United States Public Health Service*, 53.
40. Mullan, *Plagues and Politics*, 74.
41. Williams, *United States Public Health Service*, 599–600.
42. 'Florida State Board of Health Annual Report, 1918', Carlton Jackson Manuscript Collection, 'A Generation Remembers: Stories from the Flu, 1918, April 12, 1976–June 29, 1976', Box 2, File 3, Special Collections, Western Kentucky University, Bowling Green, KY. There are numerous examples of local coordination, especially in areas near military installations. For one such town, see 'Report of the Board of Health', in *Annual Reports of the Receipts and Expenditures of the Town of Ayer with Other Statistical Matter for the Year Ended December 31, 1918* (Ayer, MA: News Printing, 1919), 172.
43. 'Procedure to Establish Temporary Hospitals Under State Departments of Health', 16 October 1918, in 'Influenza Epidemic' Box 145, File 1622C, Records of the Public Health Service Central Files, 1897–1923, RG 90, NARA College Park; 'Suggested Program for Federal and State

Cooperation', 16 October 1918, in 'Influenza Epidemic' Box 145, File 1622C, RG 90, NARA College Park.

44. 'Suggested Program for Federal and State Cooperation', 16 October 1918, in 'Influenza Epidemic' Box 145, File 1622C, RG 90, NARA College Park. This cooperation was by no means uniform across states and localities. Serious, often tragic, differences in providing care were frequent across the country. See Nancy K. Bristow, Chapter 2, this volume.

45. Letter from W. S. Rankin to Hon. A. F. Lever, 29 November 1918, 'Rural Sanitation, Jan. 1918-Jan. 1919', Box 219, File 2240, RG 90, NARA College Park; 'Memorandum Relative to Estimate for Appropriation of $500,000 for Operations of the U.S. Public Health Service in "Rural Sanitation"', 2 December 1918, 'Rural Sanitation, Jan. 1918–Jan. 1919', Box 219, File 2240, RG 90, NARA College Park; Letter from Rupert Blue to W. S. Rankin, 6 December 1918, 'Rural Sanitation, Jan. 1918–Jan. 1919', Box 219, File 2240, RG 90, NARA College Park.

46. Letter from George B. Case to Rupert Blue, 1 October 1918, '803. Epidemics, 1918', Box 688, RG 200, NARA College Park.

47. Letter from J. W. Schereschewsky to Red Cross, n.d., '803. Epidemics, 1918', Box 688, RG 200, NARA College Park.

48. 'Plan for Combatting the Influenza Epidemic', 3 October 1918, '803. Epidemics, 1918', Box 688, RG 200, NARA College Park.

49. Letter from Elizabeth Ross, Director, Bureau of Nursing, to All Organizations, 3 October 1918, '803. Epidemics, 1918', Box 688, RG 200, NARA College Park.

50. 'Letter from the State of Ohio Secretary of State to the Speaker of the House of Representatives, 12 February 1919', Records of the United States House of Representatives, Petitions, Resolutions from State Legislatures, and Related Documents referred to Committee on Interstate and Foreign Commerce during 65th Congress: HR65A-H6.6 (Influenza Epidemic), RG 233, NARA DC; 'House Joint Resolution No. 12, Petitioning Congress to Take Action for the Suppression of Influenza, 4 February 1919', HR65A-H6.6 (Influenza Epidemic), RG 233, NARA DC; 'Resolution of Council of City of Cleveland, 14 February 1919', HR65A-H6.6 (Influenza Epidemic), RG 233, NARA DC; 'Resolution Transmitted by Dr. Otto Geier, Secretary, 13 June 1919', Petitions, Memorials, Resolutions of State Legislatures, and Related Documents Referred to Committee on Appropriations during 65th Congress: HR66A-H2.5 (Investigation into Causes of Influenza), RG 233, NARA DC.

51. Ibid., no page.

52. 'Statement by W. S. Rankin to State Health Officers', n.d., 'Rural Sanitation, Jan. 1919–Jan. 1920', Box 220, File 2240, RG 90, NARA College Park; Letters from towns requesting assistance from PHS, various dates, Box 246, File 2615, RG 90, NARA CP; Letter from Acting Surgeon General to Dr. Guilford H. Sumner, Iowa State Health Officer, 30 April 1919, 'State Health Activities', Box 505, File 4600, RG 90, NARA College Park.

53. 'Preparedness', Letter from Chairman, Mountain Division Influenza Preparedness Committee to J. Byron Deacon, 11 December 1919, '803. Epidemics, 1918', Box 688, RG 200, NARA College Park.
54. Letter from Charles E. Townsend to Surgeon General Rupert Blue, 28 August 1919, in 'Influenza Epidemic', Box 146, File 1622, Records of the Public Health Service Central File, 1897–1923, RG 90, NARACP.
55. Letter from Rupert Blue to Honorable Charles E. Townsend, 15 September 1919, in 'Influenza Epidemic', Box 146, File 1622, RG 90, NARA College Park.
56. Ibid., no page.
57. As Nancy K. Bristow brings out in Chapter 2, below, the perceived success in the government's response to Spanish 'flu did not match reality for many Americans. Racial and economic disparities in healthcare were plainly evident in 1918.
58. Furman, *A Profile of the United States Public Health Service*, 327; Williams, *United States Public Health Service*, 606–8. The PHS' failure to adequately care for the veterans led to this responsibility being stripped from the group in 1922.
59. Robert K. Murray, *The Politics of Normalcy: Governmental Theory and Practice in the Harding–Coolidge Era* (New York: W. W. Norton, 1973), 14, 46.
60. *Protection of Maternity and Infancy*, S. 1039, 67th Congress, 1st session, *Congressional Record* 61 (18 November 1921): H7940.
61. Duffy, *The Sanitarians*, 247–8.
62. House Subcommittee of the Committee on Interstate and Foreign Commerce, *Public Health Service: Hearing Before a Subcommittee of the Committee on Interstate and Foreign Commerce on H.R. 10125*, 69th Congress, 2nd session, 24–25 1927, 9, 12.
63. Mullan, *Plagues and Politics*, 89–90.
64. House Subcommittee, *Public Health Service: Hearing Before a Subcommittee of the Committee on Interstate and Foreign Commerce*, 1.
65. Ibid., 4.
66. Ibid., 5.
67. Ibid., 11.
68. Williams, *United States Public Health Service*, 169.
69. Mullan, *Plagues and Politics*, 104, 107, 161–2.

2

The United States in Two Pandemics: The American Century and the Costs of American Culture

Nancy K. Bristow

In the midst of the influenza pandemic of 1918, the *Baltimore Afro-American* detailed the costs of 'one of the most pitiable cases' of racism that had occurred in the crisis. The paper described struggling to find space in one of the city's overcrowded Black hospitals for an 'unknown man who was found unconscious' and sought a volunteer to take charge of his care. 'This,' the paper concluded, 'is one of the extremely sad cases that are the pitiable result of the jim crow [*sic*] policy practiced in White hospitals of the city.'[1]

Fast forward to March 2020, when Gary Fowler, a Black man living in Detroit, began feeling short of breath. With his own father suffering from COVID-19, Fowler understood that he, too, might be infected and visited three emergency rooms, pleading for a coronavirus test and help with his worsening symptoms. He was repeatedly turned away, told he was probably just suffering from bronchitis, could get better help elsewhere, or should 'go home' and 'drink water'. As it became more difficult to breathe, Fowler began sleeping in a recliner. Sometime during the night of 6 April he wrote, 'heart beat irregular' and 'oxygen level low'. The next morning his wife found him dead. Fowler was only fifty-six years old.[2]

The United States in which Fowler died was vastly different from that which suffered through the 1918 influenza pandemic. Advancements in science, medicine and public health offered new tools for combatting COVID-19 and had confirmed the efficacy of basic public health measures, providing distinct advantages to Americans in 2020. These advancements were both cause and effect of another dramatic change in American life – the expanded role of government at the federal, state and local levels, and its heightened responsibility for the welfare of the people, including their health, a change, in turn, served by a dramatically expanded public health infrastructure. In theory, too, segregation and many other forms of discrimination on the basis of race were no longer legal.

Yet as the story of Gary Fowler illustrates, racial inequities emerged during the COVID-19 pandemic, just as they did in 1918. This is not the only similarity between the two pandemics, though, a reality made particularly striking by the significant changes in American life that had emerged in the years in between. Four parallels in particular – an initial expressed over-confidence in the face of global health threats; a scattershot approach in responding to them; the politicising of the crises; and their inequitable impact based in class and racial identity – illustrate that while the role of government in preserving American health has expanded substantially over the course of the American Century, and though both federal and local governments have been armed with public health infrastructure and increasingly sophisticated science and technology to buoy their efforts, essential characteristics of American political and cultural life have remained consistent, interfering with effective pandemic management. Those four similarities are born of key elements of American culture, including hubris, resistance to federal activism, the use of crises by the powerful for their own purposes, and the unwavering force of White supremacy, aspects of the culture seemingly impervious even to the massive transformations of the American Century. All of them have continued to interfere with Americans' enjoyment of the full possibilities of a modern public health system, evidenced in the similarities in the experiences of two pandemics.

Parallel 1: American hubris

During spring 1918, the first wave of the influenza pandemic swept through the United States largely unnoticed, indistinguishable to the public from the annual 'flu. Only a handful of military epidemiologists noticed as influenza infected American training camps, in some cases bringing with it a 'virulent secondary streptococcic pneumonia'.[3] The virus attracted the broader public's attention when it travelled with American troops to the western front, soon spreading around the globe. The pandemic then exploded in its second, and worst, wave almost simultaneously in late summer in Sierra Leone, France and the United States, infecting people all over the world through the autumn. A third wave attacked in the winter as many communities were still recovering, and in early 1920, influenza struck many communities once more.

Stunningly contagious, the disease infected perhaps one-third of the global population, roughly 500 million people, while just over a quarter of Americans contracted it. In part due to secondary infections of bacterial pneumonia, its mortality rate of 2.5 per cent was twenty-five times that of other 'flu pandemics. In turn, though those who died often suffered a week or ten days of illness, it was possible to wake in the morning feeling healthy and die before nightfall. Finally, while influenza usually hits the very young and the elderly hardest, this influenza also struck with especial force among young adults, with almost half of American deaths among people aged twenty to forty. Some 675,000 Americans perished, lowering life expectancy for Americans in 1918 by twelve years.[4]

Even the most travelled military physicians were 'startled and alarmed' by what they saw, as were laypeople.[5] As family members in Chicago wrote to a relative in the Army, 'The whole world seems up-side-down.'[6] There were reasons Americans felt that way. Over the preceding half-century, the bacteriological revolution had allowed the discovery of the causal agents of several long-troubling diseases – from dysentery to yellow fever – confirming germ theory and enhancing the possibilities of prevention. By the eve of the pandemic American public health leaders were expressing increasing confidence in their ability to control disease. 'Epidemics,' they trumpeted, were 'now a thing of the past.'[7]

In the early stage of the pandemic, this confidence led some to believe they might contain the 'flu. As one local public health leader in Connecticut wrote to the state commissioner of health in mid-October, 'We ought to be in time to prevent the epidemic from assuming severe proportions if there is anything in public health education at all.'[8] In Tacoma, Washington, the city health officer reassured the public that closures and bans on public gatherings were only preventative, and suggested, 'With the precautions we've taken, I doubt that this city will be hit by the influenza as may other cities.'[9] Royal S. Copeland, health commissioner for the city of New York, was particularly prone to such optimism, suggesting on a day with 903 new cases in the city, 'We have every reason to feel encouraged and to believe that there will be no serious impairment in the health of the community.'[10] Sometimes this confidence was tinged with American exceptionalism, an evolving mythology that claims an American superiority to other nations and peoples.[11] As Copeland asked his fellow citizens when rumours of influenza circulated in mid-August, 'You haven't heard of our doughboys getting it, have you?' He rejoined, 'You bet you haven't, and you won't. But you have heard of cases in the German Army.' He concluded there was 'no need for our people to worry over the matter'.[12] Such hubris, whether tinged with exceptionalism or not, slowed public health responses as influenza soon raged across the country.

A similar sense of over-confidence was evident in the early months of COVID-19. On 24 January 2020, Robert R. Redfield, the head of the Centers for Disease Control and Prevention (CDC), told US senators, 'We are prepared for this.' At roughly the same time, Anthony Fauci, Director of the National Institute of Allergy and Infectious Disease, suggested that the coronavirus was not 'something the American people need to be worried or frightened by'.[13] As the first cases of COVID-19 appeared in the United States, many voices assumed influenza remained a more pressing and likely greater danger.[14]

Though public health officials never framed their comments in terms of American superiority and quickly shifted their stance as the threat became clearer, President Donald J. Trump continued to downplay Americans' risk, and sometimes pitched this as the result of American exceptionalism. On 29 January, with the coronavirus reported in seventeen countries, he reassured the nation, 'We have the best experts anywhere in the world, and they are on top of it 24/7!' On 24 February he told the country, 'The Coronavirus is very much under control in the USA.'[15] Though the president convened a Coronavirus Task Force and imposed a travel ban on China on 31 January, little other action followed.[16] On 2 March, he declared, 'The United States is right now ranked by far No. 1 in the world for preparedness.'[17] And a few days later, he reassured the public, 'It'll go away.'[18] Such hubris prevented the rapid mobilisation both pandemics called for.

Parallel 2: the scattershot approach to managing the pandemics

State and national borders mean nothing to a virus, and so the best way to fight a pandemic is to coordinate the responses to it across the largest area possible. Though public health knowledge had expanded exponentially between 1918 and 2020, and public health infrastructure at the municipal, county, state and federal levels had experienced complementary growth, in both 1918 and 2020 the dispersal of power to control the pandemic to state and local levels, a phenomenon of American federalism, undercut the national coordination of these efforts.

The country was not without national agencies and organisations prepared to fight the pandemic in 1918. By 1918, the United States Public Health Service (USPHS), born of the marine hospital system in the late eighteenth century, had assumed the leading role in national efforts to improve American health, mandated by Congress to prevent disease, conduct research, and maintain statistical records of health and disease across the country. When the pandemic hit, Congress appropriated $1 million to the service and charged it with combatting and suppressing the scourge.[19] As Jonathan Chilcote notes in Chapter 1, the leadership and resources of the USPHS during the pandemic enhanced its relationship with state and local public health boards and with the public, and ultimately its power.[20] The agency, led by Surgeon General Rupert Blue, played a significant role in educating the public in basic sanitary practices, offering up-to-date information through its weekly *Public Health Reports*, and deploying both its own personnel and additional physicians and nurses hired during the crisis to assist and guide local responses. It also oversaw the efforts of the Red Cross, which led efforts to solve the nursing shortage, established and supplied emergency hospitals and kitchens, provided transportation for patients and healthcare providers, offered aid to families and educated the public. Professional organisations that emerged in the nineteenth century to promote the interests of healthcare professionals, such as the American Medical Association (1847), the National Medical Association (1895) representing Black physicians excluded from the AMA, and the American Public Health Association (1872) also designed programmes for combatting influenza, promoted educational efforts, and collected and published research data.[21]

The power to determine and implement local responses to the pandemic, though, remained among municipal, county and state public health boards. The preceding half-century had seen significant growth in American public health. In the wake of the Civil War, several cities and states had established health boards, and during the Progressive Era the number and power of these boards grew, as did the stature of the Public Health Service.[22] Recognition of ongoing problems in American health revealed through conscription during the First World War, in turn encouraged both appreciation for the importance of public health and efforts to enhance its role in keeping US fighting men fit. Even so, when the pandemic struck, ultimate control over public health decision-making lay in the hands of state and local authorities, despite congressional enhancement of the role of the USPHS. The organisation and power of these local public health forces varied enormously across the United States, producing wide-ranging experiences in communities as they faced the 'flu.[23]

Some cities, like Seattle, Washington, experienced strong public health and political leadership, and created and sustained a robust response to the pandemic that served the citizenry well. On 4 October 1918, the *Seattle Post-Intelligencer* announced that 700 cadets at the naval training station located in the city were infected with influenza and one had died.[24] The next day, the city's health commissioner and its mayor moved to control the pandemic. Beginning with simple restrictions such as enforcement of the existing anti-spitting ordinance and self-quarantining, they soon drew on regulatory power to close many public amusements as well as churches and schools, and employed a new 'influenza squad' of police officers to combat resistance.

None of this was enough to stop the pandemic, leading to the local Red Cross' creation of a special influenza committee to coordinate the efforts across jurisdictions. A new emergency hospital was set up, and as cases continued to rise, public health leadership asked the police to arrest and punish those caught ignoring the restrictions. In late October, public health leadership added a masking order and shortened store hours. Influenza finally began to recede and, on 12 November, the day after the armistice, the city reopened. As was common around the country, as Seattle began to settle back into its normal routines another wave of the pandemic arrived in early December. This time leadership chose quarantining for containment, and found citizens anxious to cooperate in hopes of forestalling other restrictions. By year's end the new wave was waning. The city's early imposition of interventions, strict enforcement, and persistence in maintaining, expanding and even reimposing restrictions proved an ideal response.

Not every city or state employed such a sound programme. In some communities, such as Newark, New Jersey, handling the pandemic was complicated by tensions, even open warfare, between political and public health officials, or across levels of government, confounding the needed coordination.[25] In San Francisco, the failure of city leadership to model for citizens the importance of public health restrictions, in particular masking, encouraged massive resistance.[26] And in still other communities, political corruption interfered with the pandemic response. In Kansas City, Missouri, the public health department was loaded with those who held their positions 'by the grace of the bosses', as were both the city council and the local police. With local leadership beholden to competing political strong men, internecine warfare prevented the imposition of any effective controls for more than a week after the pandemic hit.[27] Ultimately the city was able to put in place significant restrictions aimed at slowing the pandemic, but the measures were 'poorly coordinated', 'delayed and dysfunctional'.[28]

Data from 1918 reveal that the actions of local public health leaders mattered for their communities. Seattle, for instance, fared reasonably well, its death rate for influenza and pneumonia was roughly 414 per 100,000. Alternatively, San Francisco and Kansas City, with their failures of political leadership, suffered rates of 673 and 580 per

100,000, respectively.[29] Particularly illustrative is the case of Milwau-
kee, with its exceptionally low rate of 292 per 100,000. This success
was the direct result of the public's willingness to cooperate and a
centralised coordination of the response, both made possible through
expert leadership.[30]

When the United States faced the coronavirus in 2020, it had distinct advantages over the country's circumstances in 1918 in terms
of medical and public health knowledge and infrastructure. While
scientists facing influenza in 1918 did not have the technology to
identify the virus, a century later they quickly isolated the coronavirus causing COVID-19, allowing the rapid creation of a vaccine.
Before the vaccine could be brought online, the best tools available
to control COVID remained those employed a century earlier – public health education, closures, prohibitions on large gatherings, social
distancing, masking, ventilation and quarantining. In another crucial
difference, though, data from 1918 had proven the value of these
non-pharmaceutical interventions for slowing infections and 'flattening the curve'.[31] In 2020, their employment allowed more patients
access to the lifesaving measures of ventilators and oxygen treatments unavailable in 1918.[32] Antibiotics, first employed during the
Second World War, provided another essential tool in fighting secondary bacterial infections during COVID.

These advantages reflected, in turn, the nation's much larger
scientific and public health infrastructure in 2020. Though several
Progressive Era innovations expanded the place of government in
Americans' lives prior to 1918, facilitating the federal interventions
of the war, the expanded role of the UPSHS and local mandates to
control the influenza pandemic, by 2020 the federal government's
role in protecting Americans' well-being, including their health, had
grown dramatically, particularly through programmes initiated during the New Deal of the 1930s and the Great Society of the 1960s.
Though the USPHS began conducting research through its Hygienic
Laboratory in 1887, the lab played virtually no role in the 1918 influenza pandemic. The federal role in biomedical research expanded
exponentially in the years following the Second World War, though,
as the National Institutes of Health, the Hygienic Laboratory's suc-
cessor, grew by 2020 into a massive, $42 billion biomedical research
agency.[33] Running along a parallel path, the Centers for Disease
Control and Prevention (CDC), founded in the wake of the Second
World War, by 2020, had become a global leader in disease surveillance, data collection and prevention.[34] In turn, though the surgeon
general in 1918 commanded a corps of roughly 200 officers, and
following the Congressional charge played a substantial advisory

and resource-sharing role during the influenza pandemic, by 2020, the Commissioned Corps of the USPHS had grown to 6,000 public health professionals.[35]

Despite these expanded capacities, responsibilities remained dispersed among federal agencies, while the power to implement public health mandates remained largely in the hands of state, county and municipal governments and public health boards. The result in 2020, as in 1918, was a scattershot approach to managing the pandemic that varied widely across communities and states. Though the CDC manages the nation's disease surveillance and data collection and the NIH coordinates and funds significant biomedical research, the surgeon general and the commissioned corps of the USPHS shoulder responsibility for preventing interstate and international infection. None of these, in turn, had more than the most limited power to mandate policy during the pandemic.[36] At the state level, in turn, public health management tended to be decentralised, with control over policy often situated at the local level.[37]

One result of the dispersal of power was, as in 1918, a striking unevenness in the application of measures to protect communities from the pandemic, visible, for instance, in decisions around stay-at-home or shelter-in-place orders early in the pandemic. California's order was mandated on 19 March 2020, Oregon's and Washington's on 23 March. Georgia waited until 3 April, South Carolina until 7 April. In stark contrast, Governor Asa Hutchinson of Arkansas refused to put a state-wide stay-at-home order into effect and prohibited communities from employing one.[38] North Dakota, South Dakota, Nebraska and Iowa joined Arkansas in the refusal.[39]

In Kansas, Governor Laura Kelly attempted to leave mandates in the hands of 'local health departments', but soon recognised the dangers of uneven measures, concluding, 'The reality is that the patchwork approach . . . is a recipe for chaos.'[40] Unfortunately, this chaos continued. From closures to the process of reopening, from masking mandates to vaccination requirements, there was no consistent policy across the United States. As one group of scholars explained in the *Journal of the American Medical Association*'s 'Health Forum', 'During an emergency, when the health of the nation depends on acting with coordination and cooperation, the failures of federalism come into sharp relief.'[41] Indeed, many communities in the United States suffered their worst losses from COVID from late November 2020 to late January 2021, many months after the effectiveness of public health measures had once again been proven, a circumstance that speaks directly to the costs of failing to implement public health protections in those areas.[42]

Parallel 3: the costs of politicisation

This failure to put in place scientifically proven protections suggests the price of the politicisation of public health. Though the reasons for the use of the pandemics for political purposes was quite different, in both cases it had costly consequences.[43] In 1918, it was the war that led most directly to the politicisation of the pandemic. When influenza struck in autumn 1918, the United States was in the closing months of the First World War, and public health leadership often used the war to raise the power of their appeals. Public health messages compared germs with the weapons of war, or the German enemy, and a person's duty to obey mandates to military service.[44] As the mayor of San Diego declared, 'I cannot see a particle of difference between the invasion of France by the heartless, lustful Huns and the invasion of our homes by some epidemic permitted by greed and politics.'[45] Those who refused to wear masks were sometimes deemed 'slackers'.[46] Public health leadership used the circumstances of the war to convince Americans that they had a role to play in fighting the epidemic, a patriotic duty in a time of crisis to acquiesce to public health rules.

Though using the war to sell public health may have aided the struggle against the pandemic by transforming it into a national emergency with patriotic undertones, in other ways the politics of the war interfered, as national and local leadership placed war interests ahead of public health. President Woodrow Wilson, on the advice of his Treasury Secretary William McAdoo, had chosen to fund the war in part through the selling of government bonds – Liberty Loans – and citizens faced significant pressure to show their support for the war through purchases. Despite the pandemic, the Fourth Liberty Loan drive went forward.[47] Cities and towns across the country, anxious to demonstrate patriotism and meet quotas, used public events to kick off local drives.

Philadelphia provides a cautionary tale of the costs of that choice. On 28 September the city hosted a massive parade through downtown, as the city's director of public health and the local press ignored local infectious disease experts who warned that such a gathering constituted 'a ready-made inflammable mass for a conflagration'.[48] In the event, 200,000 people turned out. Three days later, the city's hospitals were overwhelmed, foreshadowing what would prove to be Philadelphia's catastrophic encounter with the pandemic.[49] The city lost 17,500 people over the six months of crisis and suffered one of the highest excess death rates in the country at 748.4 per 100,000.[50]

In turn, placing the war ahead of the pandemic in policymaking, President Wilson refused to halt troop shipments to Europe, siding with Peyton C. March, Chief of Staff of the Army against advocates from the Army's Medical Department, facilitating the spread of influenza across the nation and among the troops.[51] During the worst three months of the pandemic, 20–40 per cent of US soldiers and sailors contracted either influenza or its sequela, pneumonia, halting stateside training and disrupting the American Expeditionary Force's Meuse-Argonne offensive. Some 30,000 American troops died before reaching Europe, and deaths from influenza and pneumonia outnumbered battlefield casualties.[52]

Perhaps most shocking, Wilson never spoke publicly of the pandemic.[53] Ever. While 25 million Americans took sick and more than half a million died, he offered no words of guidance or sympathy, apparently preferring to keep the nation focused on the war and the peace.

Though in 2020 the United States was not involved in a world war, this did not prevent the pandemic from quickly becoming politicised, this time to serve partisan interests. The politicisation of mask-wearing offers an obvious and early example. From the beginning, Democratic leaders were more likely to appear in face masks and to implement masking mandates, and a Pew poll published in June 2020 suggested their constituents were, in turn, more likely than Republicans to say they wore masks regularly.[54] Though many Republicans also supported mask-wearing, others refused to wear them and were outspoken in their opposition to masking mandates. Though Democratic presidential candidate Joe Biden declared early on that, if elected, he would 'do everything possible to make it required that people have to wear masks in public', President Trump chose to express doubt about the value of masks, to appear without one at White House events, and refused to be photographed wearing one.[55] When asked about masking at his rallies he suggested, 'I recommend people do what they want.'[56] On 3 April, he suggested that, when it came to donning a mask, 'I don't think I'm going to be doing it . . . I don't see it for myself.' Though by late summer evidence confirmed the value of masking, on 13 August he suggested, 'Maybe they're great and maybe they're just good. Maybe they're not so good.'[57] Certainly resistance to mask-wearing had many sources, including mixed messaging by public health leadership, masculine notions that wearing a mask was somehow 'shameful, not cool, a sign of weakness, and a stigma', and Americans' persistent preoccupation with individual liberties.[58] But it was in precisely this context that the president's example mattered, fostering mask resistance that was highest among his followers.[59]

The resurgence of the COVID-19 pandemic with the emergence of the Delta variant that spread through the United States in the late spring and summer of 2021 brought renewed debates and illustrated how far resistance to masking reached. On 27 July 2021, the CDC urged Americans in regions facing a renewal of the virus to return to wearing masks indoors, regardless of vaccination status. By 14 September 2021, ten states had implemented new masking mandates. All of those states had Democratic governors.[60] Conversely, by late August eight Republican-led states had prohibited local governments from imposing mask mandates, and six limited or prohibited schools from doing so.[61]

Debates over vaccination, too, illustrated how politicised, and polarised, the debates over public health responses to the pandemic had become. Though experts agreed unequivocally on the safety and effectiveness of the COVID-19 vaccines, by late summer 2021 a sizeable number of Americans were hesitant about, or entirely opposed to, vaccination. Though President Trump supported the development of a vaccine through his Operation Warp Speed, vaccine hesitancy remained strongest among Republicans, and again, particularly among the former president's supporters.[62]

The cause for that opposition was hotly debated. Some suggested the opposition was born of deep-seated beliefs, for instance, Americans' strong streaks of libertarianism and individualism, or by distrust in the federal government, a point well illustrated by the belief of some opponents that the vaccines contained tracking chips.[63] The perpetuation of misinformation and conspiracy theories by many in the leadership of the Republican Party and their media partners, though, suggest partisan politics played a significant role in fostering suspicion about the vaccine and opposition to vaccine mandates.[64] The costs of this politicisation is tragically best measured, again, in unnecessary deaths.

Parallel 4: identity matters

The 1918 influenza and COVID-19 have both brought immense trauma, suffering and death, around the globe and to American communities. Importantly, though, as the *Baltimore Afro-American* and the story of Gary Fowler suggest, that suffering has been differentially distributed not only according to local public health policies or by one's political beliefs, but also by social identity.

In 1918, despite the massive disruption of American life caused by the pandemic, the class hierarchy and systemic White supremacy survived largely unchallenged, creating experiences of the crisis that were divergent and inequitable. For the poorest families, the health crisis of the epidemic was worsened by material need. With no financial cushion, lost wages, even for a short time, might mean hunger, cold or even homelessness.[65] Such circumstances became even more precarious for families that suffered the death of an adult wage-earner, sending children to orphanages or into the workforce.[66]

For people of colour, the circumstances were still more difficult, their experiences framed by the disadvantages of racial prejudice and the broader poverty and segregated healthcare it produced. African Americans, for instance, struggled against White supremacy even as they fought the 'flu. In Miami, the city's health officer, though aware that the Black neighbourhood of Overtown would face a particular threat from influenza due to overcrowding and poor housing, did nothing to provide for the district's residents. The new Miami City Hospital did not accept Black patients, who instead were cared for in a hotel owned by the city's first Black millionaire.[67] Such discrimination was not isolated to the South. In Philadelphia, with hospitals filled to capacity and doctors and nurses overwhelmed, medical students were called into service and the city opened several emergency hospitals to deal with the legions of the ill. None of those hospitals were open to the city's African American citizens. As in Miami, it was up to the Black community to find leadership and resources to care for them.[68]

Other communities of colour suffered as well. Though death rates varied among tribal nations, in Arizona, Colorado, Mississippi, New Mexico and Utah 4–6 per cent of the Indigenous population perished. Alaska Natives suffered particularly horrific rates of morbidity and mortality.[69] At the Inupiat village of Brevig Mission, Alaska, 90 per cent of the residents, seventy-two of eighty, died in five days in November 1918.[70] Destitution, inadequate and crowded housing, lack of healthcare resources and aid, a long history of poor health conditions, and failures by the Indian Service to identify the threat in a timely manner all contributed to these outcomes.[71]

The Indian boarding schools brought their own unique tragedies.[72] At Chemawa Indian School in Salem, Oregon, for instance, students suffered from a range of health problems in the months preceding the epidemic.[73] When the pandemic hit, hundreds of children at the school became ill and several died, leaving family members devastated and without the opportunity to tend to them in either sickness or death.[74]

Today the racial and economic disparities of 1918 have not disappeared, but have been highlighted by the COVID-19 pandemic. Put simply, people of colour have died from COVID-19 in unconscionably high numbers. Using age-adjusted data, the Brookings Institute reported in June 2020 that African Americans were dying at 3.6 times the rate of White people, Latinx Americans at 2.5 times the rate. Disparities in healthcare are, as the report suggested, 'an enduring fact' of American life, one that sickens and kills people of colour every day. COVID simply offered 'the latest proof'.[75] Despite awareness of this crisis early in the pandemic, it continued. The CDC reported on 6 September 2021 that Black people had, to that point, died at twice the rate of White people, Hispanic and Latinx people at 2.3 times the rate.[76]

Indigenous communities, too, reeled from the pandemic, facing losses more than double those of the White community.[77] At one point in mid-May 2020, the Navajo Nation had the highest infection rate in the United States. Without adequate healthcare facilities or infrastructure, the community faced a high death rate as well.[78] The loss of elders, carriers of language, culture and memory, struck a particularly devastating blow for many Native communities.[79]

Poverty, with its terrible health costs, was one contributor to the dire circumstances of many communities of colour. Before the pandemic began, some scholars noted a 14.6-year difference in life expectancy between rich and poor men in this country, and a 10-year gap for women.[80] Being poor increased dramatically the likelihood that an individual entered the pandemic with pre-existing health conditions that increased the risk of severe illness and death. In turn, being poor also enhanced the chances of exposure – in overcrowded housing and workplaces with inadequate safety precautions.[81]

Unlike in 1918, there were some federal efforts to respond to the economic crisis of the pandemic, but here, too, because of the long-standing inequities in the American economy and the resultant inequality of wealth, the limitations of those attempts were felt most acutely in communities of colour. Though unemployment skyrocketed in the early months of the pandemic, passage of the $2.2 trillion economic stimulus, the Coronavirus Aid, Relief, and Economic Security (CARES) Act, passed by Congress in late March 2020, which included direct payments to individuals, initially succeeded in keeping the poverty rate below pre-pandemic levels. When the benefits of the Act began to wear off in late summer 2020, though, the poverty rate again began to climb, and did so faster among Black and Hispanic Americans.[82] Data on 'key hardship indicators' – hunger, unpaid rent and unemployment – suggest that circumstances improved after

December 2020, with the greatest improvement coming in the immediate wake of the American Rescue Plan of March 2021, a second
federal stimulus. As of October 2021, though, millions of Americans
continued to suffer food insecurity, including some 5–9 million children, or were behind on their rent. Again, communities of colour
suffered harsher economic impacts than did the White community.[83]

Conclusion: the limits of the American Century

The two pandemics offer only snapshots of the American public health
system, two moments of medical crisis in which that system and Americans' relationship to it were profoundly tested. The circumstances of
the American people in these two instances were vastly different, the
result of advancements in technology, science, medicine and public
health, as well as the significantly expanded role of the government
at the federal, state and local levels. All of these gave Americans in
2020 a meaningful advantage over their predecessors as they faced a
pandemic. Crucial aspects of US culture, however – hubris, distrust of
government, a willingness to politicise crises, and White supremacy
and class inequities – have meant that Americans in 2020 made many
of the same mistakes and experienced many of the same problems as
those who faced the influenza pandemic a century earlier.

What, then, do these parallels tell us about public health in the
United States over the course of the American Century? Despite
significant scientific advancement and the growth of governmental
and public health infrastructure, American responses to pandemics
retain many features that undercut the nation's capacity to effectively
manage these crises. The over-confidence that created a profound
sense among Americans in 2020 that *this should not be happening
to us* suggests that they have not yet come to terms with their hubris,
with their over-confidence in the face of evidence to the contrary that
science and American know-how will somehow exempt the nation
from the shared crisis of a global pandemic. This belief facilitates the
ongoing acceptance of a decentralised approach to American public
health, an approach that also suggests a deep distrust of government,
particularly at the federal level, and an ongoing unwillingness to
accept the vital role political and public health leadership should play
in the face of a global pandemic. The politicisation of both pandemics, in turn, suggests public health is an arena that people of power
will manipulate for other purposes, including political advantage,
at horrific costs to the public. And, finally, the racial and economic
disparities that this pandemic has highlighted make it clear that the

United States still has hard and crucial work to do to deal with its systemic and institutionalised White supremacy and its willingness to allow millions of its citizens to live in poverty. Until Americans confront these deep cultural tendencies, the expansive promise of public health as it developed over the American Century will remain only partially realised.

Notes

1. 'Influenza and Pneumonia Claims Many Victims', *Baltimore Afro-American*, 18 October 1918, 1.
2. Kristen Jordan Shamus, 'Family Ravaged by Coronavirus Begged for Tests, Hospital Care, but was Repeatedly Denied', *Detroit Free Press*, 19 April 2020, available at: https://www.freep.com/story/news/local/michigan/wayne/2020/04/19/coronavirus-racial-disparity-denied-tests-hospitalization/2981800001.
3. Chief Medical Officer at Camp Funston, quoted in Carol R. Byerly, *Fever of War: The Influenza Epidemic in the US Army during World War I* (New York: New York University Press, 2005), 70.
4. Jeffery K. Taubenberger and David M. Morens, '1918 Influenza: The Mother of All Pandemics', *Emerging Infectious Disease* 12:1 (2006), 15, 19; David M. Morens, Jeffery K. Taubenberger and Anthony S. Fauci, 'Predominant Role of Bacterial Pneumonia as a Cause of Death in Pandemic Influenza: Implications for Future Influenza Preparedness', *Journal of Infectious Disease* 198:7 (2008), 962–70, doi: 10.1086/591708; John F. Brundage and G. Dennis Shanks, 'Deaths from Bacterial Pneumonia during 1918–1919 Influenza Pandemic', *Emerging Infectious Diseases* 14:8 (2008), 1194; Jeffery K. Taubenberger and David M. Morens, 'Influenza: The Once and Future Pandemic', *Public Health Reports* 125 (S3) (2010), 17; Andrew Noymer and Michel Garenne, 'The 1918 Influenza Epidemic's Effects on Sex Differentials in Mortality in the United States', *Population and Development Review* 26:3 (2004), 568.
5. Rufus Ivory Cole, 'The Etiology and Prevention of Influenza' (lecture), 1 February 1946, Rufus Cole Papers (B/C671), American Philosophical Society.
6. Letter from Sam and Clara, 20 October 1918, Herbert Greenfelder Collection, HQ Company, 325th Field Artillery, 84th Division, War Experiences Questionnaire Collection, World War One Research Project, US Army Military History Institute.
7. 'Guarding Against Infection from War Epidemics', *Review of Reviews* 51 (1915), 231.
8. Letter unsigned to Dr John T. Black, Commissioner of Health, State of Connecticut, 17 October 1918, File 68-0921 – Connecticut Department of Health: Correspondence, 1916–1918, Box 68, Series III, Charles-Edward Amory Winslow Papers, Yale University.

9. 'Two Cases of "Flu" Reported in City', *Tacoma News Tribune*, 10 October 1918, 5.
10. Royal S. Copeland quoted in 'Gains Slightly Here', *New York Times* (hereafter *NYT*), 3 October 1918, 24.
11. Ian Tyrell, *American Exceptionalism: A New History of an Old Idea* (Chicago: University of Chicago Press, 2022), 3–4 (Kindle edition).
12. 'No Quarantine Here against Influenza', *NYT*, 15 August 1918, 6.
13. Both quoted in Lawrence Wright, *The Plague Year: America in the Time of COVID* (New York: Knopf, 2021), 41.
14. Lenny Bernstein, 'Get a grippe, America', *Washington Post*, 1 February 2020, available at: https://www.washingtonpost.com/health/time-for-a-reality-check-america-the-flu-is-a-much-bigger-threat-than-corona-virus-for-now/2020/01/31/46a15166-4444-11ea-b5fc-eefa848cde99_story.html.
15. Aaron Blake and J. M. Rieger, 'Timeline: The 201 times Trump has Downplayed the Coronavirus Threat', *Washington Post*, 3 November 2020, available at: https://www.washingtonpost.com/politics/2020/03/12/trump-coronavirus-timeline.
16. Operation Warp Speed, initiated on 15 May, would be an important exception.
17. Linda Qiu and Mikayla Bouchard, 'Tracking Trump's Claims on the Threat from Coronavirus', *NYT*, 5 March 2020, available at: https://www.nytimes.com/2020/03/05/us/politics/trump-coronavirus-fact-check.html.
18. Daniel Wolfe and Daniel Dale, '"It's going to disappear": A Timeline of Trump's Claims that Covid-19 Will Vanish', *CNN*, 31 October 2020, available at: https://www.cnn.com/interactive/2020/10/politics/covid-disappearing-trump-comment-tracker.
19. Fitzhugh Mullan, *Plagues and Politics: The History of the United States Public Health Service* (New York: Basic Books, 1989), 74.
20. See also Jonathan Chilcote, Chapter 1, this volume.
21. Ibid.; Nancy K. Bristow, *American Pandemic: Lost Worlds of the 1918 Influenza Epidemic* (New York: Oxford University Press, 2012), 88–93.
22. Chilcote, Chapter 1, this volume, 00–00.
23. Ibid., 00–00, 00–00.
24. All information on Seattle comes from 'Seattle, Washington and the 1918–1919 Influenza Epidemic', *The American Influenza Epidemic of 1918: A Digital Encyclopedia*, available at: https://www.influenzaar-chive.org/cities/city-seattle.html.
25. 'Newark, New Jersey and the 1918–1919 Influenza Epidemic', *The American Influenza Epidemic of 1918*, available at: https://www.influ-enzaarchive.org/cities/city-newark.html.
26. 'Ringside Picture Reveals Maskless Fans to Police', *San Francisco Chronicle*, 20 November 1918, 9; 'New Cases of Influenza at Low Record', *San Francisco Examiner*, 26 January 1919, 12.

27. Susan Debra Sykes Berry, 'Politics and Pandemic in 1918 Kansas City', Master's thesis, University of Missouri-Kansas City, 2010, 20–4, 34; David S. McKinsey, Joel P. McKinsey and Maithe Enriquez, 'The 1918 Influenza in Missouri: Centennial Remembrance of the Crisis', *Missouri Medicine* 115:4 (2018), 319–24, available at: https://www.ncbi.nlm.nih.gov/pmc/articles/PMC6140242.
28. Eric Adler, 'A Coronavirus Lesson? How KC's Response to 1918 Flu Pandemic Caused Needless Death', *Kansas City Star*, 17 March 2020, available at: https://www.kansascity.com/news/business/health-care/article241058181.html.
29. Howard Markel et al., 'Nonpharmaceutical Interventions Implemented by US Cities during the 1918–1919 Influenza Pandemic', *Journal of the American Medical Association* 298:6 (2007), 647.
30. Judith Walzer Leavitt, 'Pandemics and History: Context, Context, Context', *American Journal of Public Health* 111:6 (2021), 996.
31. The efficacy of non-pharmaceutical interventions such as these had been demonstrated by scholars using data from the 1918 pandemic. Markel et al., 'Nonpharmaceutical Interventions', 644–54.
32. Maria Godoy, 'Flattening a Pandemic's Curve: Why Staying Home Now Can Save Lives', *NPR – Shots*, 13 March 2020, available at: https://www.npr.org/sections/health-shots/2020/03/13/815502262/flattening-a-pandemics-curve-why-staying-home-now-can-save-lives.
33. Victoria A. Harden, 'A Short History of the National Institutes of Health', National Institutes of Health – Office of NIH History and Stetten Museum website, available at: https://history.nih.gov/display/history/A+Short+History+of+the+National+Institutes+of+Health; Andrea Peterson, 'Final FY20 Appropriations: National Institutes of Health', *FYI Bulletin: Science Policy News from AIP* (4 February 2020), available at: https://www.aip.org/fyi/2020/final-fy20-appropriations-national-institutes-health#:~:text=The%20National%20Institutes%20of%20Health%20is%20receiving%20a%20%242.6%20billion,agency%20a%20multibillion%20dollar%20boost.
34. 'Historical Perspectives History of CDC', *Morbidity and Mortality Weekly Report* 45:25 (1996), 526–30, available at: https://www.cdc.gov/mmwr/preview/mmwrhtml/00042732.htm#top.
35. Mullan, *Plagues and Politics*, 74; 'History of the Office of the Surgeon General', US Department of Health and Human Services, available at: https://www.hhs.gov/surgeongeneral/about/history/index.html. See also Chapter 1, Jonathan Chilcote, this volume, esp. 00, 00–00.
36. Sarah H. Gordon, Nicole Huberfeld and David K. Jones, 'What Federalism Means for the US Response to Coronavirus Disease 2019', *JAMA Health Forum* 1:5 (2020), DOI: 10.1001/jamahealthforum.2020.0510.
37. 'Health Department Governance', Public Health Professionals Gateway, CDC website, available at: https://www.cdc.gov/publichealthgateway/sitesgovernance/index.html.

38. 'Arkansas Gov. Asa Hutchinson on Why He Hasn't Issues a Stay-At-Home Order', *PBS News Hour*, 8 April 2020, available at: https://www.pbs.org/newshour/show/arkansas-gov-asa-hutchinson-on-why-he-hasnt-issued-a-stay-at-home-order.
39. Sarah Mervosh, Denise Lu and Vanessa Swales, 'See Which States and Cities Have Told Residents to Stay Home', *NYT*, last updated 20 April 2020.
40. Ibid; Tara Bubramaniam and Veronica Stracqualursi, 'Facts First: Fact Check: Georgia Governor Says We Only Just Learned People Without Symptoms Could Spread Coronavirus', *CNN Politics*, 3 April 2020, available at: https://www.cnn.com/2020/04/02/politics/fact-check-georgia-gov-brian-kemp-coronavirus-no-symptoms-stay-at-home/index.html.
41. Gordon, Huberfeld and Jones, 'What Federalism Means for the US Response to Coronavirus Disease'.
42. E. Thomas Ewing, 'Public Health Responses to Pandemics in 1918 and 2020', *American Journal of Public Health* 111:10 (2021), 1716.
43. Ibid.
44. Illustration from *Illinois Health News*, October 1918, included in Karen A. Walters, 'McLean County and the Influenza Epidemic of 1918–1919', *Journal of the Illinois State Historical Society* 74 (1981), 130.
45. Quoted in Richard H. Peterson, 'The Spanish Influenza Epidemic in San Diego, 1918–1919', *Southern California Quarterly* 71 (1989), 96.
46. 'Ten Mask Slackers Get 10-Day Sentences', *San Francisco Examiner,* 2 November 1918, 11.
47. John M. Barry, *The Great Influenza: The Epic Story of the Deadliest Plague in History* (New York: Viking, 2004), 207–8.
48. Howard Anders quoted in Barry, *The Great Influenza*, 208.
49. Kenneth C. Davis, 'Philadelphia Threw a WWI Parade That Gave Thousands of Onlookers the Flu', *Smithsonian Magazine*, 21 September 2018, available at: https://www.smithsonianmag.com/history/philadelphia-threw-wwi-parade-gave-thousands-onlookers-flu-180970372.
50. Markel et al, 'Nonpharmaceutical Interventions'.
51. Byerly, *Fever of War*, 105–8.
52. Carol R. Byerly, 'The US Military and the Influenza Pandemic of 1918–1919', *Public Health Reports* 125, (S3) (2010), 83, 89.
53. Tevi Troy, *Shall We Wake the President: Two Centuries of Disaster Management from the Oval Office* (Guilford, CT: Rowman & Littlefield, 2016), 4–5, 198 (Kindle edition).
54. Ruth Igielnik, 'Most Americans Say They Regularly Wore a Mask In Stores in the Past Month; Fewer See Others Doing It', *Pew Research Center,* 23 June 2020, available at: https://www.pewresearch.org/fact-tank/2020/06/23/most-americans-say-they-regularly-wore-a-mask-in-stores-in-the-past-month-fewer-see-others-doing-it.
55. Lauren Aratani, 'How Did Face Masks Become a Political Issue in America?' *The Guardian*, 29 June 2020, available at: https://www.theguardian.com/world/2020/jun/29/face-masks-us-politics-coronavirus.

56. Aaron Blake, 'Trump's Dumbfounding Refusal to Encourage Wearing Masks', *Washington Post,* 25 June 2020, available at: https://www.washingtonpost.com/politics/2020/06/25/trumps-dumbfounding-refusal-encourage-wearing-masks.

57. Noah Higgins-Dunn, 'Trump Calls Biden's Coronavirus Plan Unscientific', *NBC,* 13 August 2020, available at: https://www.cnbc.com/2020/08/13/trump-calls-bidens-coronavirus-plan-unscientific-rejects-call-for-national-mask-mandate.html.

58. Zeynep Tufekci, 'Opinion: The CDC Needs to Stop Confusing the Public', *NYT,* 4 August 2021, available at: https://www.nytimes.com/2021/08/04/opinion/cdc-covid-guidelines.html; Valerio Capraro and Helene Barcelo, 'The Effect of Messaging and Gender on Intentions to Wear a Face Covering to Slow Down COVID-19 Transmission', *PsyArXiv,* 11 May 2020, DOI: 10.31234/osf.io/tg7vz; Jessica Flanigan, 'Bioethicist on Libertarian Views Toward Face Mask Laws', *All Things Considered,* 19 July 2020, available at: https://www.npr.org/2020/07/19/892855760/bioethicist-on-libertarian-views-toward-face-mask-laws. For an excellent discussion of the interplay between American notions of individualism and masculinity both historically and during COVID-19, see Olga Thierbach-McLean, Chapter 12, this volume.

59. Leo H. Kahane, 'Politicizing the Mask: Political, Economic and Demographic Factors Affecting Mask Wearing Behavior in the USA', *Eastern Economic Journal* (5 January 2021), 1–21, available at: https://www.ncbi.nlm.nih.gov/pmc/articles/PMC7783295.

60. 'State-Level Mask Requirements in Response to the Coronavirus (COVID-19) Pandemic, 2020–2021', *Ballotpedia,* available at: https://ballotpedia.org/State-level_mask_requirements_in_response_to_the_coronavirus_(COVID-19)_pandemic,_2020-2021.

61. Alison Durkee, 'Montana Becomes Latest State to Restrict School Mask Mandates', *Forbes,* 31 August 2021, available at: https://www.forbes.com/sites/alisondurkee/2021/08/31/montana-becomes-latest-state-to-restrict-school-mask-mandates---heres-the-full-list/?sh=288f324444a1.

62. Jennifer Kates, Jennifer Tolbert and Kendal Orgera, 'The Red/Blue Divide in COVID-19 Vaccination Rates is Growing', Kaiser Family Foundation (KFF) website, 8 July 2021, available at: https://www.kff.org/policy-watch/the-red-blue-divide-in-covid-19-vaccination-rates-is-growing.

63. Maria Carrasco, 'Libertarian Students Fight Campus Vaccine Mandates', *Inside Higher Ed,* 9 September 2021, available at: https://www.insidehighered.com/news/2021/09/09/young-libertarians-protest-vaccine-mandates-campus; Susan Milligan, 'A Deadly Political Divide', *US News and World Report,* 23 July 2021, available at: https://www.usnews.com/news/the-report/articles/2021-07-23/coronavirus-vaccines-highlight-a-deadly-political-divide.

64. Lisa Lerer, 'How Republican Vaccine Opposition Got to This Point', *NYT,* 17 July 2021, available at: https://www.nytimes.com/2021/07/17/us/politics/coronavirus-vaccines-republicans.html.

65. Case #13906, Reel #197, Family Welfare, Minneapolis Family and Children's Service Case Records, 1895–1945, Social Welfare History Archives, University of Minnesota Libraries.

66. 'Spanish Stonecutter's Widow', in 'Four Women', American Life Histories, Manuscripts from the Federal Writers' Project, 1936–1940, American Memory Project, Library of Congress, available at: https://www.loc.gov/resource/wpalh3.38041005/?st=pdf; Melvin Lynn Frank, 'Reminiscences: "Sawmill City Boyhood"',' 83, undated, Minnesota Historical Society.

67. 'A Historical Snapshot of Miami During the 1918 Flu Pandemic', *WLRN 91.3 FM*, 6 April 2020, available at: https://www.wlrn.org/local-news/2020-04-06/a-historical-snapshot-of-miami-during-the-1918-flu-pandemic.

68. Vanessa Northington Gamble, '"There Wasn't a Lot of Comforts in Those Days": African Americans, Public Health, and the 1918 Influenza Epidemic', *Public Health Reports* 125 (S3) (2010), 119.

69. Benjamin R. Brady and Howard M Bahr, 'The Influenza Epidemic of 1918–1920 among the Navajos: Marginality, Mortality, and the Implications of Some Neglected Eyewitness Accounts', *American Indian Quarterly* 38:4 (2014), 459, 461.

70. '1918–19: "Spanish Influenza" claims Millions of Lives', *Native Voices: Timeline*, National Library of Medicine website, available at: https://www.nlm.nih.gov/nativevoices/timeline/420.html.

71. Brady and Bahr, 'The Influenza Epidemic of 1918–1920', 469–74.

72. Brenda J. Child, *Boarding School Seasons: American Indian Families, 1900–1940* (Lincoln: University of Nebraska, 1998), 55, 60–8.

73. Hospital Record, 1917–1924, Chemawa Indian School, Box 134, Record Group 75, National Archives, Pacific-Alaska Region.

74. Student Files, Chemawa Indian School, Box 66, Record Group 75, National Archives, Pacific-Alaska Region.

75. Tiffany N. Ford, Sarah Reber and Richard V. Reeves, 'Up Front: Race Gaps in COVID-19 are Even Bigger than They Appear', *Brookings*, 16 June 2020, available at: https://www.brookings.edu/blog/up-front/2020/06/16/race-gaps-in-covid-19-deaths-are-even-bigger-than-they-appear.

76. Center for Disease Control, 'COVID-19 Infection, Hospitalization, and Death by Race/Ethnicity', updated 9 September 2021, available at: https://www.cdc.gov/coronavirus/2019-ncov/covid-data/investigations-discovery/hospitalization-death-by-race-ethnicity.html.

77. Ibid.; Mark Walker, 'Pandemic Highlights Deep-Rooted Problems in Indian Health Service,' *NYT*, 29 September 2020, https://www.nytimes.com/2020/09/29/us/politics/coronavirus-indian-health-service.html?action=click&module=RelatedLinks&pgtype=Article.

78. Alexandra Sternlicht, 'Navajo Nation Has Most Coronavirus Infections Per Capita in US, Beating New York, New Jersey', *Forbes*, 19 May 2020, available at: https://www.forbes.com/sites/alexandrasternlicht/2020/05/19/

navajo-nation-has-most-coronavirus-infections-per-capita-in-us-beating-new-york-new-jersey/?sh=3f9825ac8b10.

79. Jack Healy, 'Tribal Elders are Dying From the Pandemic, Causing a Cultural Crisis for American Indians', *NYT*, 19 January 2021, available at: https://www.nytimes.com/2021/01/12/us/tribal-elders-native-americans-coronavirus.html.

80. Raj Chetty, Michael Stepner and Sarah Abraham, 'The Association between Income and Life Expectancy in the United States, 2001–2014', *Journal of the American Medical Association* 315:16 (2016), 1750–66.

81. Caitlin Brown and Martin Ravallion, 'Poverty, Inequality, and COVID-19 in the US', *Center for Economic and Policy Research, Vox-EU*, 10 August 2020, available at: https://voxeu.org/article/poverty-inequality-and-covid-19-us.

82. Priyanki Boghani, 'How COVID Has Impacted Poverty in America', *PBS FRONTLINE*, 8 October 2020, available at: https://www.pbs.org/wgbh/frontline/article/covid-poverty-america.

83. 'COVID Hardship Watch: Tracking the COVID-19 Economy's Effects on Food, Housing, and Unemployment Hardships', Center on Budget and Policy Priorities, available at: https://www.cbpp.org/research/poverty-and-inequality/tracking-the-covid-19-economys-effects-on-food-housing-and, updated October 2021.

3

The Politics of Public Health: Disease and Medical Authority in Twentieth-Century America

Naomi Rogers

How do we reckon with the lessons of pandemics past? Living through the COVID pandemic has raised questions about the meaning and scope of public health in ways that have not been experienced since the AIDS crisis of the 1980s.[1] The 1918–1919 influenza pandemic – a horrifying threat to health that entangled medical care by military institutions and efforts to prevent and treat civilian communities terrified by the likely spread of the disease – has been consistently used as a critical historical parallel to COVID. Allusions to the ordering of American civilians to stay at home in a strategy called 'home quarantine', with local health departments placarding houses warning outsiders not to enter and residents not to leave, have been irresistible. So, too, have the iconic century-old masking practices, as well as the attendant scepticism regarding these preventive practices and perceived government over-reach.[2]

The history of disease offers important insights into public views of the proper use of state power. Epidemic disease and efforts to fight it have tested existing infrastructure and claims to authority. In twentieth-century America during times of crisis members of the public accepted some public health measures as temporarily legitimate, but also interpreted them as a threat to individual liberty. Fundamental to such struggles were efforts to determine who was a legitimate source of expertise and who should have the power to dramatise the dangers of disease and to prescribe preventive measures. With the expanding role of federal government in matters of health and well-being, those who claimed authority over health governance were increasingly and visibly immersed in political and ideological struggles around the rights of citizens and the power of experts. The threat to health, as was true in earlier eras, provided opportunities to expand state power. But at the same time public scepticism to government over-reach and the authority of health officials led to popular resistance to many public health measures in ways that frustrated and puzzled health officials and scientific researchers.

My focus is not on influenza, but rather polio, another frightening disease that engaged widespread cultural and medical resources in twentieth-century America. Efforts to define and control this disease occurred both inside and outside formal public health departments. The history of polio in the twentieth century exemplifies a particular moment in American health politics: polio policy was shaped by the power of a president and a philanthropic organisation he founded and promoted that used his name and reputation in its fundraising, its political influence and its assumption of leadership in scientific research. This organisation – the National Foundation for Infantile Paralysis or March of Dimes – was readily identified as part of the health establishment as a wealthy, powerful institution allied with the medical profession, the federal government and research scientists. To understand the history of polio it is crucial to explore the contested power of public health and underscore the consistent politicising of government health measures.

American officials in the past, as well as the present, claimed that they were 'following the science', and were quick to explain popular dissent as a result of scientific ignorance and misinformation. Health teaching in schools and universities, based on the discoveries of laboratory science, blossomed in the mid-twentieth century, as did a wider fascination with medical heroes. But popular eagerness to embrace scientific solutions and scientists as experts was frequently undermined by frustration when answers were not clear or were seen as not immediately efficacious. Many reporters observing recent resistance to COVID vaccines have assumed that such issues are novel and a sign of twenty-first-century social media culture. They have sought a previous 'golden age' with the development of the polio vaccine, but, as I shall argue here, even in the 1950s, a time when becoming a doctor was the loftiest dream for many students and their parents, many Americans remained sceptical of the efficacy of vaccines and medical research, and rejected the expertise of health officials and scientists. Indeed, health departments struggled to convince the public that their pronouncements were the sole authority in determining how to respond to the threat of disease. During polio epidemics fearful parents continued to seek out ways to protect their children, no matter whether experts saw such precautions as effective, or sensible or science-based.

Presidential power and polio policy

In twentieth-century America, public health as a field and a profession constantly struggled for prestige and power. Epidemics have often, but not always, provided opportunities to expand that power, gain health officials greater public esteem, and led to the tighter integration of departments within political systems. In the case of polio and tuberculosis, though, public health departments did not realise such achievements; they became partners, but secondary partners, to such voluntary health organisations as the March of Dimes and the National Tuberculosis Society (later the American Lung Association), which were far more influential in shaping political and social responses to disease. For the March of Dimes, polio care included crisis programmes in which physicians, nurses, iron lungs and crutches were sent to communities in need and year-long programmes of professional training. The National Tuberculosis Society initiated preventive campaigns and encouraged communities to alter germ-spreading behaviour and establish sanatoria for the care of tubercular patients. Both groups developed sophisticated ways to channel public fear into political action, raising awareness and funds for tackling their specific diseases, making them visible and culturally significant and ameliorating gaps in the funding and availability of medical facilities, professionally trained providers and research.[3] Both organisations integrated some of their efforts with local and state government agencies, but only tuberculosis – long recognised as a 'social disease' responsive to improvements in housing and nutrition – became fully integrated in a wider public health network.

By the late 1940s, polio was a familiar recurring epidemic threat. As its epidemiology took many decades to decipher polio was difficult to predict and treat. Yet while it was a frightening disease and the subject of many media stories, it was never a significant cause of morbidity or mortality.[4] While private physicians and public health officials were important figures in the response to polio epidemics, the March of Dimes claimed special authority backed by the imprimatur of the White House.[5]

During the 1920s and 1930s Franklin Delano Roosevelt's own experience of polio paralysis had led him to become a founder and patron of the March of Dimes. It was a sign of Roosevelt's wealth and family isolation that, unlike most Americans, he was not exposed to the polio virus until 1921 when he was in his late thirties. His legs were paralysed and remained paralysed for the rest of his life. A lawyer and aspiring politician, throughout the 1920s Roosevelt sought ways to return to public life. He visited and then bought Warm Springs, Georgia, a mineral springs health resort, and turned it into a polio rehabilitation centre. At Warm Springs, Roosevelt allowed others to see his leg braces, but outside that community he pretended that he was not disabled as he did not believe that he could be elected governor or president as a disabled man.[6] Polio historian Hugh Gallagher has called Roosevelt's efforts to conceal his disability his 'splendid deception'. He used a long cigarette holder and a cape in order to draw the public's eye to his shoulders and head. When he visited public buildings with front steps, the Secret Service would build a temporary ramp so that his car could drive up to the entrance allowing him to be carried from the car into the main part of the building. Any reporter who tried to take pictures of that process had their cameras knocked from their hands and destroyed. Once Roosevelt left the building, the ramps were taken down.[7] This was a performance of disability hidden in plain sight and denied, as temporary infrastructure was removed with the blessing of a disabled president.

In the 1930s, after he became president, Roosevelt became the patron of polio fundraising, a symbol of someone who had 'conquered' the disease. By his second term Roosevelt began to face political attacks on his expanding New Deal policies. In response to claims that Warm Springs was a politicised institution too close to the Democratic Party, he and his advisers decided to set up a separate charity, known as the National Foundation for Infantile Paralysis or the March of Dimes, which became America's largest disease philanthropy. The March of Dimes provided services during polio outbreaks and ongoing programmes of training and care in rehabilitation, as well a small programme funding scientific research. Its rehabilitative services merged well with New Deal programmes, especially as the new 1935 Social Security Act established a government-funded social safety net that expanded public health departments and services for 'crippled' children.[8]

After Roosevelt died in 1945 his legacy in the history of polio lingered with the director of the March of Dimes who had been a close friend and ally of Roosevelt's since the 1920s. Born into a working-class family Basil O'Connor was an Irish Catholic at a time when someone of that ethnicity and religion usually had little chance to succeed in elite society. With the aid of a donor, he attended Dartmouth College and then, with an additional scholarship, he entered Harvard Law School. As a lawyer he practiced first in Boston and then in New York City, and became wealthy from his work with oil and real estate companies. An ambitious man, O'Connor wanted to practice law in a partnership with a prominent member of the New York establishment and met Roosevelt in the mid-1920s. They became friends and partners. O'Connor was appointed a trustee of Warm Springs and, in 1937, at Roosevelt's request, had become president of the March of Dimes, a position he held until his death in 1972.[9]

The March of Dimes, like all American health organisations, operated in a racist world. Physicians, policymakers and civic leaders –

frequently members of March of Dimes chapter boards – defended segregated medical training and limited access to hospital care with assertions about the inferiority of Black bodies and minds. Trying to remain impartial amid the contested civil rights tensions of the New Deal was no easy task. The March of Dimes at first tried to ignore paralysed Black patients and then sought to design campaigns that recognised Black children as visible and vulnerable polio victims, promoting the organisation as both race aware and race neutral.[10] Still, until the late 1940s, the March of Dimes largely presented polio as a White disease. Warm Springs, centred in the heart of Georgia, was a segregated institution: all patients, physical therapists, physicians, nurses and pool attendants were white. Its laundry, cleaning and janitorial work, in contrast, was done by Black men and women.[11] Civil rights protesters raised this issue, reminding Roosevelt and other Democrats of the growing importance of Black voters. It was clear that to have Roosevelt's own Warm Springs centre remain a white, segregated facility was terrible optics. However, the conservative, White trustees of Warm Springs and powerful White southern Democrats in Congress were unyielding. In a tactic O'Connor hoped would appease both sides, the March of Dimes financed the construction of a Black polio hospital at the Tuskegee Institute in Alabama. This opened in 1941 alongside a programme that offered fellowships to Black nurses, doctors and physical therapists around the country to visit the hospital and learn the latest polio treatments. It was a very small institution and did not transform the care of polio for most Black Americans.[12] Indeed, a photograph found in the March of Dimes archives, probably from around 1950, depicted the White patients and the White staff at Warm Springs watching a movie along with some of the Black staff, separated by an interior white picket fence.[13]

In 1944, the March of Dimes hired its first 'inter-racial' official, Charles Bynum, a Black educator and administrator whose task was to reach out to middle-class Black communities and raise money for the March of Dimes. The March of Dimes poster child campaign, which began after the Second World War, featured its first Black child in 1947. But polio care for most Black Americans was the kind experienced by the Olympic athlete Wilma Rudolph. Rudolph, born in 1940, was paralysed by polio as a young girl and wore a leg brace. She was treated at a clinic at Meharry Medical College in Nashville, Tennessee, some 50 miles from her home. Reflecting the inadequate number of Black physicians with experience in treating polio, Rudolph and her mother took the long bus ride two or three times a week to attend this clinic. She wore a leg brace for around seven years

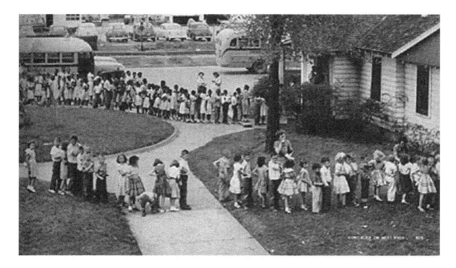

Figure 3.1 Black elementary schoolchildren being bussed to a White public school to gain access to the Salk vaccine, 1955

and, as she recalled later: 'My doctor told me I would never walk again. My mother told me I would. I believed my mother.' In 1960, she won three gold medals in track and field in the Summer Olympics at Rome.[14] Throughout the 1950s, March of Dimes posters, reflecting the continuing racial segregation in American medicine, depicted Black children cared for by a Black physician and Wwhite children cared for by a White physician.[15]

The March of Dimes also played an outsize role in shaping federal policies around polio. After the Second World War, there was a massive expansion in the federal National Institutes of Health as Congress funded institutes of heart disease, mental health, arthritis, neurological disease, blindness and allergy.[16] Congress did not establish a National Polio Institute, although one was proposed during hearings in Congress during the late 1940s. Basil O'Connor rejected this proposal. Despite pressure to make medical research the responsibility of the federal government, he preferred research funded by voluntary health agencies like the March of Dimes in which, as he argued in a speech on 'The American Way', 'individuals . . . join together for the common good . . . without any sort of emolument in terms either of money or privilege'.[17]

In 1948, O'Connor sent March of Dimes officials to testify to Congress and warn that if the March of Dimes research programmes were taken over by the government, the organisation would lose its public appeal. This was a moment when the March of Dimes moved visibly away from the federal expansionist ideology of Roosevelt's

New Deal. O'Connor's brother, John J. O'Connor, who had been a New York Democrat congressman until 1939 and was now a March of Dimes official, appeared at the congressional hearings to tell the story of his son, a graduate from Harvard Medical School who had recently been paralysed by polio. John O'Connor declared that 'I did not want then, and I do not want now any Government representative whether he is a scientist or a doctor, treating me or my people under such circumstances. I want to get the best private treatment. And this proposed research by the Government is bound to develop to the Government taking over completely.' Even a 'government research bureau' which just collected data, he argued, 'is the proverbial camel getting its nose under the tent and from that time on you have the whole animal, and the whole carcass, right in the centre of the ring'.[18] Reflecting early Cold War suspicions of Soviet-style planning which were rapidly casting a shadow over New Deal programmes, John O'Connor also articulated the long-standing fear among conservative physicians that government intervention in medicine would lead to a government-run healthcare system. 'The government taking care of the personal disease of our people,' was, he argued, 'a completely totalitarian idea that was never intended in America.'[19] With such arguments, proposals for a polio institute were soundly defeated. The March of Dimes, a private organisation established by Roosevelt and integrated into New Deal programmes, now articulated a stance against government intervention in medical care and health policy.

Vaccine strategies

The pivot to vaccine development as a strategy to defeat polio drew on wider enthusiasm for such public health measures. In 1947, for example, New Yorkers were horrified to learn that there were a few cases of smallpox in their city, a disease that by the 1940s had begun to be seen as one of those old-fashioned problems which science had largely solved. The city's commissioner of health immediately urged New Yorkers to get vaccinated and members of the public lined up at health department offices in every borough to follow his advice. As a result, there was no epidemic of smallpox in 1947.[20] Yet, while many ordinary Americans sought out vaccination from their health department for a disease that they recognised as scary and deadly, others remained sceptical of new polio vaccines available only a few years later.

By the late 1940s, the March of Dimes began to focus on the hope that medical science, developed by its own researchers, would conquer the disease. Indeed, until the 1960s the March of Dimes provided more money to fund virology research than the National Institutes of Health, and this research led to significant success. In 1954, virologist Jonas Salk developed a polio vaccine based on a killed or inactivated poliovirus. With the encouragement of Basil O'Connor, the March of Dimes set up the world's largest clinical trial to test the vaccine on American schoolchildren around the country, a massive event that resulted in Salk being featured on the cover of *TIME* magazine. Relying on schools, including the many segregated by race, the March of Dimes made sure that Black children participated in the trial by either bringing the vaccine to their separate schools or bussing them to a White school to receive the vaccine. But in May 1954, the Supreme Court's decision in *Brown* v. *Board of Education*[21] raised new public awareness of the damaging effect of racism in elementary schools. Photographs of Black children being vaccinated outside White schools, forbidden to use the schools' restrooms or entering White schools through a separate door now appeared as disturbing images of America's segregated medical and educational systems.[22]

To promote the Salk vaccine the March of Dimes partnered with public health departments. Famously it used the 1950s celebrity Elvis Presley, who was photographed in 1956 being given a shot by the Assistant Commissioner of the New York City Health Department backstage before he performed on the Ed Sullivan Show.[23] Health

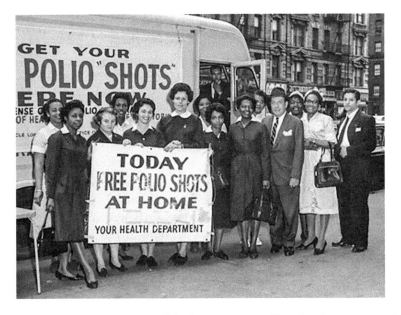

Figure 3.2 New York City health department staff and volunteers outside mobile vaccine station on 84th Street and Amsterdam Avenue in 1961

officials directed the vaccination rollout around the country, emphasising the vaccine's availability without charge at public clinics and school auditoriums. The vaccination was also presented as being accessible to all children, whatever their race or ethnicity. The New York City Health Department distributed a Spanish-language pamphlet and recruited schoolchildren to parade through Harlem wearing sandwich boards that urged 'Get your free polio shots now.' A department mobile van staffed with Black nurses travelled around Harlem offering the Salk vaccine.[24]

In the late 1950s the March of Dimes began to recognise the problems of reaching children in inner city and isolated rural communities, as well as adults who were often unwilling to accept the required three shots over a series of weeks. This was the moment when Albert Sabin, another virologist funded by the March of Dimes, began to test his own distinctive polio vaccine, a live, attenuated vaccine given not by injection but by mouth. Sabin tested his oral vaccine in the Soviet Union and in 1961 it was licensed by the US Public Health Service.[25] Seen as more effective than the Salk vaccine, this vaccine was also much easier to disseminate as it was given in a small amount of fluid which could be dropped on a sugar cube and thus did not have to be given by a doctor or a nurse, which made it an appealing technology for use in the developing world as well. Public health departments quickly shifted to promoting 'Sabin Sundays' for entire communities, attracting not only children but also their parents and other adults. In 1991, the last known case of polio in the Western Hemisphere was a boy in Peru and polio is now close to being eradicated across the globe.[26] The victory over polio by the March of Dimes, in a way, resulted in the end of the polio-centred March of Dimes, but by the mid-1960s its philanthropy switched to tackling birth defects and today plays an important role in combatting infant and maternal morbidity and mortality.

The anti-vaccine impulse and erosions of authority

The announcement of the COVID vaccines in 2021 was hailed as a major turning point in efforts to control the recent pandemic. Yet protests against vaccine mandates have been audible throughout the pandemic in the United States and around the world. Similarly, during the 1950s many Americans, inspired by the announcement of the Salk vaccine, hoped that this would be the beginning of a vaccine victory over other diseases. In 1954, a *Miami Daily News* cartoon personified cancer, heart disease and other diseases wondering 'when will our vaccines come?'[27] But vocal anti-vaccination advocates made it clear that safeguarding the public's health in the Cold War would not be achieved by such technical fixes. Instead, resistance to the Salk vaccine became part of a broader movement targeting a range of government health programmes which were supposedly anti-American, perhaps pro-Soviet, as well as incredibly dangerous.

Drawing on allegations from the nineteenth-century anti-vaccination movement, antagonists warned that the new vaccine was dangerous and that mandating vaccination was an attack on individual liberties, a potent combination of medical and political arguments.[28] Health officials had long protested that anti-vaccinationists were driven by lies, misinformation and bigotry.[29] Yet it was clear that their popularity reflected a wider lack of trust among many Americans. In the 1940s and 1950s, for example, the public paid no attention to March of Dimes researchers and health experts who claimed that insects did not spread polio. Consumers not only bought domestic fly sprays but also pressured their city and state sanitation agencies to spray DDT and other pesticides to make sure that their homes and streets were polio safe.[30]

In the 1950s anti-vaccinationists focused on the new Salk polio vaccine, arguing that compulsory vaccination laws, despite their long-standing support by the Supreme Court, were anti-American. Nor were they convinced that research funded by the March of Dimes was accurate, suggesting that the polio virus might not in fact cause the symptoms of polio paralysis. Perhaps polio was instead the result of parental neglect, a clinical condition caused by parents who allowed their children to eat ice-cream and other poor nutritional choices. Various small anti-vaccination groups published pamphlets attacking the Salk vaccine and sent them to polio experts and health departments around the country, as well as to ordinary Americans. These pamphlets urged the public to pressure their senators and congressmen to hold open hearings in order to learn 'the truth' about polio and to make sure that doctors of 'every healing profession' were invited. Perhaps the March of Dimes, anti-vaccinationists warned, was too beholden to the American Medical Association. Surely, once March of Dimes 'poliophobia' was exposed and replaced with the truth, no polio vaccine would ever be licensed.[31]

In the early 1950s, Dion Miller, a Florida cosmetic manufacturer and one of the major instigators of these anti-polio vaccine messages, challenged Basil O'Connor, Jonas Salk and the Public Health Service. He proposed that polio patients from any 'designated hospital' be treated by 'chiropractic methods of polio care' in front of reporters from *Life* magazine, the Associated Press and television networks to show how much better such methods were than those the March of Dimes was funding. Convinced that the polio virus was not the cause of paralysis, Miller offered to serve as a human guinea pig and have blood from a new polio patient injected into his bloodstream or taken orally, taunting O'Connor by asking if he was 'man enough' to 'accept these challenges for the good of little children everywhere'.[32] O'Connor made sure that the March of Dimes ignored these attacks and continued to promote the Salk vaccine through posters, pamphlets and the work of sympathetic journalists.

Public scepticism of public health measures and medical experts was reinforced by the idea of government health services being a sign of an expanding communist plot. Another pamphlet produced by the anti-Communist group Keep America Committee [sic] warned of 'The Unholy Three', linking together polio vaccines, fluoridated water and the expansion of mental health services. The March of Dimes 1955 vaccine drive, it warned, was the entering wedge for nationwide socialised medicine to be instigated by the Public Health Service, an organisation that the Committee maintained was heavily infiltrated by Russian-born doctors; in enemy hands such a government campaign could 'destroy a whole generation'.[33]

The Public Health Service and local health officials were prominently identified with the fluoridation movement by the early 1950s. In 1945, with the agreement of the Grand Rapids, Michigan, city council, federal health officials had poured sodium fluoride into the city's waterworks so that citizens could drink artificially fluoridated water and thereby prevent dental cavities. School children then had their saliva tested and their teeth examined regularly as part of this project. In 1951, after researchers observed significant decrease in tooth decay surrounding cities began to demand fluoridated water as well.[34] Health officials supported by city councils frequently asked local residents to approve these projects and fund them. But despite the strong endorsement of the Public Health Service and the American Public Health Association many communities refused, influenced by anti-fluoridation campaigns urging them to 'get the poison out of our drinking water'; between 1954 and 1955 around 60 per cent of local referenda rejected fluoridation.[35]

Congress debated this issue in 1954. Miss Florence Birmingham, head of a conservative women's political club, testified that fluoridation destroyed 'human tissues, health, life, and the constitutional rights of millions'. It was, she argued, an example of human experimentation, analogous to the criminal acts recently exposed during the Nuremberg trials, and was the result of a conspiracy among

At the Sign of THE UNHOLY THREE

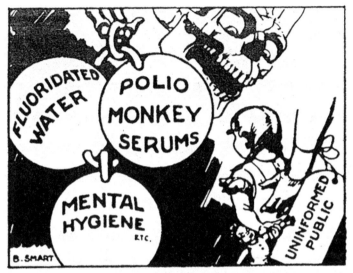

Are you willing to PUT IN PAWN to the UNHOLY THREE all of the material, mental and spiritual resources of this GREAT REPUBLIC?

FLUORIDATED WATER

1—Water containing Fluorine (rat poison—no antidote) is already the only water in many of our army camps, making it very easy for saboteurs to wipe out an entire camp personel. If this happens, every citizen will be at the mercy of the enemy—already within our gates.

POLIO SERUM

2—Polio Serum, it is reported, has already killed and maimed children; its future effect on minds and bodies cannot be guaged. This vaccine drive is the entering wedge for nation-wide socialized medicine, by the U. S. Public Health Service, (heavily infiltrated by Russian-born doctors, according to Congressman Clare Hoffman.) In enemy hands it can destroy a whole generation.

MENTAL HYGIENE

3—Mental Hygiene is a subtle and diabolical plan of the enemy to transform a free and intelligent people into a cringing horde of zombies.

Rabbi Spitz in the American Hebrew, March 1, 1946: "American Jews must come to grips with our contemporary anti-Semites; we must fill our insane asylums with anti-Semitic lunatics."

FIGHT COMMUNISTIC WORLD GOVERNMENT by destroying THE UNHOLY THREE !!!   It is later than you think!

KEEP AMERICA COMMITTEE
Box 3094, Los Angeles 54, Calif.   H. W. Courtois, Secy.   May 16, 1955

Figure 3.3 Pamphlet published by Keep America Committee on 16 May 1955

public officials who falsely claimed that there was scientific proof
of fluoride's therapeutic value, a claim based on 'unproven, miscon-
strued, misinterpreted, and superficial facts'.[36] Birmingham speculated that these officials might be in league with chemical and drug
companies, but other anti-fluoridation proponents went further.
The *Dan Smoot Report*, a right-wing newsletter that chronicled
alleged communist infiltration in various parts of the government,
cited Aldous Huxley's *Brave New World* in which the government had mandated drugs to pacify the population. 'How could
ruling authorities ever manage to give drugs to an entire population?' asked Smoot, and his answer was via drinking water, just
like fluoridation.[37] Pressured by Birmingham and other anti-fluoridation advocates, including some physicians and dentists, Congress
chose not to either ban or support fluoridation. The politicising of
these public health measures left health officials frustrated at the
spotty acceptance of fluoridation across the country. But there was
no dental March of Dimes to combat these claims with posters or
pamphlets, and the American Dental Association's muted support
of fluoridation did not stop a vocal number of dentists and doctors
from offering their own clinical 'evidence' as part of anti-fluoridation campaigns. Medical experts disagreed, reinforcing the public's
scepticism about government public health measures.

Conclusion

From the influenza pandemic to polio to even fluoride and, certainly,
COVID, the question of state responsibility and authority remained
central. In times of crisis, like a global pandemic, what special powers are seen as legitimate by the public? When are public health measures seen as a threat to individual liberty? Or as critical for global
and national security? When are they considered undemocratic or
un-American? And whose vision of citizenship do they embody?
Individualism has long been central to American identity. Citizens
are expected to be cautious, yet strong and self-reliant; committed to
family and community, yet quick to exclude those seen as outsiders.
Who gets to define those boundaries? Who determines the tactics
of dramatising the consequences of disease by depicting patients on
a ventilator or on crutches? What about the dangers of contagion,
perhaps dangerous germs or poisoned drinking water, or dangerous
ideas undermining the healthy body politic? And what happens to
these potent images and ideologies when disease threats fade?

During COVID the American public demanded guidance from
non-partisan public health experts and has been frustrated to find
inconsistent and unclear messaging. In the 1940s and 1950s scientists

and physicians were celebrated as heroes and discoverers. Yet, simultaneously, these experts were also seen as misguided and untrustworthy; the government agencies with which they were affiliated, including health departments, were maligned as allied with powerful insidious forces such as pharmaceutical and chemical companies. Indeed, the COVID pandemic has largely created health villains rather than heroes. And even notions of health have been unstable. The public has demanded protection from deadly infection, but without a consensus around the extent to which practices intended to ensure this protection should limit social and economic life. Despite the many pronouncements of public health and medical experts, there continues to be a long-standing faith in the individual control of health, although this is rarely commensurate with the notion of social determinants in shaping health. Such tensions can in extreme cases lead to the idea of 'doing your own research' to assess the safety of vaccines or other health measures.

Throughout American history, the work of a health official has often been neither easy nor widely respected. In 2021, the *New York Times* featured Dr Allison Berry, a health officer for a Washington state county, who was depicted being escorted to her car by a local sheriff after she attended a COVID briefing. Berry had proposed mask mandates and proof of vaccination, measures supported by the CDC and the Public Health Service. In response she received death threats to her family, as well as herself.[38] Berry's promotion of public health measures was seen by some of her neighbours as a threat to individual liberty and a sign of government over-reach. This reaction reflected the weaponising of COVID public health measures as groups of Americas resisted claims for government special powers to prevent the epidemic's spread and to protect the uninfected. This pandemic – like others in the past – challenged the US government and efforts to expand its authority to deal with the crisis. Public resistance to government health infrastructures is based on long-standing popular scepticism of medical experts and the fear that nefarious motivations – not objective scientific facts – are at the heart of the promotion of measures that potentially threaten individual liberty and American patriotic ideals.

Notes

1. I would like to thank the organisers and participants of the Roosevelt Institute for American Studies 2021 conference 'Public Health and Disease in the American Century' for their insights and enthusiasm; Melissa Grafe, Kayleigh Larsen and Shiliu Wang for their help with research and logistics; and Kelly O'Donnell for close editing and support.

2. 'Three Shot in Struggle with Mask Slacker', *San Francisco Chronicle*, 29 October 1918; Francesco Aimone, 'The 1918 Influenza Epidemic in New York City: A Review of the Public Health Response', *Public Health Reports* 25 (S3) (2010), 71–9; John M. Barry, *The Great Influenza: The Story of the Deadliest Plague in History* (New York, Penguin, 2004); Nancy K. Bristow, *American Pandemic: Lost Worlds of the 1918 Influenza Epidemic* (New York: Oxford University Press, 2012); Alfred W. Crosby, *America's Forgotten Pandemic: The Influenza of 1918*, 2nd edn (Cambridge: Cambridge University Press, 2012); Diane M. T. North, 'California and the 1918–1920 Influenza Pandemic', *California History* 97 (2020), 3–36; Laura Spinney, *Pale Rider: The Spanish Flu of 1918 and How It Changed the World* (London: Jonathan Cape, 2017); Nancy Tomes, 'Destroyer and Teacher: Managing the Masses During the 1918–1919 Influenza Pandemic', *Public Health Reports* 125 (2010), 48–62.

3. Richard H. Shryock, *National Tuberculosis Association, 1904–1954: A Study of the Voluntary Health Movement in the United States* (New York: National Tuberculosis Association, 1957); Scott Cutlip, *Fund Raising in the United States* (New Brunswick, NJ: Rutgers University Press, 1965); Richard Carter, *The Gentle Legions* (New York: Doubleday, 1961); Olivier Zunz, *Philanthropy in America: A History* (Princeton, NJ: Princeton University Press, 2012).

4. On the history of polio in the United States, see David M. Oshinsky, *Polio: An American Story* (New York: Oxford University Press, 2005); John R. Paul, *A History of Poliomyelitis* (New Haven, CT: Yale University Press, 1971); Naomi Rogers, *Polio Wars: Sister Kenny and the Golden Age of American Medicine* (New York: Oxford University Press, 2014).

5. Naomi Rogers, *Dirt and Disease: Polio before FDR* (New Brunswick, NJ: Rutgers University Press, 1992).

6. Daniel Holland, 'Franklin D. Roosevelt's Shangri-La: Foreshadowing the Independent Living Movement in Warm Springs, Georgia, 1926–1945', *Disability & Society* 21 (2006), 513–35; David W. Rose, *Friends and Partners: The Legacy of Franklin D. Roosevelt and Basil O'Connor in the History of Polio* (Cambridge, MA: Academic Press, 2016); Turnley Walker, *Roosevelt and the Warm Springs Story* (New York: A. A. Wyn, 1953).

7. Hugh Gregory Gallagher, *FDR's Splendid Deception* (New York: Dodd, Mead, 1985); see also Amy L. Fairchild, 'The Polio Narratives: Dialogues with FDR', *Bulletin of the History of Medicine* 75 (2001), 488–534; Davis W. Houck and Amos Kiewe, *FDR's Body Politics: The Rhetoric of Disability* (College Station, TX: Texas A & M University Press, 2003); Naomi Rogers, 'Polio Chronicles: Warm Springs and Disability Politics in the 1930s', *Asclepio: Revista de Historia de la Medicine y de la Ciencia* 61 (2009), 143–74.

8. Oshinsky, *Polio*; Rogers, *Polio Wars*; Edward D. Berkowitz, *Disability Policy: America's Programs for the Handicapped* (Cambridge: Cambridge

University Press, 1987); Glenn Gritzer and Arnold Arluke, *The Making of Rehabilitation: The Political Economy of Medical Specialization, 1890–1980* (Berkeley: University of California Press, 1985).

9. Alden Whitman, 'Basil O'Connor, Polio Crusader, Dies', *New York Times*, 10 March 1972, p. 40; Rose, *Friends and Partners*.

10. Naomi Rogers. 'Race and the Politics of Polio: Warm Springs, Tuskegee and the March of Dimes', *American Journal of Public Health* 97 (2007), 2–13; Stephen E. Mawdsley, '"Dancing on Eggs": Charles H. Bynum, Racial Politics, and the National Foundation for Infantile Paralysis, 1938–1943', *Bulletin of the History of Medicine* 84 (2010), 217–47; David B. Smith, *Health Care Divided: Race and Healing a Nation* (Ann Arbor: University of Michigan Press, 1999).

11. Rogers, 'Race and the Politics of Polio'.

12. Ibid.; see also David B. Smith, *Health Care Divided: Race and Healing a Nation* (Ann Arbor: University of Michigan Press, 1999).

13. Rogers, 'Race and the Politics of Polio'.

14. Amy Ruth, *Wilma Rudolph* (New York: Lerner Publications, 2000); Maureen Margaret Smith, *Wilma Rudolph: A Biography* (Westport, CT: Greenwood Press, 2006).

15. On one such poster campaign, see Naomi Rogers, 'Resistance to Polio Vaccines in mid-Twentieth-Century America: The Role of the March of Dimes, Community Skepticism, Racial Inequalities, and Medical Politics', *Nursing History Review* 31 (2022), forthcoming.

16. On NIH expansion, see, for example, Judith Robinson, *Noble Conspirator: Florence S. Mahoney and the Rise of the National Institutes of Health* (Washington, DC: Francis Press, 2001).

17. Basil O'Connor, 'The American Way', 7 June 1947, Public Relations File, American Medical Association, March of Dimes Archives, White Plains, New York; see also Rogers. *Polio Wars*, 307–10; Oshinsky, *Polio*, 80–1.

18. John J. O'Connor, 13 May 1948, *Hearings before the Committee on Interstate and Foreign Commerce, House of Representatives*, 80th Congress, 2nd session on N.H. 977. . ., H.R. 3257 . . . H.R. 3464 . . . May 13, 14 and 19 1948 (Washington, DC: Government Printing Office, 1948), 41, 49–50.

19. John J. O'Connor, ibid. See also Roger L. Geiger, *Research and Relevant Knowledge: American Research Universities Since World War II* (New York: Oxford University Press, 1993); Steven Strickland, *Politics, Science and Dread Disease: A Short History of United State Medical Research Policy* (Cambridge, MA: Harvard University Press, 1972); Jessica Wang, *American Science in an Age of Anxiety: Scientists, Anticommunism, and the Cold War* (Chapel Hill: University of North Carolina Press, 1999); John Harley Warner, 'The Doctor in Early Cold War America', *Lancet* 381 (2013), 452–3.

20. Judith Walzer Leavitt, 'Public Resistance or Cooperation? A Tale of Smallpox in Two Cities', *Biosecurity Bioterrorism* 1 (2003), 185–92; Brendan Gill and Spencer Klaw, 'New York City's Smallpox Scare',

New Yorker, 16 May1947; James K Colgrove, *State of Immunity: The Politics of Vaccination in Twentieth-Century America* (Berkeley: University of California Press, 2006).

21. *Brown* v. *Board of Education of Topeka* 347 US 483 (1954).
22. Oshinsky, *Polio*, 198; Rogers, 'Resistance to Polio Vaccines'.
23. Stephen Mawdsley, '"Salk Hops": Teen Health Activism and the Fight against Polio, 1955–1960', *Cultural and Social History* 13 (2016), 249–65; 'Presley Receives a City Polio Shot', *New York Times*, 29 October 1956.
24. James K Colgrove, *Epidemic City: The Politics of Public Health in New York* (New York: Russell Sage Foundation, 2011); Colgrove, *State of Immunity*, 134–6.
25. Oshinsky, *Polio*, 243–68.
26. Deepak Sobti, Marcos Cueto and Yuan He, 'A Public Health Achievement Under Adversity: The Eradication of Poliomyelitis from Peru, 1991', *American Journal of Public Health* 104 (2014), 2298–2305; Oshinsky, *Polio*, 287–8.
27. Anne Mergen, 'Giving Them Something to Think About', *Miami Daily News*, 14 April 1954.
28. The anti-vaccination movement which emerged in the United States in the late nineteenth century was influenced by British anti-vaccinationists; see Nadji Durbach, *Bodily Matters: The Anti-Vaccination Movement in England* (Durham, NC: Duke University Press, 2004); and see Robert D. Johnston, 'Contemporary Anti-vaccination Movements in Historical Perspective', in Robert D. Johnston (ed.), *The Politics of Healing: History of Alternative Medicine in Twentieth-Century North America* (New York: Routledge, 2004), 266–82; James Colgrove and Sara J. Samuel, 'Freedom, Rights, and Vaccine Refusal: The History of an Idea', *American Journal of Public Health* 112 (2022), 234–41.
29. American Public Health Association, *Health in Pictures: A Collection of Cartoons Illustrating the Fundamental Principles of Personal and Public Health* (New York: American Public Health Association, 1930); see also Colgrove, *State of Immunity*; James Colgrove, 'Science in a Democracy: The Contested Status of Vaccination in the Progressive Era and the 1920s', *Isis* 96 (2005), 167–91.
30. Heather Green Wooten, *The Polio Years in Texas: Battling a Terrifying Unknown* (College Station, TX: Texas A&M University Press, 2009), 72–5; and see, for example, the 1946 news reel, 'City Gets DDT Treatment', from San Antonino, Texas, Universal Newsreels, National Archives and Records Administration, available at: https://unwritten-record.blogs.archives.gov/2014/05/19/this-week-in-universal-news-spraying-ddt-to-prevent-polio-1946; and 'DDT Use of Started Here to Curb Polio', *Houston Chronicle*, 18 November 1946.
31. *Murder Inc.* (Coral Gables, FL: Polio Prevention Inc.), 25 March 1955; see also Elena Conis, *Vaccine Nation: America's Changing Relationship with Immunization* (Chicago: University of Chicago Press, 2014).

32. Dion Miller. *Double Polio Challenge* (Coral Gables, Fl: Polio Prevention Inc.), November 1954; 'Duon H. Miller, 75, Cosmetic Manufacturer', *Miami Herald*, 28 November 1969.

33. *At the Sign of The Unholy Three* (Los Angeles, CA: Keep America Committee), 16 May 1955.

34. Catherine Carstairs, 'Debating Water Fluoridation Before Dr. Strangelove', *American Journal of Public Health* 105 (2015), 1559–69; Gretchen Ann Reilly, 'Not a So-Called Democracy: Anti-Fluoridationists and the Fight over Drinking Water', in Robert D. Johnston (ed.), *The Politics of Healing: History of Alternative Medicine in Twentieth-Century North America* (New York: Routledge, 2004), 132–50; Alyssa Picard, *Making the American Mouth: Dentists and Public Health in the Twentieth Century* (New Brunswick, NJ: Rutgers University Press, 2009).

35. Washington State Council against Fluoridation, 'Vote Against Fluoridation', pamphlet cover, circa 1951; Fluoridation Files, Series 254, Seattle-King County Department of Public Health, box 3, Campaign for Fluoridation Scrapbook, Section 11, Material Distributed by the Opposition, Fluoridation, King County Archives, Seattle, Washington State, available at: https://archivesearch.kingcounty.gov/SCRIPTS/MWIMAIN.DLL/128818095/1/2/246?RECORD&DATABASE=DESCRIPTION.

36. Miss Florence Birmingham, United States Congress, House of Representatives, Committee on Interstate and Foreign Commerce, *Hearings on a Bill to Protect the Public Health from the Dangers of Fluoridation of Water* (Washington, DC: Government Printing Office, May 1954), 83rd Congress, 2nd session, 48–51.

37. 'Facts on Fluoridation', *The Dan Smoot Report* 5:39 (28 September 1959), 1; see also Nicole Hemmer, *Messengers of the Right: Conservative Media and the Transformation of American Politics* (Philadelphia: University of Pennsylvania Press, 2017).

38. Mike Baker and Danielle Ivory, 'Threats, Resignations and 100 New Laws: Why Public Health is in Crisis', *New York Times*, 29 October 2021.

4

From the 'Lung Block' to the 'China Virus': Public Health, Xenophobia and US Identity Formation over the American Century

Stefano Morello and Kerri Culhane

> The sickness of the world is also our sickness . . . And nowhere in the world have man's failures been so little excusable as in the United States of America. Nowhere has the contrast been so great between the reasonable hopes of our age and the actual facts of failure and frustration.
>
> Henry R. Luce, 1941[1]

The American Century, the time in which the United States pursued worldwide political, economic and cultural hegemony, has been bracketed by two gilded ages – one forged in late nineteenth-century capitalist industrialism and the other in late twentieth-century global techno-capitalism. Each age was marked by gross and growing inequalities, racial, class and identity conflict, and cultural agendas largely set and reinforced by mass media: the mass circulation of books, newspapers and magazines then, media conglomerates and a largely unregulated social media apparatus today. Global public health crises, a century apart – rampant tuberculosis that was only beginning to be managed in the late nineteenth century and now the COVID-19 pandemic – also draw parentheses around this era in which the United States both exerted its power outwards and asserted its global gravitational pull.[2] This chapter focuses on the role of public health crises (and the policies that ensued) in defining US identity, and especially the iterative reassertion of whiteness in the face of a diversifying demographic. We emphasise the case of the 'Lung Block' at the turn of the twentieth century on New York's Lower East Side and efforts by Progressive reformers to cast it and its inhabitants as a threat to the city and to the established social order.[3]

Perceived threats to US fundamental racial hierarchy invigorated racial resentment both then and now. In the late nineteenth century, White Anglo-Saxon Protestant leadership was confronted with a newly free African American citizenry, and millions of immigrants troubling the colour line and bringing with them new languages, customs and religions. Yet, as historian Erika Lee has recently reiterated, anti-immigrant sentiment 'has been neither an aberration nor a contradiction' in US history – it is fundamental to the American project.[4] During the late nineteenth century, Chinese immigrants in San Francisco were singled out by local public health officials as dangerous vectors of smallpox and other ills, despite the fact that statistical data showed White people, and in particular the Irish (the primary antagonists of the Chinese) to be far more represented in both cases and mortality.[5] In the first decade of the twentieth century, it was Italian immigrants, in particular those residing on New York City's 'Lung Block', who were rendered by Progressive reformers and the popular press as tuberculosis bogeymen, and by extension, an existential threat to the moral and social fabric of the city. As Alan M. Kraut has demonstrated, the characterisations of the Chinese in San Francisco and the Italians in New York City are but two examples of a larger phenomenon of racialising disease, or pathologising race.[6] The nation's perennial struggles to manage foreign bodies, not only bacteriological or viral pathogens but the non-White and the immigrant, have served to reinforce a White, and White supremacist, identity.[7]

The Progressive movement emerged in large part to assert a code of practice and an understanding of modernity based on White, Protestant culture and morality that required an adoption of accepted norms to maintain a White supremacist cultural and social order.[8] Today, due in large part to its liberalised immigration policies in the post-war era, the United States is headed for a 'minority majority' within decades, a projection by the US 2020 Census that actualises the demographics long feared by the White ruling classes.[9] While the course of the American Century also coincided with increasing precision of medical diagnosis and scientific specificity, the murky association of disease with those perceived as non-normative subjects, of which the figure of the immigrant is a chief example, remains a potent tool of political rhetoric.[10] The discourse around the COVID-19 pandemic, therefore, echoes a familiar pattern: Donald J. Trump's 'China Virus' recalls a long history of associating disease with foreign people or places for baldly political purposes. If, as Howard Markel and Alexandra Minna Stern have suggested, US popular discourse has always prioritised ideology over evidence – sentiment over science – especially during public health crises, it has perhaps never proven as deadly as during the most recent pandemic.

A nation of immigrants?

Since the days of early European settler colonialism, the United States has been the living definition of, as John F. Kennedy (notably the first Irish Catholic president) put it in the title of his 1958 book, *A Nation of Immigrants*, a fact at best evoked selectively in the current political discourse. The inclusion of this expression in the US Citizenship and Immigration Service's mission statement under the George W. Bush administration, and its removal under Donald Trump's presidency, suggest the conditional nature of the national narrative that casts the country as a promised land.[11] Yet, throughout the past two centuries, for many immigrants who have 'made it' in the United States, becoming American has been consistently synonymous with becoming 'white'.

Of course, as the likes of David Roediger, George Lipsitz, Matthew Frye Jacobson and Ruth Frankenberg remind us, the contest over whiteness has always been critical to the nation's identity formation, and yet a messy and invisible affair that points to a logic of race that is both seemingly natural and exceptionally unstable.[12] Thinking of whiteness in the context of immigration – whereby it is conflated with 'Americanness', as made evident by the Trump administration's immigration policy and the precedents in US history that inspired it – requires us to think about both the *assimilated* and the *unassimilable*. Italian Americans and Asian Americans are two examples worth considering in this context. As a number of contemporary public figures have demonstrated – think, for instance, of the way the recent shenanigans of Andrew Cuomo and Rudy Giuliani were associated, blamed and socially sanctioned, with, on and through their Italian heritage – Italian Americans have (and have been) integrated into a somewhat precarious (and at times hyperconservative) whiteness. On the other hand, Asian Americans, despite their upward mobility, accedence to many American cultural norms, and even an increasing political conservatism, have been and still are perceived as foreign by a nation that imagines itself as white.

US xenophobia is a form of self-othering – whereby US citizens disassociate themselves from a large part of their history, ethnicity or racial identity to iteratively affirm their own whiteness, with the inevitable consequence of creating a unified front against those who cannot 'belong' (that is, 'be white'). The reification of whiteness justifies structures of racial and economic inequality, which over time have grown more entrenched. This holds true for Americans of Anglo-Saxon descent, whose very national identity has been shaped in part by unacknowledged contributions of non-White people, and it is especially true for Italian Americans and other White-passing ethnic populations for whom assimilation entailed a negation of their own ethnicity, conforming and reshaping it into a White or 'less ethnic' version of their own native culture.

The association between the immigrant and disease persists throughout contemporary history, whereby the latter has been used as the justification for this process of othering, and for the exclusion of vulnerable members of society from entry to the United States or full citizenship. Disease works as an especially powerful metaphor that suggests immigrants, like germs and other vectors of disease, are external agents attacking the body from within. Such exclusionary logic creates a sense of cohesion on the part of the perpetrators and is further driven by cultural, social and political agendas informed by the demands of capitalism. For instance, at the turn of the twentieth century, the US Public Health Service (PHS) enforced the biopolitics of a nation seeking a workforce able to fulfil its needs for cheap manual labour. The PHS held the sovereign right to seize, repress and destroy immigrants' lives, often under the guise of preserving American life. Conducted at the ports of entry on both coasts and at the borders with Mexico and Canada, medical inspection consisted of both physical and attitudinal tests used to examine thousands of immigrants, lined up and passing through stations within a PHS facility – a process that quite literally applied Frederick Taylor's 'principles of scientific management' to public health, creating standards (concerning both process: the assembly line; and product: the subjects passing through the assembly line) that sought to maximise efficiency.[13]

PHS' interpretation of its own mission often exceeded its charge of 'preventing the entrance of disease to the nation', and was generally understood (by both its practitioners and politicians) as preventing the entrance of undesirable people and weeding out 'bad seeds': carriers of chronic disease and disability, and those 'who would not make good citizens'.[14] As Alison Bateman-House and Amy Fairchild have noted, the eugenics agenda in service of capitalism, hidden behind the scarecrow of disease, is especially evident from the fact that of the few 'who were denied entry, most were certified, not with "loathsome and dangerous contagious diseases", but with conditions that limited their capacity to perform unskilled labour'.[15] Unsurprisingly, Bateman-House and Fairchild continue, 'non-Europeans faced more considerable medical obstacles to entry at the nation's Pacific Coast and Mexican border immigration stations. Disease, health officials argued, was not so easily 'read' in the 'inscrutable' Asians, particularly the Chinese.[16]

Of course, the association of Asian people and disease is not a relic of history. Since the very start of the COVID-19 pandemic and extending to the present moment, the rise in anti-Asian violence in the United States can be directly linked to the association of China and Chinese people with the novel coronavirus. On 19 March 2020, after the unpreparedness and negligence of both local and national government allowed COVID-19 to proliferate throughout the United States, Trump wilfully edited his speech to the nation about 'corona virus [sic]' to read 'Chinese virus'. In an instant, and through Trump's endless repetition in the following months, Asian Americans were (again) cast as an undifferentiated internal enemy as alleged vectors of 'the China Virus' or the 'Kung Flu'.[17] In doing so, Trump reified the American tradition of casting non-White populations as vehicles of disease – external agents to the nation's otherwise allegedly whole-some body, a rhetorical strategy that he also deployed both pre- and mid-pandemic to target Mexican immigrants.[18] The relentless associ-ation of Asian bodies with the deadly pandemic produced immediate and violent results across the United States and, as Kim Yi Dionne and Fulya Felicity Turkmen have observed, across the majority of the Western world as well.[19] In the United States, victims of the ensu-ing anti-Asian violence include people of Chinese, Korean, Japanese, Thai or other Asian diasporic descent, most of whom are, in fact, US citizens; physical assault is often accompanied by an aporic order to 'go back to where [they] came from'.

Coming at a moment when the country's own identity seemed to be especially fractured, Trump's ploy was part of a larger strategy to treat disease as a sociological problem and use it as a metaphor to other and scapegoat marginalised communities. Despite Luce's emphatical assertion that, during the American Century, 'the sickness of the world is also our sickness', the tendency to associate the other with disease has been repeatedly extended to any social formation that does not conform to the hegemonic values that inform the US national project.[20] Luce was writing met-aphorically, of course, but the notion of an American global, let alone domestic, empathy is easily disproved. For instance, we have seen similar othering processes at play during the AIDS crisis of the 1980s, when the disease was wrongly and uniquely associated with the queer community. Queerness was also identified as a threat against the nuclear family, one of the pillars of the neo-conservative Reagan vision for a white(r) heteronormative America. At the turn of the twentieth century, the same mechanism was used to vilify Italian (and other othered) immigrants, including those living in New York City's Lung Block.

The Lung Block

In 1903, the area bounded by Monroe, Catherine, Cherry and Market Streets, a former merchant enclave turned sailortown turned tenement district, became the epicentre of both the local debate and the national discourse on public health, immigration and housing reform. In many ways, this particular block was indistinguishable from the rest of the Lower East Side – a bustling, immigrant stronghold characterised by five- and six-storey brick tenements and the occasional old house. During the 1880s and early 1890s, the block had already been the object of inquiry for missionary Helen Stuart Campbell in *Darkness and Daylight* (1892), and for muck-raking journalist Jacob Riis, who documented and dramatised its residents' living conditions in *How the Other Half Lives* (1890).[21] Looking at different immigrant enclaves across the Lower East Side, Riis judged each according to popular stereotypes. The Italian was 'picturesque', but 'content to live in a pig-sty'. Riis ascribed to the Italians a general propensity for 'destitution and disorder' that was a 'danger' to the 'American community'.[22] The combination of allegedly poor housekeeping with abysmal housing conditions together enabled the conditions for disease – and fear of the diseased – to proliferate. Riis' exposé ultimately cast the entire block under the shadow of a sinister narrative: that death was embedded in the very walls of its buildings, and that it might escape the boundaries of the slums.

One memorable piece of visual propaganda from 1901, titled 'The Tenement: A Menace to All' (Figure 4.1) depicts a range of common ethnic and cultural stereotypes (the prostitute, the sick, the gangster, the drunk, the gambler, the opium addict) emanating, with death, like ghosts or miasmas, from a tenement house.[23] The caption – 'not only an evil in itself, but the vice, crime and disease it breeds invade the homes of rich and poor alike' – speaks of the agenda behind what Riis had called 'The Battle with the Slum'.[24] Indeed, in New York City, the Progressive reformers' noble goal of tenement house reform – the improvement of housing standards of the immigrant poor – can be better understood as a containment strategy, a means of keeping the poor and 'their' alleged diseases and vices from spreading to better neighbourhoods uptown.

In turn-of-the-century New York, the concurrent emergence of a coordinated public health response to the eternally simmering tuberculosis pandemic, in which the city's public health authorities were pioneers, intertwined with the Progressive social reform agenda to cure the perceived moral, social and physical ills of the immigrant, while maintaining established social and racial hierarchies exacerbated

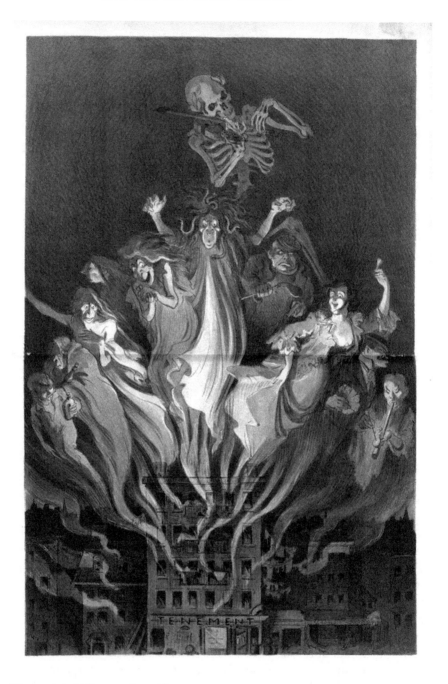

Figure 4.1 Udo Keppler, 'The Tenement: A Menace to All', 1901

by public health crises.[25] Before the acceptance of germ theory in the mid-nineteenth century, it was believed that sensory evidence such as visible filth or noxious smells were reliable indicators and even vectors of disease. Germ theory proved that the enemy microbe was invisible to the naked eye, yet this revelation did not stop reformers and others from looking for visible signs. The Victorian pseudoscience of eugenics and scientific racism – the classification and regulation of people based on visible difference – also came to prominence in this period.[26] As Victoria Rosner has observed, under the tyranny of a modernity informed by a new understanding of hygiene, 'dirt and dust functioned as metonyms for the invisible disease carrying germs'.[27] So, too, were race and its culturally constructed and often unintelligible sensorial markers – as represented by the stereotypes of the 'dirty' Italian, the 'drunken' Irish, or the 'rat-eating' Chinese – used as a proxy for dissipation or threat of disease. In that context, sanitary and purification trends in building interiors – promoted by housing and public health reformers through tenement reform and evidenced by white plastered walls and gleaming white tiles – mirror the alleged purity and privileging of racial whiteness.

Yet science *was* at the root of reformers' efforts to manage disease, despite abuses in its name. One of New York City's pioneers of public health practice, Dr Hermann Biggs, initiated compulsory reporting of disease in the mid-1890s, which enabled government officials as well as reformers to track and visualise the spatial distribution of disease city-wide. Citing immigrants as the 'poorest and most ignorant classes', and unwilling to assimilate into American customs and language, Biggs felt the 'sanitary surveillance of infectious diseases in the overcrowded, tenement house districts of New York City' to be his ultimate challenge.[28] In 1899, housing reformer Lawrence Veiller, on behalf of the Charity Organization Society (COS), the leading Progressive charitable institution in the city (for which Biggs was an adviser), overlaid the spatialised Board of Health data, population statistics and charity cases on hand-drawn neighbourhood maps compiled through house-to-house research. These maps, designed to show the correlation of congestion, poverty and disease, were presented during the Tenement House Exhibition of 1900. The exhibition, a public demonstration of the need for housing reform, led to the New York State Tenement House Act of 1901, the first successful attempt at banning lightless and poorly ventilated tenement buildings in the state.[29] Robert De Forest, then COS president and soon to be New York City's first Tenement House Commissioner, declared the block bounded by Catherine, Monroe, Cherry and Market streets, as the worst, most dense and tubercular of the city. According to the wealthy White Progressive reformers, this 'lung block' represented a threat not just to its struggling working-class immigrant residents, but to the city at large.[30]

The Lung Block appeared especially threatening to White America because of the increasingly unintelligible immigrant and non-White communities that, beginning in the mid-1880s, had been proliferating within its boundaries and in their surroundings. In 1789, George Washington's first executive mansion stood just a block to the west on what later became known, through Riis' narratives, as the infamous Cherry Hill. This once upper-class residential area began attracting suspicion and curiosity during its days as a mid-nineteenth century sailortown, when the houses of well-to-do merchants had given way to boarding houses, brothels, saloons and an ecosystem that served sailors in port. It held a racially, religiously and ethnically diverse residential population, and was visited by the middle- and upper-classes who found in the downtown slums an outlet for their vices at once geographically close and yet far removed from their uptown homes.[31] If the moral character of this sailortown concerned Protestant reformers, the influx of new waves of immigrants, together with the ongoing discourse about public health in immigrant quarters, focused unprecedented attention on the neighbourhood by both settlement workers and the popular press.

Of course, like the majority of Lower Manhattan at the time, the Lung Block was mostly populated by a struggling (and eventually up and coming) working class, made up of first- and second-generation migrants from Italy, Ireland and Eastern Europe. Around the turn of the twentieth century, a majority of the block and the wider neighbourhood had become home to a thriving Italian community; census data shows that by 1905, Italians made up nearly 50 per cent of the block's population. The block was, in fact, a pan-Italian enclave, populated by people from districts culturally and geographically far apart from one another: eastern Sicilians coexisted with Abruzzesi, Piacentini, western Sicilians and Tuscans. Although popular narratives treated the Lung Block as a discrete entity, its residents participated in a larger community that extended well beyond its borders. As chronicled in articles such as Kelly Durand and Louis Sessa', 'The Italian Invasion of the Ghetto' (1905), the expansion of the 'Italian quarter' was one very much feared by anglophone newspapers and publications. Southern Italians in particular were perceived as a much more threatening population than the majority Jewish population of the adjacent neighbourhood.[32]

Housing conditions, admittedly poor in a block mostly constituted by old tenement buildings, improved after the enforcement of the New York State Tenement House Act of 1901, but also during the concurrent period of increasing Italian ownership and building occupation.[33] Despite a marked improvement, reformers engaged in an effort, spearheaded by University Settlement, a local progressive social service organisation, and volunteer settlement worker Ernest Poole, to raze the block and build a park in its place.[34] It was indeed Poole, journalist and future Pulitzer prize-winning author, in his short essay 'The Plague in Its Stronghold' (1903) who indelibly applied the term 'Lung Block'. 'The Plague', therefore, was not only an attempt to shape public opinion and gain support for the crusade against the slums, but it was specifically a propaganda tool to make the case to replace the Lung Block with a public park to provide 'light and air' to the tenement district. Like Riis before him, Poole's work was part of a tradition of journalistic exposés of the slums and popular culture pulp writing advancing the cause of the Progressive reform movement. While not all of the Lung Block residents are depicted as innately bad in Poole's eyes, all of them appear to be doomed.

Regardless of ethnicity or nationality, and in accordance with the popular views of the Progressives, all the immigrants in Poole's narrative are cast as inherently flawed. In particular, the Irish are both perpetrators and victims of vice (especially alcohol consumption), while the Italians are depicted as especially hopeless, passive and dirty – signifiers for pauperism, the great fault of the poor since the Victorian era. It should not go unremarked that both the Irish and Italians were predominantly Catholic, a significant defect in the eyes of the majority Protestant Progressives. Through the critical lens of the reformers, steeped in the Christian notion of progress from sin to salvation, Italian cultural and social practices – including housekeeping and culinary habits – were deemed to be superstitious, inferior and suspect.[35] The presumed capacity of Italian (and Chinese) immigrant populations to thrive in lower standards of living was perceived as a threat to a notionally high American standard of living and, as such, to the way (white) America saw itself. While Poole does not direct his contempt solely towards the Italian residents of the block, his unflattering depictions further reinforce stereotyped narratives built upon the frugality of Italian immigrants that tapped into pre-existing discourses ranging from charitable writing (such as Riis' infamous remarks about Italians being 'content to live in a pig-sty') to melodramatic narratives perpetuated by nativist and popular culture representations that cast the Italian as particularly susceptible to disease for both genetic and cultural reasons.[36]

Southern Italians in particular were believed to be genetically predisposed to tubercular disease, a condition exacerbated by what White reformers saw as poor housekeeping practices by an immigrant group from a pre-industrial society. Further raising suspicion, southern Italians troubled the colour line with their darker complexion and alarmed Reformers with their 'problematic' relationship with Catholicism (as Henry J. Browne would later have it).[37] The economy of their lives – per Samuele Pardini, 'based on the Southern Italian notion of *rispetto* that prioritises cooperation, mutuality, the primacy of the public space, the recognition of the other, and inclusive social relations over the logic of monetary profit' – also undermined the fundamental dictates of capitalism.[38]

The fight for the Lung Block, therefore, was little concerned with facts, but largely based on fear that disease, and the diseased, could spread throughout the city, especially above 14th Street, the imaginary line separating the working class from the upper classes. Apart from Poole's exposé, this fear of moral and medical contamination emanating from the slums also emerges in a number of Progressive publications and contemporary newspaper articles raising social anxiety about the spread of disease through prostitution, vice, and especially food and goods manufactured in tenement districts, such as garments, artificial flowers and cigars.[39] Italian doctor Antonio Stella, a member of COS' Tuberculosis Committee, documented that the living (and even more so the working) conditions of Italian women and children, rather than their genetic traits, were to be blamed for the rates of contagion in Italian quarters. Stella's findings found no room in American newspapers and, as such, had little impact on popular opinion. Neither did the statistics from the Board of Health, which showed that the death rate from tuberculosis among Italians in New York was among the lowest in the city.[40]

As Alan Mayne and others have convincingly argued, turn-of-the-century slums were products of cultural and political discourse rather than actual demographic or geographical realities. Focusing on middle-class writings by anglophone reformers and journalists, Mayne has concluded that the slum was a myth that fed on the ideology of its perpetrators. The universal application of the term slums, he writes, 'subsumed the innermost working-class districts of every city into one all-embracing concept of an outcast society'.[41] The discrepancies between scientific data and the narratives of the reformers involved in the crusade against the Lung Block testify to our claim that the latter reflect the social anxieties of the middle and upper classes at a specific historical conjuncture, more so than their concerns for the well-being of the immigrant working classes. Not once in Poole's narrative do we hear the local population's voice, unless it is through racialised and ridiculous caricatures. Poole and many of his predecessors affirm Christian and bourgeois – thereby 'American' – values by presenting characters leading lives in clear opposition with them as 'others'. Yet slums as constructs have important consequences in terms of both urban policies and the otherness cast inevitably upon the residents.

In 1904, a year after COS president Robert DeForest was installed as the head of New York City's newly formed Tenement House Department, the Lung Block was one of the first blocks to receive departmental attention. By 1907, DeForest declared that due to his department's interventions, the so-called Lung Block was no longer a threat to its residents or the city. Though DeForest's observations were confirmed in a feature article about its 'redemption' that appeared in COS' journal a year later, the narrative around the Lung Block would persist through the 1920s, by which time the Italian Americans of the block had managed to acquire a majority of the buildings, and the emerging Italian American rentier class lived alongside their working-class tenants.[42] Redeemed, and at the edge of the booming financial district, the Lung Block was now prime real estate.

Towards the end of the decade, real estate mogul Fred F. French, developer of New York City's Tudor City, successfully revived the spectre of the Lung Block by republishing the anti-Lung Block pamphlets that circulated at the beginning of the century in order to make a case for replacing the entire block with a large-scale, middle- and upper-middle class development. French's neighbourhood-scale project, to be called Knickerbocker Village (its name evoking the early White settlers of New York), was designed to cater to White Wall Street workers, 'a class of people' French felt should not be inconvenienced by riding the subway to work.[43] While his full vision was not realised, the one block that was demolished and replaced was the Lung Block.

Conclusion

Though Progressive reformer narratives remind us that it was not that long ago that the Italians (and the Irish) were not quite white, Trump's redemption of Italy (rendered 'a beautiful place') and the simultaneous association of China with disease, speaks of the instability of America's racial imaginary. During the post-war era and throughout the American Century, Italian Americans – perhaps more than any other White ethnic group – have embraced and have been accepted into whiteness.[44] As Fred L. Gardaphé has observed, 'Italian Americans have become whites on a leash. And as long as they behave themselves (act white), as long as they accept the images of themselves as presented in the media (don't cry defamation) and as long as they stay within corporate and cultural boundaries (don't identify with other minorities) they will be allowed to remain white.'[45]

Italians' assimilation has won them not only respectability, but also centre stage in national and local politics, as well as in US culture. While the loyalty oath Italian Americans took during the Second World War, their upward mobility and the domestication of at least part of their perceived exoticism were key to their becoming white, their pigmentation (notwithstanding its ambiguity), represented the condition of possibility for this process of assimilation.[46] Yet US citizens of Asian descent remain the unassimilable other. Asian Americans, like other Black, indigenous and other people of colour (BIPOC), are unable to conceal their non-whiteness, and, as the Trump administration's rhetorical choices before and especially during the pandemic made clear, are still subject to the kind of racial othering that *makes* whiteness.

America's public health triumphs at the start of the American Century – including controlling and eventually curing tuberculosis – are commensurate with its failures at the end. Among the United States' great failures is its inability to accept itself as a nation of immigrants. Markel and Stern, writing in 2002, presciently warned that we need to understand the US tendency to associate immigrants with disease in order to deal with future health crises and avoid the 'scapegoating of a particular group'.[47] In 2020, nativism and nationalism prevented the United States from dealing effectively with the COVID-19 public health crisis, reducing public health guidance to a matter of politics, and scapegoating anyone perceptibly Asian as a threat.

Luce defined an end to isolationism as the start of the American Century. In the post-war era, liberalised US immigration laws, including the end of Chinese exclusion and the expansion of immigration eligibility from Asia and other non-western countries, offered a virtuous vision of America as a multicultural democracy. There is no better symbol of renewed isolationism, and US anti-immigrant doctrine that brings the American Century to a close than the southern border wall. Two political cartoons featuring the wall illuminate the ironies of the United States' conflicted consciousness regarding the country's permeability to contagion. The first, 'Immigration Disease' by Rick McKee, originally published in *The Augusta Chronicle* in August 2014, depicts brown-skinned immigrants trying to scale a wall marked 'US Border', approached by three anthropomorphic viruses – a filovirus, a rhabdovirus and, indeed, a coronavirus – carrying a bindle unambiguously labelled 'DISEASE'. Echoing Trump's later rhetoric, McKee's depiction reinforces the persistent association between non-White migrants and disease, and relies on the unstable and yet recurring metaphor of migrants *as* disease, symbolising whiteness' fear of contamination.[48] The second cartoon (Figure 4.2), by Signe Wilkinson, was published in the *Philadelphia Inquirer* at the end of April 2020, when the United States already countenanced the most cases of COVID-19 globally. It depicts the United States as a nation that has sealed itself off behind an iron-clad wall posted with 'Do Not Enter' signs – a clear reference to Trump's unfulfilled promises for a hermetic wall between the United States and Mexico, and an end to non-White immigration.[49] Wilkinson's cartoon inverts the perspective typically associated with immigration and disease, thus highlighting the artificial nature of both categories of analysis. Far from being a wholesome body subject to a virulent external attack by (non-white) immigrants, the United States is trapped within its own wall, which acts as a means of containment for the rampant virus that the Trump administration failed to control within its own borders. As the coronavirus proliferates within the wall, two external characters comment approvingly: 'Fine. As long as *they* can't leave.'

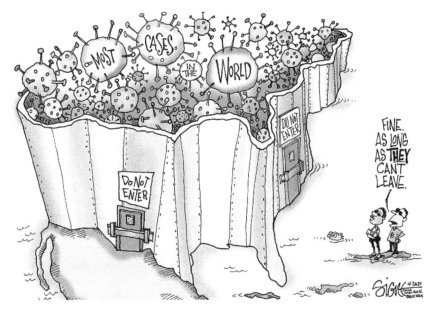

Figure 4.2 Signe Wilkinson, *Philadelphia Inquirer*, 26 April 2020

Notes

1. Henry R. Luce, 'The American Century', *Diplomatic History* 23:2 (1941), 160.
2. See for just one example Michel Gobat, *Empire by Invitation: William Walker and Manifest Destiny in Central America* (Cambridge, MA: Harvard University Press, 2018).
3. The' Lung Block', an expression that became a generic term for urban housing where tuberculosis proliferated, was originally coined by social worker, journalist and novelist Ernest Poole to describe this Lower East Side tenement district populated by a majority Italian working-class population.
4. Erika Lee, *America for Americans: A History of Xenophobia in the United States* (New York: Basic Books, 2019), 7.
5. Linnea Kell, 'The "Regulars" and the Chinese: Ethnicity and Public Health in 1870s San Francisco', *Urban Anthropology* 12:2 (1983), 185.
6. See Alan M. Kraut, *Silent Travelers: Germs Genes and the 'Immigrant Menace'* (Baltimore, MD: Johns Hopkins University Press, 1995).
7. Alison Bashford, *Imperial Hygiene: A Critical History of Colonialism, Nationalism and Public Health* (New York: Palgrave Macmillan, 2004).
8. Shannon L. Walsh, *Eugenics and Physical Culture Performance in the Progressive Era: Watch Whiteness Workout* (New York: Springer, 2020); Roy Lubove, 'The Progressives and the Prostitute', *The Historian* 24:3 (1962), 308–30; Paul Boyer, *Urban Masses and Moral Order in America, 1820–1920* (Cambridge, MA: Harvard University Press, 1992).
9. Jonathan Vespa, Lauren Medina and David M. Armstrong, 'Demographic Turning Points for the United States: Population Projections for 2020 to 2060', US Bureau of the Census, 2020, available at: https://www.census.gov/library/publications/2020/demo/p25-1144.html, last accessed 5 December 2021.
10. Howard Markel and Alexandra Minna Stern, 'The Foreignness of Germs: The Persistent Association of Immigrants and Disease in American Society', *Milbank Quarterly* 80:4 (2002), 780–1.
11. See, for example, Woody Holton, *Liberty is Sweet: The Hidden History of the American Revolution* (New York: Simon & Schuster, 2021); Jill Lepore, *These Truths: A History of the United States* (New York: W. W. Norton, 2018).
12. David R. Roediger, *The Wages of Whiteness: Race and the Making of the American Working Class* (London: Verso, 1991); George Lipsitz, *The Possessive Investment in Whiteness: How White People Profit from Identity Politics* (Philadelphia, PA: Temple University Press, 1998); Matthew Frye Jacobson, *Whiteness of a Different Color: European Immigrants and the Alchemy of Race* (Cambridge, MA: Harvard University Press, 1999); Ruth Frankenberg, *White Women and the Social Construction of Whiteness* (London: Routledge, 1993).

13. Frederick Winslow Taylor, *The Principles of Scientific Management* (New York: Harper, 1900).
14. Alison Bateman-House and Amy Fairchild, 'Medical Examination of Immigrants at Ellis Island', *Virtual Mentor* 10:4 (2008), 235–41.
15. Nearly 1 in 5 immigrants underwent further medical examination in a PHS facility; fewer than 1 per cent were barred entrance into the country. The number grew exponentially after the restrictive National Origins Quota of 1924; in 1925, it reached 5 per cent.
16. See Kell, 'The "Regulars" and the Chinese'.
17. This recalls the history of ill-treatment of Chinese immigrants in America since the mid-nineteenth century. Perceived as a threat to white labour, the Chinese were recast as a moral and sanitary threat to the nation, inspiring the US' first race- and class-based immigration restrictions, the Chinese Exclusion Act of 1882, and its subsequent renewals. See Andrew Gyory, *Closing the Gate: Race, Politics, and the Chinese Exclusion Act* (Chapel Hill: University of North Carolina Press, 1998); Nayan Shah, *Contagious Divides: Epidemics and Race in San Francisco's Chinatown* (Berkeley: University of California Press, 2001).
18. Rupert Neate and Jo Tuckman, 'Donald Trump: Mexican Migrants Bring "Tremendous Infectious Disease" to US', *The Guardian*, 6 July 2015, available at: https://www.theguardian.com/us-news/2015/jul/06/donald-trump-mexican-immigrants-tremendous-infectious-disease. last accessed 11 September 2022; Antonio De Loera-Brust, 'As the US Exports Coronavirus, Trump is Blaming Mexicans', *Foreign Policy*, 14 July 2020, available at: https://foreignpolicy.com/2020/07/14/as-the-u-s-exports-coronavirus-trump-is-blaming-mexicans, last accessed 11 September 2022.
19. Kim Yi Dionne and Fulya Felicity Turkmen, 'The Politics of Pandemic Othering: Putting COVID-19 in Global and Historical Context', *International Organization* 74:1 (2020), E213–E230.
20. Luce, 'American Century', 160.
21. Helen Stuart Campbell, *Darkness and Daylight, or, Lights and Shadows of New York Life: A Woman's Narrative of Mission and Rescue Work in Tough Places, with Personal Experiences Among the Poor in Regions of Poverty and Vice* (Hartford, CT: A. D. Worthington, [1891] 1897); Jacob A. Riis, *How the Other Half Lives: Studies Among the Tenements of New York* (New York: Charles Scribner's Sons, 1890), 42–4.
22. Riis, *How the Other Half Lives*, 48.
23. Udo J. Keppler, 'The Tenement: A Menace to All', *Puck* 49 (20 March 1901), centrefold. Retrieved from the Library of Congress at: www.loc.gov/item/2010651390, last accessed 25 January 2022.
24. Jacob A. Riis, *The Battle with the Slum* (New York: Macmillan, 1902).
25. Katherine Ott, *Fevered Lives: Tuberculosis in American Culture Since 1870* (Cambridge, MA: Harvard University Press, 1996), 111–13.

26. Shah, *Contagious Divides*, 5.
27. Victoria Rosner, *Machines for Living: Modernism and Domestic Life* (New York: Oxford University Press, 2020), 101. Tyranny in that the aggressive reform campaigns of the reformers were intended to force compliance with their norms (modern cultural and sanitary practices) to extirpate cultural norms in conflict with the reformer's 'civilising' mission.
28. Herman Biggs, 'Administrative Control of Tuberculosis', *Public Health Journal* 3:11 (1912), 613.
29. Charity Organization Society Collection, 'Map Showing Over-Crowding of Buildings on Lots and Consequent Lack of Light and Air Space, Also the Prevalence of Tuberculosis, Typhoid Fever, Scarlet Fever and Diphtheria in the Tenement House District Bounded by Division Street, East River, Catharine, Rutgers Streets', prepared for the Tenement House Committee of the Charity Organization Society, under the direction of Lawrence Veiller, 1899, New York Historical Society; Robert DeForest and Lawrence Veiller (eds), *The Tenement House Problem*, vols 1 and 2 (New York: Macmillan, 1903). See also Richard Plunz, *A History of Housing in New York City* (New York: Columbia University Press, 1990), 21–49.
30. The data, however, was less conclusive; Veiller's maps showed that blocks in nearby Chinatown and Little Syria had far greater incidences of disease, congestion and conditions of poverty.
31. The cultural and racial diversity of the neighbourhood is addressed in W. T. Lhamon, *Raising Cain: Blackface Performance from Jim Crow to Hip Hop* (Cambridge, MA: Harvard University Press, 1998), 1–55. For more on the neighbourhood's decades as sailortown, see Johnathan Thayer, 'Merchant Seamen, Sailor Towns, and the Shaping of US Citizenship, 1943–1945', PhD Dissertation, City University of New York, 2018. On slumming in Lower Manhattan, see Chris J. Westgate, *Staging the Slums, Slumming the Stage: Class, Poverty, Ethnicity, and Sexuality in American Theatre, 1890–1916* (New York: Palgrave Macmillan, 2014); Robert M. Dowling, *Slumming in New York: From the Waterfront to Mythic Harlem* (Urbana: University of Illinois Press, 2007).
32. Kellogg Durland and Louis Sessa, 'Italian Invasion of the Ghetto', *University Settlement Studies* 1 (1905/6), 106–17; New York, State Census, 1905, A.D. 2 (vols 13, 14, 15), A.D. 4 (vols 1, 2, 3, 8).
33. By 1905, Italians represented nearly 50 per cent of the residents of the Lung Block. By 1910, two-thirds of block residents were either first- or second-generation Italian immigrants, and a growing number of Italians began buying or leasing tenements. By 1929, Italians occupied 97 per cent of the housing on the Lung Block and owned over 75 per cent of its buildings. See Stefano Morello, 'A New York City Slum and Its Forgotten Italian Immigrant Community', MA thesis, University of Naples, L'Orientale, 2015; Kerri Culhane and Stefano Morello, 'A New York City Slum and Its Forgotten Italian Immigrant Community', available at: tinyurl.com/lungblock, last accessed 5 December 2021.

34. Though neither addresses the Lower East Side Lung Block, Dorceta E. Taylor, *The Environment and the People in American Cities, 1600s–1900s: Disorder, Inequality, and Social Change* (Durham, NC: Duke University Press, 2009), chs 7–9; Rachel E. Iannacone, 'Open Space for the Underclass: New York's Small Parks (1880–1915)', PhD dissertation, University of Pennsylvania, 2005, offer important context on the urban parks movements.

35. On the ideological and theological origins of the Progressive movement in urban areas, see Boyer, *Urban Masses and Moral Order in America*; on the standards of living of Italians and their housekeeping practices, see Lillian W. Betts, 'The Italian in New York', *University Settlement Studies* I (1905), 90–104; Lillian W. Betts, 'Italian Peasants in a New Law Tenement', *Harper's Bazaar* 38 (1904), 802–5; on the stigmatisation of Catholicism, see the manifold political cartoons that populated the pages of *Harper's Weekly* post-1850, especially those by Thomas Nast.

36. Edward Alsworth Ross, *The Old World in the New: The Significance of Past and Present Immigration to the American People* (New York: Century, 1914); Alan M. Kraut, 'Southern Italian Immigration to the United States at the Turn of the Century and the Perennial Problem of Medicalised Prejudice', in Lara Marks and Michael Worboys (eds), *Migrants, Minorities and Health: Historical and Contemporary Studies* (New York: Routledge, 1997), 228–249.

37. Henry J. Browne, 'The "Italian Problem" in the Catholic Church of the United States, 1880–1900', *United States Catholic Historical Society Historical Records and Studies* 35 (1946), 46–72.

38. Samuele F.S. Pardini, *In the Name of the Mother: Italian Americans, African Americans, and Modernity from Booker T. Washington to Bruce Springsteen* (Hanover, NH: Dartmouth College Press, 2017), 18. See also Robert Orsi, *The Madonna of 115th Street: Faith and Community in Italian Harlem, 1880–1950* (New Haven, CT: Yale University Press, 1985), 92–103.

39. Ernest Poole, *The Plague in Its Stronghold* (New York: Committee on the Prevention of Tuberculosis of the Charity Organization Society of the City of New York, 1903), 28; Mary Sherman, 'Manufacturing of Foods in the Tenements', *Charities and The Commons* 15 (1906), 669–73; Annie S. Daniel, 'The Wreck of the Home: How Wearing Apparel is Fashioned in the Tenements', *Charities and the Commons* 14 (1905), 624–29; Lawrence Veiller, 'To Restrict Work in the Tenements', *Charities and the Commons* 12 (1904), 529–33.

40. Antonio Stella, 'The Prevalence of Tuberculosis among Italians in the United States', *Transactions of the Sixth International Congress on Tuberculosis, September 28 to October 5, 1908*, Department of Health of the City of New York, 1915, Annual Report.

41. Alan J. C. Mayne, *The Imagined Slum: Newspaper Representation in Three Cities, 1870–1914* (Leicester: Leicester University Press, 1993), 1.

42. Emily Wayland Dinwiddie, 'The Redemption of the Lung Block', *Charities and the Commons* 19 (1908), 579–81.
43. Fred F. French, 'Slum Clearance and Knickerbocker Village', 7–8, Box 3, Folder 2, Fred F. French Companies Records, New York Public Library, Rare Books and Manuscripts; Louis Heaton Pink, 'Old Tenements and the New Law', *University Settlement Studies* (1907), reprinted by the Fred F, French Companies, 1932, Box 3, Folder 2, Fred F. French Companies Records, Rare Books and Manuscripts, New York Public Library; Culhane and Morello, 'A New York City Slum and Its Forgotten Italian Immigrant Community'.
44. Noel Ignatiev, *How the Irish Became White* (New York: Routledge, 2009); Jennifer Guglielmo and Salvatore Salerno, *Are Italians White? How Race is Made in America* (New York: Routledge, 2003).
45. Fred L. Gardaphé, 'We Weren't Always White', *Literature Interpretation Theory* 13:3 (2002), 189.
46. Thomas A. Guglielmo, *White on Arrival: Italians, Race, Color, and Power in Chicago, 1890–1945* (New York: Oxford University Press, 2020).
47. Markel and Stern, 'The Foreignness of Germs', 781.
48. The authors were not granted permission to include the cartoon in this publication. See Rick McKee, 'Immigration Disease', 25 August 2014, *Political Cartoons*, available at: https://politicalcartoons.com/sku/151877, last accessed 20 August 2022.
49. In 2018, Donald Trump famously asked for more Norwegian immigration to the United States, rather than immigrants from 'shithole countries', by his definition, Haiti and majority non-white countries in Africa. See Julie Hirschfeld Davis, Sheryl Gay Stolberg and Thomas Kaplan, 'Trump Alarms Lawmakers with Disparaging Words for Haiti and Africa', *New York Times*, 11 January 2018, available at: https://www.nytimes.com/2018/01/11/us/politics/trump-shithole-countries.html, last accessed 25 January 2022.

5

Oil, Progress and Public Health in the Early Twentieth Century

Gaetano Di Tommaso

In January 1924, a local New Jersey newspaper printed a heartfelt appeal to Congress, urging them to take oil pollution seriously and pass legislation to curb it. The author, Republican state Senator J. S. Frelinghuysen, had delivered the same impassioned statement in person to the nation a few days earlier during a Senate hearing in Washington, DC. 'The menace of oil pollution is widespread . . . It is so great,' he explained, 'that it is affecting the life, health and property of everybody along the coasts.' From Long Island to New Jersey shores, waters were almost everywhere 'coated with a thin, sticky substance which adheres to the bodies of bathers, affects the eyes and health, and makes bathing practically impossible'. Blazing fires along the coast were common too, due to the oil that covered harbours and 'soaked' wooden piers. In the nightmarish scene Frelinghuysen described, everything was oil-smeared, both above and below the water, where tar covered oyster beds, suffocating life and posing unprecedented challenges to the fishing and seafood industry.[1]

A few months later, in October 1924, New Jersey newspapers reported on another health and safety hazard that suddenly caught people's attention in the state and beyond. At the Bayway plant of the Standard Oil Company of New Jersey, located just outside Elizabeth and across from Staten Island, at least five people had died, and more than thirty were hospitalised within a matter of days. They all worked in manufacturing a new type of fuel, a product whose name – 'ethyl gasoline' – skilfully hid its key ingredient: lead. The accidents marked the first visible consequences of the introduction of leaded gasoline to the market, which General Motors' chemical engineers had successfully achieved just a few months earlier. The first newspaper articles covering the accidents at the petrochemical plant repeated reports of mysterious deaths due to a 'looney gas' that made men severely and violently ill, to the point where they often needed to be confined in a straitjacket.[2]

The mobilisation against oil pollution in water and the fear of chemical poisoning following the introduction of leaded gasoline may seem different at first sight. The 'blackening' of the American landscape was a personal experience for many citizens who could see, touch and smell (sometimes even taste) the contaminating effects of unabated oil pollution on the country's lands, rivers and waters. Furthermore, petroleum-induced environmental degradation began in the late nineteenth century and continued practically unchecked for decades. Leaded gasoline, on the other hand, appeared suddenly to US consumers. Unlike oil spills and discharges, which were unpleasant yet familiar occurrences in many parts of the country, tetraethyl lead (TEL) was the latest result of industrial research and innovation unknown to most. Americans were supposed to consume the product as a fuel without even realising what made it different. Significantly, TEL was different from oil at the sensory level as well. As a colourless liquid with a pleasant, sweet odour, it had little that could point even those most exposed to it – like the workers involved in its manufacturing – to its poisonous nature.

Despite these differences, the growth of oil pollution and the roll-out of leaded gasoline have numerous, deep and multifaceted connections beyond the shared timing and location. Oil spills, chemical poisonings in refineries and accidents in petrochemical plants were not unforeseeable events at the time, given companies' heedlessness of their limits and risks. Instead, they were intrinsic and, in many respects, complementary components of the development of the petroleum industry in the United States in the early twentieth century. The continuous growth of petroleum-based products available to consumers and the rapid increase in their economic value marked the expansion of the 'oil industrial complex' as much as the increase of environmental hazards and public health threats it generated. Looking at how public officials adjusted and responded to hazards of an incipient petromodernity, from the slow but mounting contamination of US waters to the lethal decision to market an unsafe product like leaded gasoline, opens a unique perspective on the relationship between business, society and the state.

This chapter focuses on how the oil-fuelled prosperity companies were busy building for the nation clashed with broader conceptions of the common good. It discusses American authorities' early struggles to strike a balance between tangible progress and people's safety through two emblematic cases – the rise of oil pollution and the introduction of leaded gasoline – in which federal officials eventually failed to enact legislation strict enough to match the danger. Not doing so highlights Washington's long-standing difficulties in regulating business, even in the face of potential public health crises, and its limits in managing the evolving and often conflicting needs of economic prowess and social well-being. The prevention of public health risks linked to the growth of oil companies' operations presented a significant opportunity for the expansion of federal regulatory powers, especially considering how limited were the tools available to individual states to confront such threats, which often originated from commercial enterprises whose scale and reach went well beyond their territory and control. In the early twentieth century, however, the outcome, rather than the empowerment of federal agencies, was the delegation – or the surrender – to private actors of the search and implementation of mitigating actions. This course of action represented a version of the public–private dynamic that would remain central throughout the century and would often lead to overlooking public health priorities for economic gain and productivity's sake. The foundations of the American Century, then, lay firmly in oil companies' continuous experimentation, audacious marketing, undue political influence, and inherent disregard for the health and safety of those working in the industry or otherwise exposed to its operations. In the following decades, the tradeoff between health and industrial might that the oil companies forced on the country became only more urgent, as US power – and global ambitions – grew.

Plentiful, wasteful and threatening

Petroleum began its commercial career in the 1860s as nothing more than a cheap fuel for lamps and lanterns. Kerosene, extracted from crude oil's lighter fractions (or 'cuts'), was the only component actively marketed.[3] By the turn of the century, however, the types of derivative being sold ranged from distillates of oil's most volatile fractions like gasoline and naphtha to heavier byproducts like paraffin wax, lubricants, fuel oil, and 'bottom of the barrel' residues like tar and asphalt. In just a few decades, oil came to permeate Americans' daily life and found application virtually everywhere. In one form or another, refined petroleum became essential for things as varied as healing cuts and burns, greasing mechanical joints, anesthetising people, manufacturing candles and chewing gums, producing paints and dyes, and powering lamps and engines.

The frantic pace at which the oil business moved left little room for caution. Companies continuously chased innovation to fend off competition and worked aggressively to create new outlets to market the growing quantity of oil extracted.[4] Risk was an in-built feature of an industry characterised (and shaken) by tremendous boom and bust cycles from the beginning. Rashness and wastefulness were hall-marks of the way in which wildcatters and operators extracted and refined oil in the early stages of the industry, as evidenced by the experiences of the 'oil rushes' that upended life in several American communities between the late nineteenth and early twentieth centuries – first in Pennsylvania (1870s–1880s), then in Texas (1900s–1930s) and California (1910s–1930s) – leaving trails of environmental degradation and human exploitation in their wake.[5]

Over-production and pollution remained inevitable corollaries to oil exploration. The structure of mining and mineral rights in the United States did not help in this respect since the so-called rule of capture on which the system was based (and is, to some extent, still based) encouraged competition, 'forcing' drillers to extract as much petroleum as they could before other oilmen could tap into the newly discovered reservoir and drain it themselves.[6] In such a context, companies' eagerness to profit, obvious gaps in scientific knowledge on the adverse health effects of hydrocarbons and still poor technical expertise in operating oil wells combined to make toxic contamination inescapable. A deadly mix of lack of awareness, unskilfulness and unwillingness on the companies' side condemned the country to environmental degradation and chemical exposure. It was not unusual, for instance, to see wells flowing wide open, with oil and brine pouring directly into waterways or accumulating in large and highly flammable pools on the ground.[7] Similar problems were present in other processing stages. Once extracted, crude oil went through transporting methods with equal (dis)regard for people's safety. The example of the first pipelines – hailed as a break-through in the oil business when they appeared in the late nineteenth century – shows the industry's fixation on economic growth. The new installations were not spill-proof, but those operating them soon realised that losing part of the fluid load they carried was more con-venient than spending money to fasten miles of ducts and joints. As a result, segments of this expanding web of oil conduits criss-crossing the country leaked easily and often burst, sometimes causing raging fires that lasted for hours.[8] As for refining, the thick residue left after the distillation of the lighter and most valuable petroleum cuts was usually considered 'useless' (that is, not profitable enough) in the early stages of the industry and thus were allowed to 'run to waste'.[9] It formed lakes of petroleum, 'which were often set on fire to get rid of them or carried off by pipes into the sea'.[10] Finally, when local communities tried to make oil operators liable for their oil spills, authorities' narrow understanding of petroleum toxicity could easily preclude any meaningful actions. Suits and requests for regulation could be brushed off with a simple justification: 'matter floating on top of water does not kill fish'.[11]

Standard of living versus quality of life

The success of companies in modernising and motorising society, as well as fuelling the rise of the United States to global superpower status, indirectly legitimised the inherently exploitative nature of petroleum extraction and production.[12] Between 1900 and 1920, US annual oil production increased from around 65 million barrels to over 440 million, accounting for about 65 per cent of all the oil extracted in the world.[13] In the same period, the number of motor vehicles (cars, buses and trucks) in the country rose from about 8,000 to over 9 million.[14] Meanwhile, the number of people engaged in petroleum refining (excluding those involved in operations at the well) grew from 15,000 to about 75,000, and the total value of petroleum products (including gasoline, illuminating oils, lubricants, paraffin wax, greases and others), which was $175 million in 1904, reached $1.6 billion by 1919.[15] Although oil did not overtake coal as a primary energy source in the country until the 1940s, the aggregate commercial value of petroleum surpassed that of coal as early as 1925.[16] As a result, petroleum quickly assumed the status of a strategic and economic asset. Its penetration into American society (and minds) was due not only to the tremendous practical and technical advantages it provided as an energy source, but also to its versatility as a product. Its commodification was extreme and extremely successful. As a symbol of the dramatic change that American industry and economy underwent during those years, petroleum embodied the promise of a type of modernity that, from the 1910s onward, following the conversion of the US Navy from coal to oil, combined consumerism with military preparedness.

Companies' public image suffered during the transition from the Gilded Age to the Progressive Era. However, what came under Washington's scrutiny was the monopolistic conduct of oil magnates rather than the toxic features of their businesses. John D. Rockefeller's predatory price-cutting and aggressive commercial tactics became the quintessential symbol of the corruption and inequality that engulfed the country in the late nineteenth century, and was a catalyst for the widespread anti-big business sentiment that emerged as a response. The popular characterisation of Standard Oil as a predatory trust and a 'soulless corporation' had little to do with the way in which the industry exposed people to teratogens like crude oil and its carcinogenic components (such as benzene).[17] Indeed, the resulting legal battle that state and federal authorities waged against trusts and business concentration at the turn of the century, which aimed at (and succeeded in) breaking up Standard Oil in 1911, affected corporate structures but left the oil industry's production, refining and transportation methods, as well as safety standards, practically untouched.[18]

The oil industry's socio-political clout and economic weight made it extremely difficult to establish legal (or scientific) grounds for a regulatory framework to restrict hazardous activities.[19] Throughout the early twentieth century, nuisance laws, which in common law allowed individuals to seek legal recourse against something – an activity or condition – that interfered with the use and enjoyment of their property, remained the only tool for citizens to tackle pollution.[20] Their use became widespread, but it remained largely ineffective as legal recourse in practice. First, this kind of litigation tended to deliver compensation rather than injunctions, meaning courts assigned money damages to plaintiffs instead of ordering industrial plants to eliminate the 'nuisance' or shut down their activities altogether.[21] The reasoning was that doing otherwise would have placed too heavy an economic burden on the business entity and, in situations where the defendant was a large enterprise of significant public value, on the community as a whole. A second obstacle when trying to obtain legal remedy was that regulations dealing with water quality were usually local ordinances with limited jurisdiction and thus had little effect on refineries and other factories that affected water quality downstream. In some instances, to make matters worse, the polluting plants or activities were located outside the state whose citizens were seeking relief. Approving similar legislation in nearby cities (or states) would have obviously addressed the issue. However, fears of industrial flight worked against this solution, accounting for the third main obstacle. Stringent rules that exposed companies to litigation encouraged businesses to leave, relocate or not invest in the first place – a risk that many officials were not willing to take.[22]

The lack of nationwide legislation on industrial pollution during those years was a blind spot amid the proliferation of public health practices and policies at the state and federal levels. A limited number of local health departments were operating in the northeast of the country as early as the eighteenth century, and state-level agencies multiplied in the second half of the nineteenth century.[23] In 1912, the old system of US Marine Hospitals was transformed (and renamed) into the US Public Health Service, marking the beginning of a greater degree of federal intervention. These institutional attempts at reform became more structured as progress in medicine and epidemiology transformed experts' understanding of how pathogens spread. The

attention to bacterial agents, however, meant that the agencies identified and targeted sewage, rather than industrial pollution, as the
real public health hazard.[24] The treatment of drinking water to prevent waterborne diseases such as cholera and typhoid remained the
primary concern of public health workers for decades with regard to
water quality. Consequently, public interventions focused on water
filtration and chlorination while overlooking the toxicity of chemicals released by refineries, mines, tanneries, canneries, paper mills,
textile factories, sawmills and alcohol-manufacturing plants, among
others.[25] By the end of the First World War, the situation was so
dramatic that in some parts of the country, waterways were so acidic
they corroded steel ships and killed vegetation.[26]

Toxic waste and health hazards were issues that affected all
industrial sectors to varying degrees. However, petroleum pollution
presented a unique challenge due to the socio-political-cultural significance of the industry and the nature and extent of the health risks
its operations posed (and still pose) to society. Petroleum pollution
stood apart from other forms of toxic contamination not only for
its economic impact, but also for its striking visual aspect. The oleaginous nature of crude oil, its blackish colour, and the slimy, sticky
consistency of its residues, which coated an increasing number of
American cities, riverbanks and coasts, made the fossil fuel's threat
appear both inescapable and exceptionally vivid. Consequently, it
was no coincidence that the first piece of federal legislation concerning environmental health – aimed at protecting public health by
addressing factors in the environment that could negatively impact
human well-being – was enacted in the 1920s and specifically targeted the issue of oil pollution in American waterways.

Federal intervention on oil pollution

Americans' perception of oil contamination worsened rapidly in the
first two decades of the twentieth century. US newspapers reflected this
change, as reporting on oil spills and the fire hazards associated with
handling petroleum products shifted from discussing 'nuisances' –
sometimes conceding that standard industry practices were, in fact, a
'problem' – to extensively covering (and receiving complaints about)
petroleum as a 'polluting' element.[27] Along with oil terminals and
refineries, one of the leading causes of water contamination, particularly in coastal areas, was the extraordinary growth of oil-burning
vessels and cargo ships transporting petroleum products that characterised the First World War and immediate post-war years.[28] The
worsening of conditions along the American coast was due to the

practice of dumping 'oil-contaminated ballast water and bilge water' directly at sea, close to the shore, as ships approached their terminals for loading and discharging.[29] More generally, unregulated cleaning procedures led tanker operators to discard everything, including oil sludge, from oil storage tanks or compartments.

Pressure on Congress to act began to mount in 1921 when a first draft bill was introduced by T. Frank Appleby (Republican, NY) in the House and Frelinghuysen (Republican, NJ) in the Senate. In the hearings that followed, oil pollution was not only described as a catastrophe for waterside property, but also as a threat to public health. In fact, it was 'first of all a menace to health', according to David Neuberger, who testified on behalf of an interstate committee on pollution prevention in New York and New Jersey coastal waters. The conditions in some locations along the US coast, he reported, had become 'such that they were absolutely intolerable, a menace to health, a sanitary menace, absolutely destructive of sanitary conditions'. Oil pollution interfered with and affected Americans' health in two ways, according to Neuberger: directly, through contact, due to its harmful and irritating effects on the human body; and indirectly, due to its effects on people's food – fish, specifically. 'Commercial fishermen,' he claimed, 'have suffered to the point to which some of them have been nigh extinguished . . . If food be the question, the health of the nation is a question also to be determined . . ..'[30] Neuberger intervened in DC among numerous officials, experts and civic association representatives. As most Americans at the time, he had limited specific knowledge or understanding of petroleum's toxicity. However, while the exact mechanisms and extent of the health risks associated with oil pollution were not fully understood at the time, the connection between the two appeared clear. 'You ask why we are here? Why is importance attached to this situation?,' he explained, 'The importance is to you gentlemen and your families, as well as all the families in the United States. Pollution of fish brings about ptomaine poisoning and other diseases. Pollution of the beach and coast waters brings disease.' In closing his statement, he insisted that '[t]rade wastes' could not and should not 'be made superior to the public health', and stated that the unwillingness of oil executives to invest to avoid discharges of highly poisonous substances into the environment could not be an excuse to '[subject] the public to that danger'.[31]

Soon after, an interdepartmental committee was established, bringing together members from the seven departments (State, Treasury, War, Navy, Interior, Agriculture and Commerce) and the Shipping Board. The committee was tasked with studying various aspects of the problem, including the prevention of oil pollution by ships, and evaluating the extent of pollution in American waters. Their investigations focused on the sources of pollution, as well as the resulting hazards and damages to marine and shore property, waterfowl and fisheries. This comprehensive examination served as preparatory work for an international conference that the Republican-dominated Congress had requested the president convene, as indicated in a Joint Resolution, to specifically address the prevention of water pollution by 'oil waste, fuel oil, oil sludge, oil slop, tar residue, and water ballast'.[32]

Meanwhile, in the rest of the country, mobilisation took off following the creation of a national Coast Anti-Pollution League (with Neuberger as president) in 1922. The following year, a crowd of more than one hundred federal, state and municipal officials, together with businesspeople, met at the organisation's annual conference in New Jersey, where various working groups were set up.[33] Among those proposed, which dealt with the effects of oil pollution on harbour infrastructures and wildlife, there was also one entirely dedicated to public health issues, where the organisation placed representatives of the US Public Health Service, state boards of health, state sanitary engineers and municipal health officers.[34]

The League was very vocal, appearing in local and national newspapers and organising speeches around the country on the dangers of oil pollution.[35] The public campaign culminated in new congressional hearings in January 1924, where a wide range of citizens, professionals and public health officers submitted their statements.[36] The anti-oil pollution coalition included conservationists and naturalist organisations worried about the damage to American flora and fauna; landlords and developers concerned about the drop in real estate values in areas blackened by oil; fisheries in distress due to the impact of pollution on marine life; tourists and tourism businesses upset about the impossibility of using beaches for recreational purposes; and even insurance companies interested in reducing the risk of fire and thus their financial exposure. They all had very particular, often material interests and reasons to demand legislation on the issue, yet the impact of oil pollution on people's health repeatedly figured among the arguments in favour of federal intervention. In his statement, Neuberger even used dramatic stories of 'women and children' with 'skin poisoned', 'eyes ruined' and 'ears noses and throats affected by oil pollution' for added effect.[37] These stories underscored the immediate and severe health consequences faced by those living in polluted areas, further emphasising the need for urgent action and legislation to protect public health.[38] Neuberger and others' statements also stressed how fatal oil pollution proved to be to marine life and emphasised the risks associated with the consumption of contaminated seafood, highlighting the potential for illnesses linked to food poisoning due to the presence of toxic substances in fish and shellfish.[39]

A few months later, in June, Congress approved the first Oil Pollution Act 1924, prohibiting intentional fossil fuel discharges in immediate American coastal waters. However, contrary to what the bill's proponents had initially asked, the new regulations targeted only seagoing vessels, leaving out land plants. The loophole represented a welcome omission for American oil companies, which could continue to evade accountability vis-à-vis the federal government for their extractive and refining operations on land. This narrow focus on seagoing vessels left communities vulnerable to health risks from toxic chemicals released by various industries, including the oil industry, as their activities ashore remained unregulated. The legislation's outcome was not accidental and pointed instead to the industry's leverage. Federal agencies, in many cases, did not possess the expertise necessary to independently investigate, assess and give recommendations on many of the technical issues surrounding the oil industry's activities and had to rely on the only subject that had that level of scientific knowledge and type of competencies – the oil industry itself. A clear example of the relationship between public officials and business experts is the comprehensive report on oil pollution that the Bureau of Mines, a technical body of the Department of Interior, prepared in the early 1920s. To complete their study, government specialists turned for assistance to the American Petroleum Institute and the American Steamship Owners Association, the two parties directly interested – if not targeted – by the investigation. The report claimed a 'definite relationship between oil pollution and public health'.[40] Despite stating that the exact degree to which oil pollution was affecting people's health was not possible access due to a lack of sufficient information, there was little doubt about the long-term adverse effects of oil contamination.[41]

The investigation results were also published in the form of a Public Health Report drawing on observations from health commissioners in coastal states in the east, west and south. The majority reported that it was almost impossible to bathe without getting covered in oil.[42] On some beaches, the situation was so dreadful that 'shower baths were equipped with kerosene for cleaning oil from the bodies of the bathers'.[43] However, the same report pointed to cooperation between public authorities and business entities as the real answer to the problem and advised caution before considering any punitive measures for companies. The study explained that a general agreement existed among the interviewed parties (that is, federal, state, municipal and local authorities, and representatives of the various industries) that new regulations needed to be 'reasonable and practicable' to avoid imposing undue hardship on the businesses involved, particularly shipping. Federal laws, more specifically, could be effectively enforced 'only if practical, remedial and preventative methods are available to meet varying economic and operating requirements of the industries'. The report's message, which focused on cooperation instead of coercion and emphasised the need not to inconvenience businesses 'unreasonably', soon found its way into Congress. The relatively toothless piece of legislation enacted in 1924 in the form of the Oil Pollution Act effectively sealed the fate of the dispute over companies' water contamination.

Misleading the nation on lead

In the same months in which Congress was debating the passage of the original 1924 Oil Pollution Act, public health authorities discussed how to deal with the deaths due to lead poisoning at Bayway. General Motors' (GM) chemists and engineers had been researching 'anti-knock' agents for years and, by the early 1920s, had tested a series of different additives to improve engine compression and efficiency with varying degrees of success. Although known as a toxic chemical, lead was cheap, giving it an economic edge. Its use as a gasoline additive was perfected in 1923 when TEL was first introduced to the market.[44] The following year, GM (controlled by Du Pont) partnered with Standard Oil of New Jersey to create the Ethyl Gasoline Corporation and bring the revolutionary fuel to American motorists everywhere. As distribution widened, production increased, and the Bayway plant was brought into operation. That was also when Standard Oil workers began experiencing severe symptoms due to lead poisoning.

Medical scientists had raised the alarm about the manufacturing of tetraethyl lead (TEL) even before the deaths in New Jersey. The Public Health Service began to receive warnings about the possible toxicity of the product immediately after GM presented it. As a result, federal agencies – specifically the Bureau of Mines – conducted preliminary tests that had, in fact, cleared TEL for the market. However, more than providing evidence of leaded gasoline's safety, the outcome signalled the strong corporate influence over industrial review processes. Tasked with an investigation for which they had limited funds to study a product about which they knew very little, federal officials acquiesced to the company's requests for control. GM, which had offered to fund the research, managed to exercise strict supervision over it and effectively sanitised the final report.[45]

The ongoing production and marketing of TEL were clearly a public health failure. However, it is interesting to see how the debate around the issue was framed in the months that followed the deaths. Public health was front and centre in the conversation, and its safeguarding was presented as a critical policy goal, but it was not the only issue on the table. Public health competed with – and eventually lost against – the vision of an oil-fuelled civilisation that the oil industry offered to the country. Frank A. Howard, an Ethyl Gasoline Corporation spokesperson, set forth the reasoning for the continued production and use of leaded gasoline amid proliferating health concerns. In 1925, at a conference US Surgeon General Hugh S. Cumming had convened to determine whether to keep the product off the market, Howard asked, 'Is [tetraethyl lead gasoline] a public health hazard?'[46] The problem, he claimed, was not so simple. The company was engaged in activities such as the 'manufacture of automobiles and refining of oil' that were essential to the nation. It produced 'things' on which 'our present industrial civilization is supposed to depend'. Given what was at stake, business operations could not be stopped only because of the 'remote probability' that they may be harmful to humans. Brazenly turning the tables on his audience, Howard asserted that Ethyl's responsibility was to keep manufacturing leaded gasoline if the goal was to safeguard the nation's well-being. The argument elicited strong reactions from the public health experts and professionals in attendance, but it stuck. A few months earlier, due to long-standing concerns about the prospects of an impending scarcity of petroleum, President Coolidge had created the Federal Oil Conservation Board, composed of the secretaries of War, Navy, Interior and Commerce, to study the status of the domestic oil industry. The aim was to find ways to prevent possible shortages by preserving petroleum resources and reducing their profligate use. In this context, Howard framed leaded gasoline, which improved engine efficiency and naturally diminished petroleum consumption, as necessary. TEL became vital and in the words of Howard, a 'gift of God'. 'What is our duty under the circumstances?' he asked; the answer perfectly exemplified the tension between economic growth and public well-being in modern society, pitting health versus wealth. The industry representative turned the precautionary principle on its head, arguing that the continued production of leaded gasoline was the best choice from a moral perspective. 'Frankly', he said, 'we can not justify ourselves in our conscience if we abandon the thing . . . merely because of our fears'.[47] Despite the presence of authoritative

voices extremely concerned about the health dangers of leaded gasoline and in favour of direct federal intervention, the conference ended
with a call for a blue-ribbon committee to conduct another investigation of leaded gasoline, which would eventually fall short again of
stopping TEL production and marketing.[48]

Once the tragic deaths in New Jersey prompted local authorities to
ban the sale of TEL and question the safety of the product, the company jumped into action to avoid the fallout. The Ethyl Corporation
neutralised the threat of new federal regulations, swayed the debate
over the accidents and eventually obtained permission to reintro-
duce TEL to the market in 1926.[49] In that year, the report produced
by the latest committee found 'no good grounds for prohibiting the
use of ethyl gasoline . . .' provided that workers manufacturing and
handling it used forms of protection.[50] The federal government soon
after authorised its sale again everywhere in the country. Despite a
growing body of medical research on the poisoning effects of lead
exposure, especially after the Second World War, producers – particularly GM and Standard Oil – prevented the establishment of federal
regulations until the 1970s, when scientific evidence grew so overwhelming as to become undeniable, and Congress began phasing out
leaded gasoline. For decades, however, lead industries managed to
control the scientific and political debate by funding and disseminating their own research on the toxicity of lead additives and stifling
independent studies.[51] The Ethyl Corporation continued to produce
its brand of leaded gasoline until the mid-1980s, and it took until the
following decade to see the product banned altogether.

Conclusion

The oil and petrochemical industry's extremely competitive business
strategies, with their tendency to maximise profit and experiment
aggressively, contributed to turning petroleum into the lifeblood of
modern civilisation. Company practices in the United States made
them economic and political giants and powered Washington's rise
to dominance in the twentieth century. However, they also produced
widespread environmental crises, dangerous working conditions
and public health hazards – from the very beginning of the industry.
The slow reaction of public authorities to these threats represented a
blind spot in public health care and created a gap in environmental
health governance that later proved hard to close. Amid a period of
formidable industrialisation and unprecedented economic growth, US
authorities chose not to hinder the process of the oil-fuelled modernisation of the country, effectively capitulating to commercial interests.

Despite growing awareness among people and public health experts about the toxic consequences of the industry's choices and operations, the federal government failed to enact new regulatory frameworks to safeguard Americans' health and safety from new industrial menaces.

In this respect, the government's shortcomings were an illustration of the structural advantage that economic freedom had at the beginning of the century over a still inchoate notion of public good/public interest. The attempts to balance these values or, better, to redress the situation by expanding federal responsibilities fell short, failing to account appropriately for environmental and public health costs. The decisions Washington took after the First World War sealed the debate around oil pollution and leaded gasoline for roughly another half a century – a period in which the political and social clout of the oil and petrochemical industry grew even more, and in which companies maintained an advantageous position to shape the public and political discussion around the production and distribution of petroleum derivatives.

Notes

1. 'Would Stop Pollution of Coastal Waters, Legislation is Urged by J. S. Frelinghuysen', *Keyport Weekly* (New Jersey), 18 January 1924.
2. US newspapers published dozens of articles on the events in New Jerseys; see, for example, 'Fifth "Loony" Gas Victim Dies Raving in a Straitjacket', *Brooklyn Daily Eagle*, 30 October 1924; 'Lead Poison, Drove Bayway Men Crazy, Killed 5 and Sent 30 More to Hospital; Antidote Found to End Death Toll', *Brooklyn Daily Eagle*, 2 November 1924.
3. For the description of late nineteenth- and early twentieth-century refining procedures and products' composition, see Harold F. Williamson and Arnold R. Daum, *The American Petroleum Industry: The Age of Illumination, 1859–1899* (Evanston, IL: Northwestern University Press, 1959); P. H. Giddens, *The Birth of the Oil Industry* (London: Macmillan, 1938); L. Fanning, *The Rise of American Oil* (New york: Harper, 1936). For a contemporary account, see John McLaurin, *Sketches in Crude Oil: Some Accidents and Incidents of the Petroleum Development in All Parts of the Globe* (Published by the author, 1898), 16. For a focus on the southwest of the country, see Joseph A. Pratt, 'The Ascent of Oil: The Transition from Coal to Oil in Early Twentieth Century America', in Lewis J. Perelman, August W. Giebelhaus and Michael D. Yokell (eds), *Energy Transitions: Long-term Perspectives* (Boulder, CO: Westview Press, 1981), 9–34.
4. Jonathan Wlasiuk, *Refining Nature: Standard Oil and the Limits of Efficiency* (Pittsburgh, PA: University of Pittsburgh Press, 2018).

5. Brian Black, *Petrolia: The Landscape of America's First Oil Boom* (Baltimore, MD: Johns Hopkins University Press, 2000); Sarah S. Elkind, 'Oil in the City: The Fall and Rise of Oil Drilling in Los Angeles', *Journal of American History* 99:1 (2012), 82–90; Nancy Quam-Wickham, '"Cities Sacrificed on the Altar of Oil": Popular Opposition to Oil Development in 1920s Los Angeles', *Environmental History* 3 (1998), 192; Nancy Quam-Wickham, 'An "Oleaginous Civilization" Oil in Southern California', *Southern California Quarterly* 97:3 (2015), 283–95; Christopher Sellers, 'Petropolis and Environmental Protest in Cross-National Perspective: Beaumont–Port Arthur, Texas, versus Minatitlan–Coatzacoalcos, Veracruz', *Journal of American History* 99:1 (2012). 111–23; Craig E. Colten, 'An Incomplete Solution: Oil and Water in Louisiana', *Journal of American History* 99:1 (2012), 91–9; Wlasiuk, *Refining Nature*.

6. For an explanation of the 'rule' and its implications, see Terence Daintith, 'The Rule of Capture: The Least Worst Property Rule for Oil and Gas', in Aileen McHarg, Barry Barton, Adrian Bradbrook and Lee Godden (eds), *Property and the Law in Energy and Natural Resources* (Oxford: Oxford University Press, 2010); Bruce M. Kramer and Owen L. Anderson, 'The Rule of Capture: An Oil and Gas Perspective', *Environmental Law* 35 (2005), 899–954.

7. William D. Langley and Peter M. Dunsavage, 'Pollution Control in the Oil Industry: From Spindletop to Santa Barbara', paper presented at the Fall Meeting of the Society of Petroleum Engineers of AIME, Houston, Texas, October 1970; Andrew Hurley, 'Creating Ecological Wastelands: Oil Pollution in New York City, 1870–1900', *Journal of Urban History* (1994), 340–65; Kathryn Morse, 'There Will Be Birds: Images of Oil Disasters in the Nineteenth and Twentieth Centuries', *Journal of American History* 99:1 (2012), 124–34; Hugh S. Gorman, 'Efficiency, Environmental Quality, and Oil Field Brines: The Success and Failure of Pollution Control by Self-Regulation', *Business History Review* 73:4 (1999), 601–40.

8. For a contemporary account, see: P. C. Boyle, *The Derrick's Handbook of Petroleum: A Complete Chronological and Statistical Review of Petroleum Developments from 1859 to 1899* (Derrick Publishing Co., 1898)

9. Bryan Donkin, *A Textbook on Gas, Oil, and Air Engines* (C. Griffin & Co., 1896): 278.

10. Ibid.

11. 'Oil Pollution Suits Have Been Dismissed', *Morning Star* (Indiana), 11 January 1901, 2.

12. Stephanie LeMenager, *Living Oil: Petroleum Culture in the American Century* (Oxford: Oxford University Press, 2013); David Painter, 'Oil and the American Century', *Journal of American History* 99:1 (2012), 24–39; Matthew Huber, *Lifeblood: Oil, Freedom, and the Forces of Capital* (Minneapolis: University of Minnesota Press, 2013); Darren

Dochuk, *Anointed with Oil: How Christianity and Crude Made Modern America* (London: Hachette, 2019); Bob Johnson, *Carbon Nation: Fossil Fuels in the Making of American Culture* (Lawerence: University Press of Kansas, 2014); Ross Barrett and Daniel Worden (eds), *Oil Culture* (Minneapolis: University of Minnesota Press, 2014); Brian C. Black, 'Oil for Living: Petroleum and American Conspicuous Consumption', *Journal of American History* 99:1 (2012), 40–50; Karen R. Merrill, ;Texas Metropole: Oil, the American West, and US Power in the Postwar Years', *Journal of American History* 99:1 (2012), 197–207. On how the oil industry forced the economic reconversion of whole regions, see, for example, Christopher F. Jones, *Routes of Power: Energy and Modern America* (Cambridge, MA: Harvard University Press, 2014); Martin V. Melosi and Joseph Pratt, *Energy Metropolis: An Environmental History of Houston and the Gulf Coast* (Pittsburgh, PA: University of Pittsburgh Press, 2007); Martin V. Melosi, Joseph Pratt and Kathleen A. Brosnan (eds), *Energy Capitals: Local Impact, Global Influence* (Pittsburgh, PA: University of Pittsburgh Press, 2014).

13. For the data on US annual production, US Energy Information Administration (EIA), see: https://www.eia.gov/dnav/pet/hist/LeafHandler. ashx?n=pet&s=mcrfpus2&f=a. Data on world annual production from Valentín R. Garfias, *Petroleum Resources of the World* (Chichester: John Wiley, 1923), 225.

14. Data are from the US Department of Transportation, available at: http://bit.ly/2IHIPQ2.

15. All data from the US Bureau of the Census, *Fourteenth Census of the United States, 1920*, vol. 5, Manufactures – 1919, section on Petroleum Refining (Washington, DC: US Government Printing Office, 1922). By the end of the war, more than twice as many people were working in this field than in the other long-established manufacturing activities such as pottery (about 30,000), soap (28,000) or cane sugar (27,000), and about the same number as those employed in the popular leather industry (80,000).

16. Smiley, Gene, 'US Economy in the 1920s', *EH.Net Encyclopedia*, Robert Whaples (ed.), 29 June 2004, available at: http://eh.net/encyclopedia/the-u-s-economy-in-the-1920s; Peter O'Connor and Cutler Cleveland, 'U.S. Energy Transitions 1780–2010', *Energies* 7:12 (2014), 7955–7993; Historical Statistics of the United States, 1976.

17. How the expression 'soulless corporation' became popular at the turn of the century is described in Roland Marchand, *Creating the Corporate Soul: The Rise of Public Relations and Corporate Imagery in American Big Business* (Berkeley: University of California Press, 2001), 7–11. At the time, it was used in several instances to refer specifically to Standard Oil. See, for example, H. H. Tucker Jr., *Standard against Uncle Sam: Exposing the Machinery of Injustice Lubricated by Standard Oil* (Published by the author, 1907), 97, 276.

18. On the way in which local authorities reacted to Standard Oil's dangerous working conditions and environmental pollution, specifically, see Wlasiuk, *Refining Nature*.

19. Sonia M. Zaide, *Oil Pollution Control*, 2nd edn (London: Routledge, 2019); Joseph A. Pratt, 'Letting the Grandchildren Do It: Environmental Planning during the Ascent of Oil as a Major Energy Source', *Public Historian* (1980), 28–61; Joseph A. Pratt, 'Growth or a Clean Environment? Responses to Petroleum-Related Pollution in the Gulf Coast Refining Region', *Business History Review* 52:1 (1978), 1–29.

20. Jouni Paavola, 'Water Quality as Property: Industrial Water Pollution and Common Law in the Nineteenth Century United States', *Environment and History* 8 (2002), 295–318; Jouni Paavola, 'Interstate Water Pollution Problems and Elusive Federal Water Pollution Policy in the United States, 1900–1948', *Environment and History* 12:4 (2006), 435–65. For a more general overview of how US cities addressed the problem of pollution from the late nineteenth century, see Martin V. Melosi (ed.), *Pollution and Reform in American Cities, 1870–1930* (Austin: University of Texas Press, 1980); Martin V. Melosi, *Effluent America: Cities, Industry, Energy, and the Environment* (Pittsburgh, PA: University of Pittsburgh Press, 2000); Joel A. Tarr, *The Search for the Ultimate Sink: Urban Pollution in Historical Perspective* (Akron: OH: University of Akron Press, 1996).

21. Christine Rosen, 'Differing Perceptions of the Value of Pollution Abatement across Time and Place: Balancing Doctrine in Pollution Nuisance Law, 1840–1906', *Law and History Review* 11:2 (1993), 303–81. On how judges across the US progressively changed their stance on the issue, see Jeff Lewin, 'Compensated Injunctions and the Evolution of Nuisance law', *Iowa Law Review* 71 (1985), 775.

22. Interstate compacts to address shared water control issues between states began to be implemented only in the 1920s, see Paavola, 'Interstate Water Pollution Problems'.

23. For a contemporary review of the public health activities at the state level, see Charles V. Chapin, *A Report on State Public Health Work* (Chicago, 1916), 175–82, 196–7. For a survey of early water pollution regulations, see Edwin B. Goodell, *A Review of Laws Forbidding Pollution of Inland Waters in the United States*, 2nd edn, Water and Irrigation Paper 152 (Washington, DC: US Geological Survey, 1905); Stanley D. Montgomery and Earle B. Phelps, *Stream Pollution: A Digest of Judicial Decisions and a Compilation of Legislation Relating to the Subject*, Public Health Bulletin 87(Washington, DC: US Public Health Service, 1918).

24. In the nineteenth century, some considered industrial wastes to be actually beneficial – a sort of 'cleansing agent' – because toxic chemicals killed germs, thus helping reduce sewage pollution and the diseases it carried, see John T. Cumbler, 'Whatever Happened to Industrial Waste: Reform, Compromise, and Science in Nineteenth-Century Southern New England', *Journal of Social History* (1995), 149–71. Very few officials had expressed concerns about industrial pollution by the early twentieth century – and, those who did confirmed that it was a second-rate issue in the country: M. O. Leighton, 'Industrial Wastes and Their

Sanitary Significance', *American Association of Public Health: Papers and Reports* 31 (1905), 29. For a deeper and more elaborate analysis of the experts' views in those years, see J. A. Tarr, 'Industrial Wastes and Public Health: Some Historical Notes, Part I, 1876–1932', *American Journal of Public Health* 75:9 (1985), 1059–67. See also Adam W. Rome, 'Coming to Terms with Pollution: The Language of Environmental Reform, 1865–1915', *Environmental History* 1:3 (1996,: 6–28.

25. On sanitation and the development of industrial hygiene as a science, see Christopher Sellers, 'Factory as Environment: Industrial Hygiene, Professional Collaboration and the Modern Sciences of Pollution', *Environmental History Review* 18:1 (1994), 55–83.

26. *Stream Pollution in Pennsylvania*, William B. McCaleb, October 22, 1919, Gifford Pinchot papers, Box 737, Manuscript Division, Library of Congress. Washington DC. See also Office of the Chief of Engineers, Memorandum to the District Engineer, Preliminary Report on Investigation of Pollution of Navigable Waters and their Tributaries, Office of Chief of Engineers, Civil Works 1923–1949 – General File 7235, NARA II, College Park, MD.

27. See, for example, 'No More Oil Will Go into the Lake – Manager Kelley Says Company Will Do the Right Thing, Ten Men Are Put to Work in Order to Abate the Nuisance', *Oakland Tribune*, 29 December 1900; 'Saving from Slime – Trying to Suppress Oil Nuisance, Council Promises Relief to Oil Soaked Citizens of the Southwest', *Los Angeles Evening Post*, 2 May 1901; 'The Petroleum Problem', *Merchants Journal* (Kansas), 18 June 1904; 'On "Oil Pollution" Letters to the Editor', *Philadelphia Inquirer*, 14 March 1914; 'San Louis Obispo Coast Will Be Surveyed to Find Cause of Pollution by Oil', *San Francisco Chronicle*, 20 July 1912; 'Kansas Water Being Polluted by Oil Wells', *Muskogee Times-Democrat* (Oklahoma), 8 May 1919; 'The Problem of Oil Pollution', *Miami Herald*, 8 November 1922.

28. Almon L. Fales, 'Progress in Control of Oil Pollution', *Journal of the American Water Works Association* 18:5 (1927), 587–604.

29. Ibid.

30. *Hearings on Pollution of Navigable Waters Held Before the Committee on Rivers and Harbors*, House of Representatives, 67th Congress, 25 October 1921, 1: 10–11.

31. Ibid.

32. *Report to the Secretary of State by the Interdepartmental Committee on Oil Pollution of Navigable Waters* (Washington, DC: US Government Printing Office, 1926), 1.

33. Fales, 'Progress in Control of Oil Pollution', 597.

34. Stream Pollution: National Anti-Pollution League, Pinchot papers, Box 737.

35. 'Prepare to Extend War on Pollution; National Conference Urges Laws to End Befouling of Waters by Oil', *NYT*, 3 October 1923, 25; 'Fears Oil Pollution, Speaker Claims Food Supply of Sea is Menaced', *St Joseph News-Press* (Missouri), 12 December 1923, 3.

36. *Pollution of Navigable Waters: Hearings Before a Subcommittee of the Committee on Commerce*, US Senate, 68th Congress, 1st session, January 1924.
37. Ibid., 24.
38. Ibid., 33, 73.
39. See, for example, ibid., 8, 23, 30.
40. *Pollution by Oil of the Coast Waters of the United States: Preliminary Report*, US DOI, Bureau of Mines (1923), 70.
41. Ibid., 23.
42. Some public health officials, remarkably, were still unconvinced about the adverse effects of oil pollution: F. W. Lane, A. D. Bauer, H. F. Fisher and P. N. Harding, 'Effect of Oil Pollution of Coast and Other Waters on the Public Health', *Public Health Reports* 39:28 (1924), 1661.
43. 'Oil Pollution at Bathing Beaches Source', *Public Health Reports* (1896–1970), 39:51 (1924), 3195–3206, 3202.
44. Dietmar Seyferth, 'The Rise and Fall of Tetraethyllead: Part 2', *Organometallics* 22:25 (2003), 5154–78; Herbert L. Needleman, 'Clamped in a Straitjacket: The Insertion of Lead into Gasoline', *Environmental Research* 74:2 (1997), 95–103; Joseph C. Robert, *Ethyl: A History of the Corporation and the People Who Made It* (Charlottesville: University Press of Virginia, 1983).
45. On the 1924 study and, more broadly, on the concerns that preceded and followed the introduction of leaded gasoline on the market, see David Rosner and Gerald Markowitz, 'A "Gift of God?: The Public Health Controversy Over Leaded Gasoline during the 1920s', *American Journal of Public Health* 75:4 (1985), 344–52; Needleman, 'Clamped in a Straitjacket'.
46. Frank A. Howard, Ethyl Gasoline Corporation, *Proceedings of a Conference to Determine Whether or not there is a Public Health Question in the Manufacture, Distribution, or Use of Tetraethyl Lead Gasoline*, Public Health Bulletin 158 (1925), 105.
47. Ibid.
48. Among them, there was Alice Hamilton, one of the most renowned experts on lead and chemical contamination in general, whose work contributed to the establishment of occupational health and medicine, see 'Tetra-Ethyl Lead', *Journal of the American Medical Association* 84:20 (1925), 1481–6.
49. For a detailed reconstruction of the lead industry's stalling (and deceitful) tactics, see Gerald Markowitz and David Rosner, *Deceit and Denial: The Deadly Politics of Industrial Pollution* (Berkeley: University of California Press, 2002).
50. 'Ethyl Gasoline Given Clean Bill Thus Far', *American Journal of Public Health* 16:3 (1926), 295–6.
51. Christian Warren, *Brush with Death: A Social History of Lead Poisoning* (Baltimore, MD: Johns Hopkins University Press, 2001).

6

Simkins v. *Cone* and the Hospital Desegregation Movement in the Long Twentieth Century

Richard M. Mizelle, Jr

The 1896 *Plessy* v. *Ferguson* decision[1] provided federal approval of de jure and de facto segregation on American soil.[1] The decision provided the imprimatur of government-sanctioned Black inferiority in every realm of public life and interaction. The relegation of Black people to the status of second-class citizenship, including in the realm of public health, had lasting consequences in the twentieth century.[2] American courts and laws were at the apex of shaping the meaning of democracy at the turn of the twentieth century. In so doing, courts reflected broader scientific theories that the intermingling of various groups were undemocratic and biologically unnatural. Blacks, Indigenous groups, Asians and Mexicans were considered to be incapable of both citizenship and carrying the burden of upholding democratic principles.

The *Plessy* decision also reflected a zeitgeist of science and politics that irreparably harmed the country's commitment to democracy by making an entire group of the population into second-class citizens. Statistician Frederick Hoffman's *Race Traits and Tendencies of the American Negro* (1896) leaned on a century of racial science to suggest that Black people were inherently prone to criminality and a host of venereal and contagious diseases rooted in their supposed biological inferiority. W. E. B. Du Bois countered Hoffman's assumptions with his *Health and Physique of the Negro American* published one year later in 1897. Rather than biological and racial differences, Du Bois argued that systematic structural and environmental inequalities resulted in poor Black health. Acknowledging the higher Black morbidity and mortality rates for most disease categories, Du Bois made the important point that stark poverty, hunger, poor sanitation, nutritional deficiencies and inferior housing caused Black people to suffer disproportionately from tuberculosis, pneumonia, whooping cough, diphtheria, scarlet fever, measles and infant mortality.[3] Using a transnational approach that was ahead of his time, Du Bois emphasised high rates of infectious disease among poor Blacks in the United States and poor residents in London slums as the result of environment and not biology. In the case of the latter, their rates were similarly dire.[4] Du Bois made this case for an international audience when he compiled 363 images into two albums for the 'American Negro Exhibit' at the 1900 Paris Exposition. These images showed thriving Black businesses, expressions of religion and leisure, and home ownership as a counter to popular domestic caricatures of Blacks as poor, diseased and uneducated. Disease was an outgrowth of racism and environment and not a natural state of Black existence, Du Bois made clear; thereby joining other Black intellectuals in refuting long-standing claims of inherent Black inferiority and immutable biological difference as a justification for segregation.[5]

With the *Health and Physique of the Negro American* and 1900 Paris Exposition, Du Bois was pointing out the contradictions of democracy before an international audience, refuting tenets of scientific racism as it appeared in publications in the United States and Europe, but also highlighting before a world audience the deplorable and abysmal physical environments in which some Black people resided. As the United States was emerging as a global power by the First World War and making claims of becoming a beacon of democracy that should be emulated by other nations, the physical and psychological violence directed towards Black Americans undermined and contradicted those expressed ideals.

The historian Mary Dudziak points out in her book, *Cold War Civil Rights: Race and the Image of American Democracy* (2011) that presidents and leaders throughout the twentieth century were concerned about racism and discrimination tarnishing America's image abroad.[6] Lynchings, the Scottsboro Nine, violence towards returning First and Second World War soldiers, housing discrimination, church bombings and water hoses used on civil rights protesters in Birmingham, among many other shameful episodes, undermined America's stated perch as a leader of democracy and equality. As Dudziak makes clear, American foreign relations during the Cold War made presidents reluctantly open to the advancement of Black civil rights between the 1940s and 1970s. Yet there was also widespread fear of civil rights demands harming America's global leadership position, leading to the attempted repression of dissent and criticism towards US policies during the McCarthy era.[7]

During the long twentieth century Black institutions and leaders pressured the federal government to protect the lives and health of Black Americans, pointing out the ways in which sickness harmed America's ability to shine a beacon of light around the world.

This chapter uses the hospital desegregation movement as a brief case study of how civil rights activists used courts and litigation to demand change, and in the process to achieve change in US politics. Historians have defined the ways in which segregation in many realms of public life were revealed as hypocritical when the United States expressed its democratic ideals to the world. Yet we have often ignored the desegregation of hospitals as an important battleground for democracy and inclusion of citizenship. Black activists during mid-century and the Civil Rights era forced American institutions to live up to the stated democratic ideals, values and capacities professed by leaders. The state, local and federal response to demands for justice and public health showed the contradictions of the United States as a global beacon of democracy. In this case study of the desegregation of hospitals during the Jim Crow era, Black activists used the same courts that penned laws excluding them from democracy to demand their inclusion.

Health activism

The Progressive Era increased surveillance of water- and airborne diseases through broad sanitary reform and cleanliness campaigns, targeting immigrant communities and the poor. Yet the Progressive Era would also increase surveillance of Black bodies under the guise of public health. In Atlanta and other cities, tuberculosis campaigns targeted Black communities under the assumption that Black washerwomen, for instance, were natural harbingers of disease and were spreading the tubercle bacillus in White households as domestic servants.[8] Racial science would also suggest that Black people were less likely to suffer from certain chronic diseases like cancer, heart disease, asthma and diabetes that supposedly afflicted civilised White groups only. Scientists, physicians and the broader public held up these ideas as truth through a dizzying combination of assumptions, thoughts, ideas and unfounded principles that served to visualise racial difference through the lens of disease.[9] The increased awareness of chronic disease in Black populations by mid-century disclosed a long history of suffering and public health invisibility.[10]

In his classic text *The Social System* (1951), sociologist Talcott Parsons defines the *sick role* as a theoretical explanation of illness and patienthood.[11] While disease and illness are part of the human condition, patienthood is a category of entitlement and access to medical and public health resources that has never been universally applied.[12] To put it more succinctly, everyone becomes sick but not everyone becomes a patient. Patienthood is an act, or rather the entitlement to an identity and performance that was reserved largely for White people during segregation. Patienthood brought temporary or permanent institutionalisation and the expenditure of medical attention and resources, space and expertise in a way that reified social worth. Perhaps most important, patienthood was a definition of time, of who could bend medicine and the healing apparatus for themselves in the form of attention from physicians, nurses and administrators. White people primarily had access to hospitals and clinics in the same way they held primary access to public schools, restaurants, theatres, parks and other public spaces. Patienthood was a right that only first-class citizens could demand. Being White and sick meant something very different to being Black and sick. Depending on status and wealth, sickness might bring empathy and the full range of medical resources to bear for Whites.[13]

Hospitals proved to be an important battleground for democracy. Black health activists waged court battles to desegregate hospitals for patients and gain access to public hospital facilities for themselves in ways that mirrored the school desegregation movement in the 1950s and 1960s. The hospital movement culminated in the landmark 1964 Supreme Court case, *Simkins* v. *Moses H. Cone Memorial Hospital* in Greensboro, North Carolina.[14] While the *Simkins* decision was an important victory for the health and public health of Black southerners during the Civil Rights era, the conservative backlash resembled tactics employed following the *Brown* decision to delay and prevent integration of public schools.

Imagined fears of Black and White children intermingling in classrooms were also reified in hospitals. Majority White hospitals and clinics also struck a nerve for segregationists who believed in the scientific construction of biological and racial difference as fundamentally immutable. Hospitals were not only places of potential cross-pollination of ideas and flow of information, but also of vulnerable open bodies. Men and women inhabiting the same space, sick bodies and healthy bodies, blood products and saliva, the naked bodies of patients and corpses to be examined and autopsied, all exhumed the worst fears of integration in the White imagination.[15] Added to this fear was the threat of Black physicians, dentists and nurses who sought to practice in hospitals where Whites were being served; that they would serve only Black patients during the era of segregation was little in question, but their presence as professionals and proximity to vulnerable White bodies was enough to stoke fear.

The *Simkins* decision did not emerge out of a vacuum, however, but instead was part of a longer history of Black activism. On the heels of the Great Depression, the election of President Franklin

Delano Roosevelt in 1932 signalled a New Deal of social and economic recovery programmes for the country that played out unevenly and in a myriad of ways. By 1933, roughly 12 million people were unemployed. Black farmers and workers continued to be marginalised and left behind in New Deal programmes, including the Civilian Conservation Corps, Works Progress Administration and the Tennessee Valley Authority. Black newspapers like the *Norfolk Journal and Guide* referred to the New Deal as 'No Deal' for Black people.[16] Responding to the lack of public health protections during the New Deal, Black public health leaders, professionals and communities mobilised in favour of their own health through 'Negro Health Week' programmes (originally started at the Tuskegee Institute in 1915) and other Progressive Era programmes. Mobile clinics and lectures addressing the health problems of a particular community were organised during the 1930s and 1940s. Rural clinics were popular and demonstrated, to the contrary of White assumptions, the concerns manifested by Black people over their own health. Black public health-focused nurses and community organisers were at the heart of this health movement. Long ignored within the history of medicine, Black nurses were important for thinking about the experience of disease and illness in the twentieth century. Particularly in the South, Black people suffering from chronic and contagious diseases were more likely to receive nutritional advice and diagnosis from a Black public health nurse than a Black or White physician. A greater number of trained Black nurses, along with their organising traditions, shaped the care that many Black people received.[17]

Facing racialised and gendered mistreatment during their training and professional lives, Black public health nurses endured unimaginable hostilities and slights in the name of public health. The number of trained Black nurses remained small in comparison with White nurses. Of the roughly 5,000 Black nurses in 1930, close to 500 worked as public health nurses in both rural and urban spaces. A decade and a half later that number would double, showing the ways in which Black nurses maintained a commitment to Black public health. Black laywomen and Black women's organisations coordinated with public health professionals to mobilise around the health of Black people as well. Though Black mobilisation around community health was considered necessary during an era of segregation, some leaders remained steadfast in their belief that the desegregation of medical institutions and public health was necessary for full equality.[18]

The end of 'Negro Health Week' in 1950 was applauded by Black physicians W. Montague Cobb and Louis Wright, who suggested that it reinforced racialised biological difference and segregation. Other

Black leaders suggested 'there is no such thing as Negro health'. Integration of hospitals, clinics and medical services, they would argue, was necessary for the country to uphold the democratic principles it professed to the world. Though the battle for integration of hospitals and clinics was spearheaded mostly by Black physicians in the 1960s, nurses and laywomen laid important foundations of health activism in the New Deal era and beyond.[19]

The road to *Simkins* v. *Moses H. Cone* (1963)

In North Carolina, South Carolina, Mississippi, Louisiana, Alabama and other southern states, some Black people went from cradle to the grave without ever seeing the inside of a hospital during the early to mid-twentieth century.[20] When defining the oppression of groups within colonised spaces, Martinique-born psychiatrist and theorist Frantz Fanon defined the use of spatial colonial occupation as a form of domination. Spatial occupation demands that oppressed groups must be here, but not there, visible in certain ways, but also invisible. The geography of space is a disciplining tool that effectively separated the colonising from the colonised, on sidewalks, parks, restaurants, schools and medical clinics. Segregated hospitals were an example of Fanon's notion of spatial occupation as Black patients were disciplined in public spaces in ways that demanded overt hierarchies. Spatial occupation meant being refused admittance or relegated to inferior service or facilities.[21] Black patients were exposed to shameful geographies of space that created vulnerability to disease and death. Eyal Weizman's theory of 'the politics of verticality' similarly reflects segregated hospitals where Black patients existed above or below White bodies.[22] Bodies existed and overlapped in the same space with barriers to isolate Black patients. Inside segregated hospitals Black patients might be relegated to attics or basements without running water, medical supplies, equipment and modern technology. Excruciatingly hot in the summer and bitterly cold in the winter, those attics and basements represented Black health as existing away from and outside the norm of White health. Fanon's theory of colonial spatialisation in segregated hospitals also engages with Achille Mbembe's 'necropolitics' where state power and institutional forces define the politics of who lives and who dies.[23]

Although there were attempts to desegregate hospitals in the first half of the twentieth century – Harlem Hospital in the 1920s, for instance – a larger national effort began in response to the 1946 Hospital Survey and Construction Act.[24] Known as the Hill–Burton Act after sponsors Lister Hill (Democrat, AL) and Harold Burton

(Republican, OH), the legislation authorised the spending of $75 million in matching federal and state grants to provide individual states (particularly in the South) with resources to assess population density and hospital bed space. The point was to provide individual states a pipeline to Congress for assistance in constructing new facilities or rebuilding older facilities to address bed shortages.[25] While Congress deliberated over the Act, the National Association for the Advancement of Colored People (NAACP) pressured federal officials to implement a non-discrimination clause that would prevent the use of public funds for segregated hospitals.[26] Using the precedence of *Plessy*, Congress would allow Hill–Burton funds to be used by public hospitals as long as 'separate but equal' facilities were provided. The result was a continuation of segregation within healthcare that had long existed in theory and practice. As one historian situated the 'separate but equal' clause of the Hill–Burton Act, 'the medical and hospital leadership gradually reversed the country's shortage of general hospital beds, but not its practices of hospital discrimination'.[27] That segregated hospital facilities for Black patients were inherently inferior, and in violation of their Fifth and Fourteenth Amendment rights, were systematically ignored by federal officials.

The hospital desegregation movement emerged out of the same pressurised spaces that produced larger sit-in movements and boycotts during the 1950s and 1960s. Howard University physician and anthropologist W. Montague Cobb established the IMHOTEP Conference on Hospital Integration in 1956, named after the ancient Egyptian physician (27th century BCE). As the historian John Dittmer writes, 'this largely black but interracial group of health care professionals met annually to discuss legal and political strategies to open up hospitals to African American patients and physicians'.[28] IMHOTEP emerged at a time when the anticipation of change from the *Brown* v. *Board of Education* decision was beginning to wane, and bus boycotts were being planned or implemented in Montgomery and Tallahassee.[29] Even as integration of public schools was proving slow, lawyers and physicians looked for cases to attack hospital segregation using the courts.

Conrad Pearson was among a cadre of lawyers that included Thurgood Marshall and Constance Motley Baker trained at Howard University School of Law under Charles Hamilton Houston. Houston served as Dean of the Law School from 1929 to 1935, and later as Special Counsel for the NAACP. Houston and his students argued important higher education desegregation cases before the United States Supreme Court in the 1940s and 1950s that set the precedent for *Brown* v. *Board of Education* (1954). *Gaines* v. *Missouri* (1938),

Sipuel v. *Oklahoma* (1948), *McLaurin* v. *Oklahoma* (1950) and *Sweatt* v. *Painter* (1950) were waged against segregation in graduate and law schools in border states.[30-4]

Born in Durham, North Carolina, Pearson returned to North Carolina to work for the NAACP-Legal Defense Fund after graduating from Howard in 1932. Pearson and the Legal Defense Fund filed the first hospital desegregation suit in 1956 in Wilmington, North Carolina. A port city, Wilmington was still recovering from the 1898 race riot that stemmed from increased Black political representation. *Eaton* v. *Board of Managers of the James Walker Memorial Hospital* was filed on behalf of three black physicians: Hubert A. Eaton, Daniel C. Roane and Samuel Gray.[35] There were two hospitals in Wilmington, the 100-bed Community Hospital which served Black patients, and the James Walker Memorial Hospital which primarily served White patients and maintained a segregated ward of twenty-five beds for Black patients. As historian Preston K. Reynolds writes, the segregated ward in Memorial Hospital 'had substandard lighting, heating and ventilation. Sadly, Dr. Eaton considered these facilities better than those available at . . . Community Hospital.'[36] Staffing privileges to Memorial Hospital were also refused to Black doctors and nurses.[37] Pearson and the NAACP argued that Memorial Hospital was in violation of the Fourteenth Amendment because of their use of public funds. In particular, they argued that 'because of the land contracts between the city and county and James Walker Memorial Hospital, contributions from the local governments to the hospital for maintenance and payment of services to the poor, and the conditions of the will of James Walker about the hospital, discrimination of the physicians was unconstitutional'.[38] The North Carolina district court disagreed, ruling that 'the act of discrimination did not constitute state action'. The US Court of Appeals upheld the ruling and the United States Supreme Court declined to hear the case.[39]

At issue was the use of public funds, particularly Hill–Burton funds. The Legal Defense fund had not proven (or could not effectively document) that Memorial Hospital received public funds and therefore should be considered a public institution. Pearson and other lawyers were nonetheless buoyed by the actions in Wilmington even though it resulted in defeat. They set out to find a test case that would allow them to take the next step to the Supreme Court.

Greensboro, North Carolina had a long history of radical Black activism.[40] At the centre of desegregation battles was George Simkins Jr., president of the Greensboro chapter of the NAACP between 1959 and 1984. Simkins was born in Greensboro and attended segregated public schools before graduating from Talladega College in Alabama in 1944. He enrolled in Meharry Dental College in Nashville, Tennessee, earning a DDS in 1948, and after a one-year internship in Jersey City, New Jersey, moved back to Greensboro in 1949 to set up a private practice.[41] The Black population in Greensboro faced a real dilemma when sick. There were three hospitals in Greensboro during segregation. Wesley Long Community Hospital was a 78-bed facility that did not admit Black patients or extend staff privileges to Black nurses, physicians or dentists. The much larger Moses H. Cone Memorial Hospital had a capacity for 300 patients and admitted a limited number of Black patients, mostly for surgery and special procedures, but also refused staff privileges to Black doctors. The so-called separate but equal facility was the 91-bed L. Richardson Memorial Hospital. Richardson was the only facility in Greensboro where Black dentists and physicians held admitting privileges.[42]

In a letter written to Benjamin Cone, chairman of the board of trustees for Cone Hospital, in March 1960, Simkins laid the foundation for a coalition against segregated medical facilities in the city. Simkins reminded Cone of the recent expansion project, when the public hospital was quoted as recognising 'the position of service which the hospital has built in the Greensboro community and in the state at large', while simultaneously admitting only a limited number of Black patients and refusing to extend staff privileges to Black doctors.[43] Simkins framed the insult largely from the perspective of Black patients: 'In considering this problem, we hope you will try to imagine how you would feel if you were required to give up the physician or dentist of your choice as a condition of admission to hospital service.' The NAACP wrote several letters to Cone and Long hospitals asking for equal treatment of Black patients and doctors, all of which were ignored.[44]

Looking for the right spark to mobilise a movement, Simkins was visited by Donald Lyons, a student at North Carolina Agricultural and Technical State College (now university) who expressed severe pain in a visibly swollen jaw and had a temperature of 103°F. Lyons needed prompt hospitalisation for antibiotics to lower his temperature, and Simkins contacted L. Richardson Hospital, which informed him of a two- to three-week waiting period for new admissions.[45] Simkins would later recall that when entering Richardson Hospital, 'there would be beds in the hallways. You'd have to walk down a narrow path through the hallways without running into the beds, because it was so crowded.' He called Cone and Long for admission, and though both had beds available, Long held fast to its position of not accepting Black patients. Cone had space in the segregated ward, but Lyons refused to be admitted if it meant being treated by a White dentist.[46]

The other contentious point for Simkins was a difference in technology available at Cone and Long that made Richardson's facilities inherently separate and unequal. In a signed affidavit that Simkins presented in anticipation of a court case, he wrote that Lyons had an 'impacted lower third molar that he wished removed at a hospital where the best dental facilities are available. In this area the only dental facilities available are at the Wesley Long Community Hospital and the Moses Cone Memorial Hospital. Both hospitals have dental X-rays and dental chairs. The Wesley Long Hospital also has a Weber dental unit with a light and a dental handpiece.'[47] Richardson had none of these technologies for dental care.

Simkins reached out to Thurgood Marshall and Jack Greenberg of the NAACP-Legal Defense Fund in New York and began the process of organising Black doctors in Greensboro. There would be eleven plaintiffs, including physicians, dentists and patients. The key for the Greensboro movement was proving the use of Hill–Burton funds in violation of the Fifth and Fourteenth Amendments of the US Constitution. Cone and Long had in fact received Hill–Burton funds in the amount of $2 million for expansion and renovation projects between 1954 and 1961.[48] The renovation projects were crucial to the NAACP's case, and provided evidence they were unable to prove a few years earlier in Wilmington.

On 12 February 1962, Conrad Pearson filed the suit, *Simkins* v. *Moses H. Cone Memorial Hospital* with the clerk of the US District Court for the Middle District of North Carolina. Nine months later District Court Judge Edwin Stanley ruled in favour of Moses H. Cone by arguing the court did not have jurisdiction over civil rights activities as they related to hospitals and healthcare. Greenberg filed an appeal of the lower court's decision on 1 April 1963, arguing the desegregation case before the Fourth Circuit Court of Appeals.[49] The circuit court ruled in favour of the plaintiffs, rendering its decision on 1 November 1963. In a majority opinion, Chief Judge Simon Sobeloff wrote that 'millions of dollars of public monies' were spent in hospital construction projects at Cone and Long Hospitals, making the segregation of facilities unconstitutional. When the US Supreme Court denied a writ of *certiorari* from Cone's lawyers on 2 March 1964, the Fourth Circuit Court's decision of the unconstitutionality of 'separate but equal' hospital facilities were upheld.[50]

As the *New York Times* reminded readers, 'the immediate legal effect will be in the Fourth Circuit, which covers Maryland, Virginia, West Virginia and North and South Carolina'.[51] The *Simkins* decision did not immediately include other southern states. In the years following the *Simkins* decision southern hospitals, taking their cue from public schools, would find infinite ways to delay the admittance of Black patients and extension of staff privileges to Black doctors.[52] Both Long and Cone attempted to circumvent the court's decision. Cone extended the Black physicians and dentists in Greensboro not among the plaintiffs an invitation to join the staff first, using the initial denial of admitting privileges to Simkins and other plaintiffs as a rebuke. Eventually, Simkins and the others secured staff privileges at Cone, but Long would prove even more difficult to penetrate. One local White doctor suggested that, like public schools, Black doctors would need federal troops to gain staff privileges at Wesley Long. The federal troops never came, and the staff privileges for Simkins and the other Black doctors were not initiated at Long for many years.[53]

The road from Cone

The *Simkins* case has been called the *Brown* decision for healthcare, but there was little of the national euphoria of optimistic change that marked the earlier decision. Jack Greenberg initially described it as an 'entering wedge' of Black physicians and patients into White health institutions that would 'put an end to keeping Negroes out of white hospitals or segregating them within the hospitals, and requiring them to give up their Negro doctors and hire white doctors if they wanted treatment'. The words were too optimistic, and he later sounded a more cautious tone: 'We wait to see whether the medical profession will voluntarily follow the law or whether a long, hard process of litigation such as we have had with schools will be necessary.'[54] Hospitals and healthcare facilities would in fact employ the strategy of indefinitely delaying integration.

By late 1965 it was clear to the NAACP that hospitals across the South would resist the *Simkins* decision and that more lawsuits might be necessary. Passage of the 1964 Civil Rights Act provided some hope that expensive and time-consuming lawsuits could be avoided.[55] Title VI of the Civil Rights Act made discrimination illegal in any programme or activity involving the federal government; complaints against hospitals by individuals and organisations could be filed with the Department of Health, Education and Welfare (HEW). But the HEW was slow to take legal action and enforce desegregation, and in many cases all that was necessary for hospitals to retain federal funds (particularly Medicare) was to sign a compliance form simply stating they would not discriminate.[56] By 1965, the NAACP, Medical Committee for Human Rights (MCHR) and the National Medical Association had lodged more than 300 complaints to the HEW. In a scathing report to HEW secretary John

Gardner the NAACP Legal-Defense team wrote: 'An end to exclusion or unequal treatment of Negro patients and physicians in the
South was envisioned when the Legal Defense Fund won a decisive victory in a suit against two North Carolina hospitals, upheld
by the U.S. Supreme Court last year, outlawing discrimination in
any institution receiving Federal aid.[57] Though HEW claimed it was
ill-equipped to undertake the massive overseeing of hospital compliance for the roughly 2,000 hospitals in the South that received
Hill–Burton funds, this was no excuse for the NAACP and MCHR
who demanded that HEW borrow or hire additional staff to deal
with the added burden.[58] They also pushed for discontinuation of
federal funding until hospitals complied with desegregation orders
and attempted to close the loopholes for avoiding compliance. This
included the strategy of hospital administrators waiting for the
threat or actual filing of a lawsuit to integrate and allowing hospitals to continue the practice of segregation while using reserve
Hill–Burton funds.[59]

Segregated entrances, wards, cafeteria facilities, refusal of staff
privileges to Black doctors and nurses outright or beyond a quota,
and relegation of Black patients to second-class status in emergency
rooms continued well into the 1970s. Complaints were handled by
HEW officials from Washington, DC or local investigators, the latter
a point of contention for the Legal Defense Fund. Most often White,
the Legal Defense Fund commented that 'Investigators drawn from
the South often fail to observe discriminatory practices which have
long represented the southern way of life. The Fund has asked that
Negro investigators be employed.'[60] The NAACP had long employed
the practice of sending undercover agents or friends into the South
to observe harsh labour conditions and accusations of Black mistreatment; these Black and White investigators would subsequently
report their findings to the organisation. They sent undercover agents
to observe Mississippi Delta levee camp conditions in the 1930s and
would do the same with hospitals in the 1960s.[61]

Between HEW investigators, NAACP agents and word of mouth
from Black doctors, patients, nurses and staff who engaged with
southern hospitals and clinics, it was clear that many southern hospitals were undermining federal law by remaining partly or completely
segregated. Complaints were very telling of ongoing conditions.
A series of complaints from February 1965 concerned the King's
Daughter Hospital in Canton, Mississippi. King's did not just refuse
Title VI compliance, but in order to avoid any form of potential
contact between Blacks and Whites, they reduced the number of
beds so less patients could be admitted (particularly Black patients).

The hospital continued to receive Hill–Burton funds.[62] The Jefferson County Hospital in Pine Bluff, Arkansas, continued to maintain a northwest 'Negro' wing. This complaint related to the experiences of two Black women who attempted to deliver their babies inside the Whites-only wing and were refused. When pressed as to why the hospital continued receiving Hill–Burton funds, the HEW responded that the 'Title VI cut-off procedure was too cumbersome to employ.'[63] At the Jones Memorial Hospital in Orange County, Maryland, the cafeteria and snack bars remained segregated, the out-patient department would treat Black patients only on Wednesdays, the emergency room treated all Whites in the waiting area before helping Black patients, there were quotas on the already small number of Black physicians, Black nurses could not supervise White nurses or personnel, and Black patients were rarely addressed with titles of respect upon entering the hospital. Jones also segregated blood and blood products. A quarter of a century after the Second World War American Red Cross controversy where blood products were segregated for surgeries and transfusions, there were still complaints of hospitals segregating so-called Black and White blood.[64] Throughout the South, some hospitals simply refused to comply with the *Simkins* decision or Title VI into the 1970s and 1980s, showing their defiance of the federal government and President Johnson's Great Society.[65]

Conclusion

The failure to protect the rights of Black people when sick is a failure of democracy. Throughout the twentieth century, public health departments, researchers, clinicians, statisticians, hospital administrators and courts of law designed a system of hyper-surveillance in the name of protecting White health on one end and hyper-disregard of Black health on the other. This chapter has briefly highlighted the ways in which grassroots organising in the 1930s and 1940s laid the groundwork for the hospital desegregation movement in the courts.

Civil rights victories of the 1950s and 1960s were important for helping shift America's moral compass. Following the landmark *Simkins* v. *Moses H. Cone Memorial Hospital* Supreme Court decision, public funds can no longer be used for the construction of hospitals that practice segregation and Black doctors and nurses can no longer be excluded from staffing privileges at public hospitals. But as legal scholar Daria Roithmayr has written, the advantages of Whiteness in public schools, housing, industry, politics and public health have become locked in through centuries of state- and government-sanctioned inequality.[66] Over the course of the last fifty years, the discourses of race and health have continuously been recast through imperceptible dimensions of access and medical citizenship that, for a host of reasons and mirroring public education, are increasingly more difficult to pin-point. Geographical and residential segregation makes it so that Black people and minorities continue to struggle with 'inalienable' rights when it comes to public health. The laws fought for and achieved during the Civil Rights Movement laid the seeds for a more equitable society, yet the realisation of those dreams continue to be an unfulfilled promise of democracy and equitable healthcare in the twenty-first century.

Notes

1. *Plessy v. Fergusson* 163 US 537 (1896).
2. Leon Litwack, *Trouble in Mind: Black Southerners in the Age of Jim Crow* (New York: Vintage, 1999).
3. For a discussion of both Hoffman and Du Bois in the period, see Khalil Muhammad, *The Race, Crime, and the Making of Modern Urban America* (Cambridge, MA: Harvard University Press, 2011). There is now a rich literature on race and medicine, for representative works, see Samuel K. Roberts, *Infectious Fear: Politics, Disease, and the Health Effects of Segregation* (Chapel Hill: University of North Carolina Press, 2009); Edward Beardsley, *A History of Neglect: Health Care for Blacks and Mill Workers in the Twentieth Century South* (Knoxville: University of Tennessee Press, 1999); Keith Wailoo, *Dying in the City of the Blues: Sickle Cell Anemia and the Politics of Race and Health* (Chapel Hill: University of North Carolina Press, 2001); Wangui Muigai, "Something Wasn't Clean": Black Midwifery, Birth, and Postwar Medical Education in *All My Babies*', *Bulletin of the History of Medicine* 93:1 (2019), 82–113.
4. Shawn Smith, *Photography on the Color Line: W. E. B. Du Bois, Race, and Visual Culture* (Durham, NC: Duke University Press, 2004); Aldon Morris, *W. E. B. Du Bois and the Birth of Modern Sociology* (Berkeley: University of California Press, 2017).
5. Smith, *Photography on the Color Line*.
6. Mary Dudziak, *Cold War Civil Rights: Race and the Image of American Democracy* (Princeton, NJ: Princeton University Press, 2011).
7. Dudziak, *Cold War Civil Rights*; Chad Williams, *Torchbearers of Democracy: African American Soldiers in the World War I Era* (Chapel Hill: University of North Carolina Press: 2013); Charles Payne, *I've Got the Light of Freedom: The Organizing Tradition of the Mississippi Freedom Struggle* (Berkeley: University of California Press, 1995); Ellen Schrecker, *Many Are the Crimes: McCarthyism in America* (New York: Little, Brown, 1998).

8. Tera Hunter, *To Joy My Freedom: Southern Black Women's Lives and Labors after the Civil War* (Cambridge, MA: Harvard University Press, 1998).

9. Keith Wailoo, *How Cancer Cross the Color Line* (New York: Oxford University Press, 2011); Anne Pollock, *Medicating Race: Heart Disease and Durable Preoccupations with Difference* (Durham, NC: Duke University Press, 2012).

10. Arleen Tuchman, *Diabetes: A History of Race and Disease* (New Haven, CT: Yale University Press, 2020).

11. Talcott Parsons, *The Social System* (Oxford: Routledge, 1951).

12. Edward Beardsley, *A History of Neglect: Health Care for Black and Mill Workers in the Twentieth Century South* (Knoxville: University of Tennessee Press, 1987).

13. Parsons, *The Social System*.

14. *Simkins v. Moses H. Cone Memorial Hospital* 323 F.2d 959 (4th Cir. 1963).

15. George M. Fredrickson, *The Black Image in the White Mind: The Debate on Afro-American Character and Destiny, 1817–1914* (New York: Harper & Row, 1972).

16. Richard M. Mizelle, Jr., *Backwater Blues: The Mississippi River Flood of 1927 in the African American Imagination* (Minneapolis: University of Minnesota Press, 2014).

17. Darlene Clark Hine, *Racial Conflict and Cooperation in the Nursing Profession, 1890–1950* (Bloomington: Indiana University Press, 1989); Susan Smith, *Sick and Tired of Being Sick and Tired: Black Women's Health Activism in America, 1890–1950* (Philadelphia: University of Pennsylvania Press, 1995), see ch. 3.

18. Smith, *Sick and Tired*.

19. Smith, *Sick and Tired*.

20. Vanessa Northington Gamble, *Making a Place for Ourselves: The Black Hospital Movement, 1920–1945* (New York: Oxford University Press, 1995); Edward Beardsley, *A History of Neglect: Health Care for Black and Mill Workers in the Twentieth Century South* (Knoxville: University of Tennessee Press, 1987).

21. Frantz Fanon, *A Dying Colonialism* (New York: Grove Press, 1994).

22. Eyal Weizman, *Forensic Architecture: Violence at the Threshold of Detectability* (New York: Zone Books, 2019).

23. Achille Mbembe, *Necropolitics* (Durham, NC: Duke University Press, 2019).

24. P. Preston Reynolds, 'Hospitals and Civil Rights, 1945–1963: The Case of Simkins v. Moses H. Cone Memorial Hospital', *Annals of Internal Medicine* 126:11 (1997): 898–906; P. Preston Reynolds, 'Professional and Hospital Discrimination and the US Court of Appeals Fourth Circuit 1956–1967', *American Journal of Public Health* 94:5 (2004): 710–20.

25. Reynolds, 'Hospitals and Civil Rights'; see also Edward Beardsley, *A History of Neglect: Health Care for Blacks and Mill Workers in the Twentieth-Century South* (Knoxville: University of Tennessee Press,

1990); Karen Kruse Thomas, *Deluxe Jim Crow: Civil Rights and American Health Policy, 1935–1954* (Athens: University of Georgia Press, 2011).

26. Reynolds, 'Hospitals and Civil Rights'.
27. Reynolds, 'Professional and Hospital Discrimination and the US Court of Appeals Fourth Circuit 1956–1967', 710.
28. John Ditmer, *The Good Doctors: The Medical Committee for Human Rights and the Struggle for Social Justice in Health Care* (New York: Bloomsbury, 2009), 12.
29. *Brown v. Board of Education of Topeka* 347 US 483 (1954).
30. *Missouri ex rel. Gaines v. Canada* 305 US 337 (1938).
31. *Sipuel v. Board of Regents of the University of Oklahoma* 332 US 631 (1948).
32. *McLaurin v. Oklahoma State Regents* 339 US 637 (1950).
33. *Sweatt v. Painter* 339 US 629 (1950).
34. Genna Rae McNeil, *Groundwork: Charles Hamilton Houston and the Struggle for Civil Rights* (Philadelphia: University of Pennsylvania Press, 1984).
35. *Eaton v. Board of Managers of the James Walker Memorial Hospital* 164 F. Supp. 191 (EDNC 1958).
36. Reynolds, 'Hospitals and Civil Rights', 900.
37. I use the term 'doctors' to make clear that I am referring to both dentists and physicians.
38. Reynolds, 'Hospitals and Civil Rights', 900–1.
39. Ibid., 901.
40. See Charles M. Payne, *I've Got the Light of Freedom: The Organizing Tradition and the Mississippi Freedom Struggle* (Berkeley: University of California Press, 2007); Clayborne Carson, *In Struggle: SNCC and the Black Awakening of the 1960s* (Cambridge, MA: Harvard University Press, 1995).
41. Interview with George Simkins, 6 April 1997, Interview R-0018, Southern Oral History Program Collection (#4007) in the Southern Oral History Program Collection, Southern Historical Collection, Wilson Library, University of North Carolina at Chapel Hill.
42. Reynolds, 'Professional and Hospital Discrimination and the US Court of Appeals Fourth Circuit 1956–1967'; Reynolds, 'Hospitals and Civil Rights'.
43. Letter from George S. Simkins, DDS, President, Greensboro Branch of the NAACP to Benjamin Cone, 14 November 1961, Box 1, George Simkins Jr. Papers, Archives Collection, F. D. Bluford Library, North Carolina Agricultural and Technical State University, Greensboro, NC.
44. Ibid.
45. Interview with George Simkins, 6 April 1997, Interview R-0018, Southern Oral History Program Collection (#4007) in the Southern Oral History Program Collection, Southern Historical Collection, Wilson Library, University of North Carolina at Chapel Hill.
46. Ibid.

47. George Simkins Affidavit, Guilford County, North Carolina, 1962, Box 1, George Simkins Jr. Papers.

48. Letter from George S. Simkins, DDS, President, Greensboro Branch of the NAACP to Benjamin Cone, 14 November 1961, Box 1, George Simkins Jr. Papers.

49. Interview with George Simkins, 6 April 1997.

50. P. Preston Reynolds, 'Hospitals and Civil Rights, 1945–1963: The Case of Simkins v. Moses H. Cone Memorial Hospital', *Annals of Internal Medicine* 126:11 (1997), 898–906.

51. 'Hospitals Built with Federal Aid Must Integrate: Ban on Separate but Equal Facilities is left Standing by the Supreme Court: Wide Impact Expected', *New York Times*, 3 March 1964.

52. Interview with George Simkins,6 April 1997.

53. Ibid.

54. 'Hospitals Built with Federal Aid Must Integrate', *New York Times*, 3 March 1964.

55. 'Report on the Implementation of Title VI of the Civil Rights Act of 1964 in Regard to Hospital Discrimination. Recommendations for 1966', submitted by NAACP Legal Defense Fund to Hon. John Gardner, Secretary, Department of Health, Education and Welfare, 15 December 1965, Ms. Coll, 641, Collection on the Medical Committee for Human Rights, 1963–2004, Program Work, Work With Other Organizations, National Association for the Advancement of Colored People Legal Defense and Educational Fund, Inc., 1965–1966, General Box 33, Folder 371, Kislak Center for Special Collections, Rare Books, and Manuscripts, Van Pelt-Dietrich Library, University of Pennsylvania, Philadelphia, PA.

56. 'Report on the Implementation of Title VI of the Civil Rights Act of 1964 in Regard to Hospital Discrimination. Recommendations for 1966', submitted by NAACP Legal Defense Fund to Hon. John Gardner, Secretary, Department of Health, Education and Welfare, 16 December 1965, Ms. Coll, 641, Collection on the Medical Committee for Human Rights, 1963–2004, Program Work, Work With Other Organizations, National Association for the Advancement of Colored People Legal Defense and Educational Fund, Inc., 1965–1966, General Box 33, Folder 371, Kislak Center for Special Collections, Rare Books, and Manuscripts, Van Pelt-Dietrich Library, University of Pennsylvania, Philadelphia, PA.

57. Ibid., 1. On the history of the National Medical Association, see Thomas J. Ward Jr., *Black Physicians in the Jim Crow South* (Fayetteville: University of Arkansas Press, 2003).

58. Ibid.

59. 'Report on the Implementation of Title VI of the Civil Rights Act of 1964 in Regard to Hospital Discrimination. Recommendations for 1966', submitted by NAACP Legal Defense Fund to Hon. John Gardner, Secretary, Department of Health, Education and Welfare, 16 December 1965, Ms.

Coll, 641, Collection on the Medical Committee for Human Rights, 1963–2004, Program Work, Work With Other Organizations, National Association for the Advancement of Colored People Legal Defense and Educational Fund, Inc., 1965–1966, General Box 33, Folder 371, Kislak Center for Special Collections, Rare Books, and Manuscripts, Van Pelt-Dietrich Library, University of Pennsylvania, Philadelphia, PA.

60. Ibid., 5.
61. Richard M. Mizelle Jr., *Backwater Blues: The Mississippi Flood of 1927 in the African American Imagination* (Minneapolis: University of Minnesota Press, 2014); Alan B. Cohen, David C. Colby, Keith A. Wailoo and Julian E. Zelizer (eds), *Medicare and Medicaid at 50: America's Entitlement Programs in the Age of Affordable Care* (New York: Oxford University Press, 2015).
62. 'Report on the Implementation of Title VI of the Civil Rights Act of 1964 in Regard to Hospital Discrimination, Recommendations for 1966', 5.
63. 'Report on the Implementation of Title VI of the Civil Rights Act of 1964 in Regard to Hospital Discrimination, Recommendations for 1966', 9.
64. 'Hospital Complaints', Ms. Coll, 641, Collection on the Medical Committee for Human Rights, 1963–2004, Program Work, Work With Other Organizations, US Department of Health, Education, and Welfare, 1965–1974, General Box 34, Folder 379, Kislak Center for Special Collections, Rare Books, and Manuscripts, Van Pelt-Dietrich Library, University of Pennsylvania, Philadelphia, PA; Keith Wailoo, *Dying in the City of the Blues: Sickle Cell Anemia and the Politics of Race and Health* (Chapel Hill: University of North Carolina Press, 2001); Spencie Love, *One Blood: The Death and Resurrection of Charles R. Drew* (Chapel Hill: University of North Carolina Press, 1996).
65. 'Report on the Implementation of Title VI of the Civil Rights Act of 1964 in Regard to Hospital Discrimination, Recommendations for 1966', submitted by NAACP Legal Defense Fund to Hon. John Gardner, Secretary, Department of Health, Education and Welfare, 16 December 1965, Ms. Coll, 641, Collection on the Medical Committee for Human Rights, 1963–2004, Program Work, Work With Other Organizations, National Association for the Advancement of Colored People Legal Defense and Educational Fund, Inc., 1965–1966, General Box 33, Folder 371, Kislak Center for Special Collections, Rare Books, and Manuscripts, Van Pelt-Dietrich Library, University of Pennsylvania, Philadelphia, PA.
66. Daria Roithmayr, *Reproducing Racism: How Everyday Choices Lock In White Advantage* (New York: New York University Press, 2014).

7

Better Dead than Red, or Not? Nuclear Physics and Public Health at the Dawn of the Cold War

Dario Fazzi

In 1954, the US Atomic Energy Commission (AEC), a civilian agency that since the signature of the 1946 Atomic Energy Act was in charge of the military, regulatory and developmental aspects of nuclear power in the United States, supervised a series of nuclear tests in the Marshall Islands.[1] The radiation released by one of these tests, in which a 15-megaton device nicknamed *Shrimp* obliterated an entire atoll, forced the evacuation of 236 Marshallese inhabitants and the withdrawal of the test's supervisory personnel.[2] In less than 24 hours, the fallout reached a Japanese fishing boat, the *Daigo Fukuryū Maru*, or *Lucky Dragon V*, exposing its twenty-three crew members to extremely high levels of ionising radiation.[3] The boat's chief radioman died a few months later from complications of radiation sickness. The *Lucky Dragon* accident ignited widespread fear of nuclear contamination and transformed nuclear fallout into a matter of global concern.[4] In the United States, the debate over nuclear radioactivity's health hazards hit the mainstream. Studies on the health hazards of nuclear fallout proliferated. Instigated by cellular biologist Barry Commoner, the Committee for Nuclear Information started disseminating information about the risks of strontium-90, a highly radioactive by-product of nuclear testing that, lodging in teeth and bones, could provoke different kinds of tumour and blood disease. Reports warning of milk contaminated by strontium-90 prompted nationwide surveys that helped to frame nuclear testing as a threat to public health.[5] Such mounting pressure induced the US Secretary of State John F. Dulles to recognise 'the dire consequences' that nuclear testing was producing on public opinion and President Eisenhower to announce a moratorium on nuclear testing from 1958 onward.[6]

The growing awareness of the consequences of nuclear fallout on public health, which in the mid- and late 1950s became part and parcel of a widening anti-nuclear conscience, had however deeper historical roots.[7] It stemmed from a debate between American nuclear scientists and medical professionals that this chapter brings to the fore. In the second half of the 1940s and up until the early 1950s, American scientists developed and consolidated a better understanding of the manifold effects of nuclear radioactivity on human health. Yet, at around the same time, the US government, and the AEC in particular, progressively sidelined public health concerns vis-à-vis the mounting exigencies and imperatives of the Cold War, which called instead for an unbounded expansion of the American nuclear programme. The advent of the atomic age, thus, and more so the launch of the nuclear arms race, ended up heralding the subordination of public health to national security. When, at the dawn of the Cold War and less than a decade after Henry Luce's famous proclamation of the American Century, nuclear weapons became the fundamental tool of US progress, development and ascendancy, as well as the main instruments through which to stymie the rise of global Communism, military, strategic and geopolitical considerations temporarily prevailed over the health of American people.

The benefits of the doubt

The Second World War brought about an unprecedented politicisation and militarisation of science.[8] In the United States, the expansion of empirical research was embedded into and intertwined with the government's overall war strategy. The architect of such a grand design, which interpreted science as an 'endless frontier' at the disposal of America's mission and at the service of its seemingly endless progress, was Vannevar Bush.[9] While chairing the Office of Scientific Research and Development (OSRD), a presidential advisory group, Bush's influence grew over the years to the point of convincing President Franklin D. Roosevelt of the necessity of expanding public investments in scientific programmes, and especially in nuclear physics, as the best guarantee to win the war.[10] At its height, OSRD's main venture, the Manhattan Project, employed roughly 125,000 scientific workers and cost more than $2 billion dollars in total.[11] When the war ended, Roosevelt's successor Harry Truman was confronted with the task of transitioning the vast, newly established scientific infrastructure to peacetime. Bush's emphasis on war mobilisation had to be replaced by a structure within which civilian and military authorities, public and private sectors could work together for the peaceful development of the country. The president's new Scientific Research Board, directed by John R. Steelman, summarised the new strategic approach in a famous 1947 report, which placed a greater emphasis upon basic and medical research and instructed the government to both manage its own scientific programmes and promote coordination between public institutes and private industry, universities and research laboratories.[12]

The concurrent advent of the nuclear era and the emergence of the Cold War transformed the relation between science and politics into mutual interdependence. On the one hand, experimental science – and nuclear physics in particular – widened its scope and breadth, kept attracting extraordinary amounts of public funds, and, above all, gained previously unthinkable levels of political influence mostly due to the crucial role that nuclear weapons were playing in America's global strategy.[13] Nuclear physicists, as historian Jessica Wang has noted, came to be integrated 'into public life beyond anything that had ever happened previously in the United States', simultaneously enriching and enlivening 'public discourse at every level of politics'.[14] On the other hand, the federal government became more and more interested in conditioning, when not openly determining, the outcomes of scientific research.[15] Waging the Cold War and engaging in its arms race, in the end, required the mobilisation of the nation's best intellectual forces, whose contributions to the advancement of such different fields as agriculture, computer sciences, geology, oceanography or seismology were crucial for and a cipher of America's success in the bipolar confrontation.[16] To this end, the government established a series of new institutions that were meant to shape the structure of science, its research agendas and its goals. Presidential scientific boards and advisers became among the most influential actors in Washington; the National Science Foundation was established in 1950 with the declared objective of simultaneously protecting national health and national security; the Joint Research and Development Board was created in 1952 to coordinate all research activities of interest to the armed forces; from 1946 onward, the Office of Naval Research was given ample powers to set up and fund new scientific and technological programmes, including nuclear ones.[17]

At the dawn of the atomic age, thus, the US government turned to scientific research, and nuclear physics in particular, to advance its Cold War political agenda. The problem, however, was that nuclear physics had not yet solved one of its most excruciating dilemmas: could nuclear radioactivity be considered safe, and if so, when? Nuclear irradiation both appealed and appalled at the same time. Nuclear radioactivity promised life-saving treatments against cancer and the control of deadly diseases and yet it simultaneously encompassed dire and still rather obscure threats of genetic mutations. For nuclear scientists, casting light on the overall impact of nuclear fall-out on human health was tantamount to mastering the energy of the atom. The Manhattan Project's scientific director, J. Robert Oppen-heimer, had been among the first to indicate grave concerns about the safety of the personnel working with plutonium, since no one knew what plutonium contamination really entailed. That element had just been discovered and synthesised by Glenn Seaborg and his team at the University of California and its effects on human health were at the time completely unknown. In 1943, Oppenheimer had greenlighted the creation of a health division within the Manhattan Project and had tasked it with both research into radiation exposure and occupational safety.[18] Stafford Warren, a professor of radiology at the University of Rochester, was appointed as the first director, and under his guidance the Manhattan Project's medical research team gave safety guidance to the workers at risk of contamination and initiated experimental research on radioactive poisoning. War-ren's staff tried for years to establish reliable levels of tolerance to exposure to ionising radiation. So urgent was the need to learn more about plutonium's dangers that the division's leaders soon authorised research with human subjects.[19]

These efforts notwithstanding, however, the goal of bomb pro-duction took precedence over research on the medical consequences of nuclear radiation. As Richard Hewlett and Oscar Anderson point out in their first-hand account of the early days of the nuclear era, biology and medicine ended up by 'having minor status in the Manhattan Project' and this inevitably affected the achievement of an immediate and comprehensive understanding of the full-scale con-sequences of nuclear contamination.[20] The death in August 1945 and May 1946 of two Los Alamos scientists, Harry Daghlian and Louis Slotin, both of whom had been exposed to lethal doses of radiation while performing experiments with plutonium, was the most imme-diate toll that that choice had implied.[21]

A sudden acceleration to the study of the consequences of nuclear radioactivity on human health was given by the atomic blasts in Japan. In the aftermath of the bombings, two medical experts, Shields Warren, a pathologist from Harvard, and Ashby Oughterson, a surgeon from Yale, coordinated a team of scientists that formed the Joint Commission for the Investigation of the Medical Effects of the Atomic Bomb in Japan (JCIMEAB). The JCIMEAB submitted its final report in September 1946. In roughly 1,300 pages, the commit-tee presented evidence taken from more than 14,000 cases of direct exposure to nuclear irradiation, but could not come to a unanimous conclusion on a direct correlation between nuclear fallout and health hazards.[22] To further clarify the matter, Congress created the Atomic Bomb Casualty Commission (ABCC), which, however, had no better success than the JCIMEAB. The scientists of the ABCC did not consider the mid- and long-term problems suffered by the survivors of the atomic blasts as an effect of over-exposure to radioactivity. Shields Warren, who took part in the works of the ABCC as well, defined the 'radiation sickness' that was haunting the *hibakusha* purely in terms of bone marrow sickness.[23]

This tendency to downplay the long-term medical consequences of nuclear radioactivity became the prevalent attitude within America's scientific community in the first years after the war. Under Shields Warren's leadership, the AEC Division of Biology and Medicine kept dismissing the long-term effects of nuclear exposure as being related to the emergence of secondary physiological failures. At the beginning of 1946, Warren went so far as to state that the A-bombs had basically had 'no residual effect of any significance' on their survivors. Likewise, he wrote, the radioactivity released by the 1946 Bikini nuclear test series could be considered just as 'a minor factor'.[24] Furthermore, Warren's division kept stressing the huge potential of nuclear energy's medical applicability and launched a wide radioisotope programme that, inaugurated exactly one year after the bombing of Japan, was meant to promote medical research into ionising radiation. The AEC oversaw such a programme with enthusiasm and made radioactive isotopes widely available for medical research, therapy and industry.[25]

Informed dissent

Within the broader American scientific community, however, not everyone approved AEC's rather dismissive attitude towards the health hazards of nuclear fallout. A few nuclear physicists and physicians in fact took a much more cautious and critical stance, and found in the Federation of Atomic Scientists (later the Federation of American Scientists, FAS) and the *Bulletin of the Atomic Scientists* two important channels through which to streamline their dissent. Both the FAS and the *Bulletin* had been set in motion between the end of 1945 and the beginning of 1946 by University of Chicago's leading biophysicist, Eugene Rabinowitch, who, foreseeing the dire prospect of a nuclear arms race, wanted to make sure that both the general public and the policymakers could grasp fully the extent of the threats to human health posed by the power of subatomic forces.[26] By December 1945, the FAS had launched a National Committee on Atomic Information with the specific goal of informing the public on the functioning and the potential risks of atomic energy. Similarly, the *Bulletin* was serving as one of the main platforms where scientists discussed the dangers of an unbounded application of nuclear power.[27] Whereas the main goal of the publication was to promote nuclear disarmament and the establishment of forms of civilian control of atomic energy, it was soon also addressing issues concerning the repercussions of nuclear radioactivity on public and environmental health.

In March 1946, from the *Bulletin*'s pages Farrington Daniels, a well-known chemistry professor from the University of Wisconsin, explained in layman's terms some of the most disturbing consequences and health risks that nuclear contamination entailed. Daniels emphasised how the fission process at the base of nuclear power production was able to generate dangerous gamma rays that, to be made innocuous, required the adoption of complex precautions, including not only adequate safety measures for the operators but also the construction of thick separation walls between the reactor and the external environments in order to avoid the contamination of the surrounding area. Such provisions, however, could not constitute per se a sufficient guarantee against nuclear contamination. In the case of an accident in a nuclear pile, the professor warned, the release of dangerous radioactive elements would be massive and their persistence in the surrounding environment would last for an extremely long period of time. Such consequences would be unavoidable and basically unstoppable, due to the fact that the core would remain unapproachable for years. To Daniels, thus, these issues should have preoccupied the government way more than the research on radioisotopes, and the AEC should have set up adequate forms of fallout prevention and control. The government's response, however, was to Daniel largely inadequate and seemingly indifferent to such urgent threats.[28]

Daniels was not alone. The *Bulletin* continued publishing research findings that highlighted the health hazards of nuclear radioactivity. One of the first physicians to ever study the effects of radioactive poisoning on human bodies, Harvard Medical School's pathologist Hermann Lisco, popularised his works through the *Bulletin*. Lisco, who left Berlin in 1936 to join first the pathology department at Johns Hopkins University and then Harvard Medical School, had been invited during the war to join the Manhattan Project. There, he had worked with a few colleagues from the University of Chicago to gauge the consequences of acute radioactive poisoning on human health, by studying the physiology of those operators who had been in close contact with radioactive materials.[29] Lisco was also the one to conduct the autopsy on the bodies of Harry Daghlian and Louis Slotin.[30] His findings were groundbreaking and represented a milestone in research on nuclear irradiation. Lisco, in fact, was among the first to study and publish extremely well-detailed accounts of the effects of radioactive poisoning on the human organism and to establish a direct causal relationship between high exposure to radioactivity and deadly mutations of human cells.[31] For the first time, Lisco's empirical observations and laboratory research proved that over-exposure to such radioactive elements as radium and plutonium actually led to the emergence of malignant tumours in human tissues. To Lisco, the 'catastrophic consequences' of radium absorption in human beings called for 'a whole justifiable conservation in our attitude toward human exposure to other radioelements'. The pathologist lamented that the discussion over atomic energy was revolving around national and international control, whereas the issue of the physical hazards of nuclear radioactivity was not being discussed adequately nor with the necessary 'frankness'. In his opinion, radiation sickness should have attracted a greater degree of public and political attention, as it could have represented a serious problem for the future of the country. Quoting John Hersey's famous reports from Hiroshima and demystifying any superficial account of the medical consequences of the US atomic bombing, Lisco said that 'in view of the rapidly expanding exploitation of nuclear fission for various purposes, clinical and laboratory investigation of all aspects of radiation sickness' should have become 'a primary concern to those responsible for the welfare of the people connected with such developments and to all physicians interested in the welfare of the population as a whole'.[32]

Anxiety about the health hazards of radioactivity surged with the expansion of AEC's nuclear programmes. Princeton University professor and renowned mathematician John von Neuman, while criticising the dangerous intermingling of science with politics in the atomic age, pointed out that nuclear physics' main goal should be the containment of radioactive hazards, while the government's should be the implementation of all the necessary 'safety and health regulations' to make that containment possible.[33] A young radiological safety officer who witnessed first-hand the explosions at Bikini, David Bradley, popularised the dangers of radioactive fallout through his best-selling book *No Place to Hide*, which came out in 1948. Bradley was much impressed by Stafford Warren's early efforts to awaken the public to the hazards of nuclear radiation and by Warren's work to preserve the health of Manhattan Project scientists. *No Place to Hide* revealed the extent of the menace posed by nuclear radiation and framed nuclear fallout as a direct threat to both human health and the environment.[34]

These pressures induced the AEC's Medical Board of Review, an advisory group comprising some of the most prominent physicians in the country including the Lambert Professor of Medicine at Columbia University, Robert Loeb, and the chairman of the National Research Council, Detlev Bronk, to call for a new approach towards the health hazards of nuclear energy. In a report that came out at the end of June 1947, the Board defined the need for further medical and biological research on the various effects of radioactive substances as 'urgent and extensive', and invited the AEC to cooperate more in this field with the US Public Health Service, the agency that from 1912 until the mid-1960s under the guidance of the surgeon general helped the US government to protect the welfare of the nation, to better investigate 'methods of protecting industrial employees and civilian populations against hazards of gases, dust, contact, effluents, and other forms of exposure to radiation'.[35] A few months later, the Board criticised the AEC publicly and condemned the agency's policies for raising 'new medical and public health problems'. The Board 'strongly recommended that research and training in all aspects of the application of atomic energy to medical and biological problems be continued' and possibly expanded, and it invited the AEC to assume 'extensive responsibility' for the study of the effects of products of atomic fission on human life.[36]

The Board hit a raw nerve and forced the AEC to respond to its recommendations. The Commission's overall attitude towards the health hazards of nuclear radioactivity seemed to change. The AEC launched a groundbreaking programme to further biological and medical research and education on nuclear fallout. It appointed a permanent Advisory Committee for Biology and Medicine. It established a Division of Biology and Medicine within its own headquarters in Washington, DC, tasking it with carrying out medical and biological research and connecting government-sponsored programmes with private laboratories' activities, including training projects. The AEC also set up a series of 'unprecedented safety measures' to protect the health of those atomic operators who were involved in atomic energy production processes.[37] The whole work of the AEC in relation to the health hazards of nuclear fallout was reorganised around four distinct pillars: the safeguard of atomic workers; the protection of environmental health, which involved the problems of waste disposal; the development of basic research on the effects of ionising radiation on human cells; and, eventually, the promotion of possible medical applications of radioactive isotopes as treatment for cancer.[38]

The renewed activism of the AEC served as a booster for further research into the medical consequences of nuclear fallout. Research in this field proliferated. William Bloom, a professor of anatomy in Chicago, collected and published a series of studies on the histo-pathology of nuclear irradiation, a work that aimed at establishing some clear 'tolerance levels' below which nuclear irradiation could be considered innocuous.[39] Carl Voegtlin, a PHS pharmacologist, and his colleague Herold Hodge from the University of Rochester published a two-volume study on the toxicology of uranium compounds, which related skin and eye intoxication to the contamination and absorption of uranium in the body.[40] Between November 1947 and November 1948, the AEC sponsored and concluded more than 2,000 research reports, 210 of which concerned biology and medicine. Such a growing body of research helped to clarify how and to what extent exposure to nuclear radioactivity could cause human cell mutations, that is, could interfere with the normal workings of heredity. Most of these studies were conducted through laboratory experiments that over-exposed guinea pigs to nuclear radioactivity. Others were grounded on analysis of animals that had been exposed to nuclear radiation in their own environment, as in the case of a herd of cattle that had been accidentally irradiated by the first atomic test in New Mexico in the summer of 1945. AEC scientists tried to gauge and assess the hazardousness of the radioactivity produced by both underwater and land explosions, the maximum threshold of radioactivity that living organisms could suffer, and its accumulation in certain parts of the human body. AEC researchers working in laboratories like Los Alamos and Argonne started studying the interaction between radiation and human tissues, focusing on the risk of elements commonly used in atomic processes like beryllium and plutonium. Lung disease, serious damage to the liver, kidney failure and bone marrow sickness entered the vocabulary of nuclear physics and started shaping its contours.[41] The AEC, eventually, accepted that advancing America's nuclear knowledge could not ignore the safeguarding of America's public health, and invested a lot of resources into learning how to forestall the many dangers of nuclear fallout.[42] Such a moment of reckoning, however, proved to be short-lived.

Security over health

The expansion of AEC medical programmes coincided with a whole reconfiguration of the role that nuclear power played in American politics, culture and society. From the late 1940s on, the public perception of nuclear power changed rapidly. Russia's first successful

atomic test had opened a new phase of the Cold War and inaugurated a dangerous nuclear arms race. The government took a clear
stance on atomic power and started portraying it as the main field of
competition with the rival superpower. Atomic superiority became
the nation's top priority, and to many it represented the nation's best
hope against the threat of Communism. The federal government
began to frame the dangers of nuclear radiation as a necessary part
of the superpower game and dismissed concerns over radioactivity
as simply exaggerated.[43] As historian David Holloway has pointed
out, the pursuit of an effective nuclear deterrence, which implied the
risk of further nuclear contamination and exposing people to serious
health hazards, became 'the organizing principle' of US domestic and
foreign policymaking.[44]

The renewed emphasis on nuclear power, which pervaded the United
States from 1949 onward, deeply affected the actions and policies of
the AEC, especially for what concerned its investments into research
concerning the harmful effects of nuclear fallout, but also in relation
to its broader military and civilian nuclear programmes. The H-bomb
project, for instance, which took off after President Truman signed
the famous National Security Council Paper 68 (NSC-68) in 1950,
monopolised the attention of the Commission for years.[45] The radioisotopes programme, which had been the AEC's flagship for the promotion of the peaceful uses and medical applications of atomic energy,
was resized and downgraded in light of the intensifying nuclear arms
race. The radioisotopes programme was split into a series of smaller
international programmes and most of its experimental research was
outsourced to Britain and Canada, which were permitted to purchase
isotopes for medical and industrial applications.[46]

Subscribing to such a new mood, AEC director David Lilienthal started popularising the idea that the expansion of the nuclear
programme was innocuous and did not contribute to an increase in
health hazards.[47] At the 1948 national convention of the American
Medical Association, Shields Warren chaired a special session on
atomic energy in which several physicists and AEC commissioners
praised the medical value of radioisotopes and defended the experimental application of nuclear radioactivity.[48] In a presentation titled
'The Medical Profession and Atomic Energy', AEC commissioner
Lewis Strauss urged physicians to help nuclear physics to overcome
a widespread 'prejudice against work on atomic energy', which was
based, according to Strauss, on purely insufficient and fragmented
information. To him, the impression that atomic energy could constitute a health hazard was misleading and physicians had to work
side by side with the AEC to assuage rising public fears about nuclear

fallout.[49] As the historian Paul Boyer has explained, 'the implicit (and often explicit) message underlying much of this medical discussion of atomic energy – that the therapeutic promise far outweighed and even cancelled out its menacing aspects – penetrated the profession very deeply'. As a result, 'with rare exceptions, all levels of organized medicine actively supported and lent credibility to the government effort to persuade the American people' of the overall soundness and harmlessness of America's nuclear expansion.[50]

Strauss, and prominent physicists such as Edward Teller, Karl Compton and Ernest Lawrence, openly called for expansion of the AEC nuclear testing programme, even if they knew that this would have entailed further emission of radioactivity and exposure to nuclear fallout. They were convinced that in the wake of the newly achieved Soviet atomic capability the United States had no choice other than to upgrade its nuclear arsenal by investing in more powerful systems, such as, for instance, thermonuclear weapons. To Teller, it was not the duty of scientists to determine whether the government should authorise the building, or even the use, of an H-bomb. Scientists, to him, were only charged with the duty of studying the technical feasibility of such programmes. Any concern that was not strictly related to the exigencies of national security, and any limitation on nuclear research – including those limitations determined by the fear of the possible impact that nuclear testing might have on public health – had to be declared illegitimate.[51]

Those who criticised such a lenient attitude towards the health hazards of nuclear radioactivity came to be perceived as a threat to national security and therefore as potentially un-American. Any form of dissent began to be progressively isolated within the AEC, when not openly ostracised. AEC scientists who showed their dissatisfaction with the new course came under increasingly intrusive Congressional scrutiny. In the summer of 1949, Republican Senator Bourke Hickenlooper, chairman of the joint Committee on Atomic Energy, asked for and received an official statement on the loyalty of AEC fellows.[52] Congress attacked AEC management of nuclear material. Throughout that year, a series of Congressional investigative hearings were held to determine whether certain shipments of radioisotopes to Norway and Finland had to be considered national security lapses.[53]

The main targets of this conservative campaign in favour of unbounded nuclear developments were the members of the General Advisory Committee (GAC) of the AEC, who reacted vehemently against the prevailing pro-nuclear mood. Chaired by Oppenheimer and composed of other prominent figures in nuclear physics such as

James Conant, Enrico Fermi, Cyril Smith, Lee DuBridge and Isador Rabi, the GAC warned against the extreme health hazards that the project of building new nuclear weapons implied. These dissenters championed another form of security and argued that nuclear deterrence could not preserve international stability and peace because it could not eliminate the risk of nuclear war. To them, the 'superbomb' represented an intolerable 'threat to the future of the human race', and its use, which would be an 'inhuman application of force', could be neither strategically justified nor ethically countenanced. In addition, the release of radioactivity related to the testing of these new devices would have provoked 'very great natural catastrophes'.[54] According to this view, the potentially harmful effects of nuclear radioactivity outnumbered any supposed military advantage.[55] These ideas were also shared by the American Institute of Physics, which expressed 'grave concerns' over the 'misleading impression on the public' resulting from Congress discrediting the AEC and lamented the substantial abandonment of research focusing on the health hazards of nuclear fallout.[56] In his testimony before Hickenlooper's commission, Alan Gregg, the head of the AEC Advisory Committee on Biology, a committee that fully aligned with the GAC's group in matters concerning nuclear fallout, condemned government's intrusion into the cause of science and stressed that such an interference was hampering the possibility of achieving superior aims such as the safeguarding of public health.[57]

No controversy, however, better exemplified the tension that was dividing the American scientific and medical community between the end of the 1940s and the beginning of the 1950s than the one between Willard Libby, the physical chemist who pioneered radiocarbon dating, and the renowned biochemist Linus Pauling, who at that time was conducting groundbreaking studies on the effects of nuclear radiation on blood cells. Both Libby and Pauling published widely circulated articles and gave numerous interviews in which both of them kept providing two distinct and conflicting interpretations of the relationship between radiation exposure and public health.[58] Libby was a staunch supporter of nuclear power and believed that the abundance it could bring about would one day make nuclear weapons superfluous. Nuclear power, to Libby, would also satisfy human 'needs for all time' and nuclear medicine would herald a disease-free world.[59] Pauling, in contrast, framed people's exposure to nuclear radiation as a violation of human rights to 'life, liberty and the pursuit of happiness'.[60] Libby was convinced that it was possible to determine a safe threshold for people's exposure to nuclear radiation and that it was therefore possible to conduct nuclear testing safely.[61] Pauling publicly opposed such an idea and stressed on multiple occasions how the simple fact that radioactivity exposure produced genetic mutations was sufficient to prove the impossibility of determining the existence of any safe threshold of nuclear fallout.[62]

Cold War medicine and the American Century

As with many other scientific fields, medicine therefore became a hot Cold War battlefield.[63] By the mid-1950s, only a few physicians in the United States remained optimistic about the chances of providing adequate medical responses to the health hazards of nuclear testing and contamination, while a few others kept working on the promising field of nuclear medicine, breaking new ground in cancer treatment and diagnosis. Such peaceful endeavours, however, were seldom disinterested. The promotion of the atom entailed, almost intrinsically and unavoidably, as historian Jacob Darwin Hamblin has recently demonstrated, the endorsement of a broader Cold War confrontation.[64] Thus, those physicians who despised the risks of nuclear fallout and warned against the jeopardisation of public health openly joined the (liberal) camp of those who were calling for a halt to both the nuclear arms race and any medical research supporting it.

The arms race and the unabated quest for nuclear supremacy ended up undermining people's health in many ways: from the militarisation of landscapes to the radioactive contamination of communities and commodities.[65] Yet America's early Cold War nuclear entanglements simply could not contemplate illness. Medical and scientific dissent was able to subvert such a narrative only when it finally converged into a broader, grassroots and transnational anti-nuclear campaign, which demanded the safeguarding of human health over political, ideological and military aims. By the early 1960s, the management of nuclear policies was framed as an issue concerning global and environmental health, and this induced the US government and its main allies to start thinking beyond the logic of the blocs. Since then, as proved by appeals like that of American paediatrician Benjamin Spock, the influential work of Hellen Caldicott, and the activism of groups such as Physicians for Social Responsibility, trading public health for national security became more difficult.[66] But, back in the late 1940s and early 1950s, when nuclear physics represented the main instrument of America's Cold War, the imperatives of national security largely overshadowed the differences of opinion within the scientific community on the importance of public health.

Notes

1. Martin V. Melosi, *Atomic Age America* (London: Routledge, 2013).
2. Castle Series, 1954, United States Atmospheric Nuclear Weapons Tests, Nuclear Test Personnel Review, prepared by the Defense Nuclear Agency as Executive Agency for the Department of Defense, 1 April 1982, available at: https://www.osti.gov/opennet/servlets/purl/16380885-g1vuWf/16380885.pdf, last accessed 5 March 2022. See also Gregg Herken, *Cardinal Choices: Presidential Science Advising from the Atomic Bomb to SDI*, rev. expanded edn (Stanford: Stanford University Press, 2000), 81–6.
3. Mark D. Merlin and Ricardo M. Gonzalez, 'Environmental Impacts of Nuclear Testing in Remote Oceania, 1946–1996', in John R. McNeill and Corinna R. Unger (eds), *Environmental Histories of the Cold War* (New York: Cambridge University Press, 2010), 167–202.
4. Petra Goedde, *The Politics of Peace: A Global Cold War History* (New York: Oxford University Press, 2019), 68–95.
5. Joseph J. Mangano, *Radioactive Baby Teeth: The Cancer Link* (La Vergne, TN: Lightning Source, 2008); Ellen Griffith Spears, *Rethinking the American Environmental Movement post-1945* (London: Routledge, 2019), 74.
6. Lawrence S. Wittner, *The Struggle against the Bomb, Vol. 2: Resisting the Bomb: A History of the World Nuclear Disarmament Movement, 1954–1970* (Stanford: Stanford University Press, 1997), 128–9.
7. Dario Fazzi, *Eleanor Roosevelt and the Anti-Nuclear Movement: The Voice of Conscience* (New York: Palgrave, 2016).
8. Richard Rhodes, *The Making of the Atomic Bomb* (New York: Simon & Schuster, 1986).
9. *Science: The Endless Frontier*, Report to the President by Vannevar Bush, Director of the Office of Scientific Research and Development, July 1945 (Washington, DC: US Government Printing Office, 1945), available at: https://www.nsf.gov/od/lpa/nsf50/vbush1945.htm, last accessed 5 March 2022.
10. G. Pascal Zachary, *Endless Frontier: Vannevar Bush, Engineer of the American Century* (New York: Free Press, 1997).
11. Paul S. Boyer, *Fallout: A Historian Reflects on America's Half-century Encounter with Nuclear Weapons* (Columbus: Ohio State University Press, 1998), 27.
12. US President's Scientific Research Board, *Science and Public Policy, Vol. 1: A Program for the Nation* (Washington, DC: US Government Printing Office, 27 August 1947). See also William A. Blanpied, 'Inventing US Science Policy', *Physics Today* 51:2 (1998), 34–40.
13. David Holloway, 'Nuclear Weapons and the Escalation of the Cold War, 1945–1962', in Melvyn P. Leffler and Odd Arne Westad (eds), *The Cambridge History of the Cold War, Vol. 1: Origins* (New York: Cambridge University Press, 2010), 376–97.

14. Jessica Wang, 'Scientists and the Problem of the Public in Cold War America, 1945–1960', *Osiri*, 17:2 (2002), 323–47.

15. Naomi Oreskes, 'Introduction' and 'Science in the Origins of the Cold War', in Naomi Oreskes and John Krige (eds.), *Science and Technology in the Global Cold War* (Cambridge, MA: MIT Press, 2014), 1–11, 12–30.

16. Brit Shields, 'Mathematics, Peace, and the Cold War: Scientific Diplomacy and Richard Courant's Scientific Identity', *Historical Studies in the Natural Sciences* 46:5 (2016), 556–91; Elena Aronova, 'Recent Trends in the Historiography of Science in the Cold War', *Historical Studies in the Natural Sciences* 47:4 (2017), 568–77; Audra J. Wolfe, *Freedom's Laboratory: The Cold War Struggle for the Soul of Science* (Baltimore, MD: Johns Hopkins University Press, 2020).

17. Philip N. Powers, 'The Organization for Science in the Federal Government', *Bulletin of the Atomic Scientists* 3:4/5 (1947), 122–3; Sarah Bridger, *Scientists at War: The Ethics of Cold War Weapons Research* (Cambridge, MA: Harvard University Press, 2015).

18. Angela N. H. Creager, *Life Atomic: A History of Radioisotopes in Science and Medicine* (Chicago: University of Chicago Press, 2013), 152–253.

19. William Moss and Roger Eckhard, 'The Human Plutonium Injection Experiments', *Los Alamos Science*, 23 November 1995; Eileen Welsome, *The Plutonium Files: America's Secret Medical Experiments in the Cold War* (New York: Dial Press, 1999).

20. Barbara Day and Howard Waitzkin, 'The Medical Profession and Nuclear War: A Social History', *Journal of the American Medical Association* 254:5 (1985), 644–51.

21. Barton C. Hacker, *The Dragon's Tail: Radiation Safety in the Manhattan Project, 1942–1946* (Berkeley: University of California Press, 1987); Alex Wellerstein, 'The Demon Core and the Strange Death of Louis Slotin', *New York Times*, 21 May 2016.

22. *Medical Effects of Atomic Bombs*, Report of the Joint Commission for the Investigation of the Effects of the Atomic Bomb in Japan, vol. 1, United States Atomic Energy Commission, 19 April 1951, available at: https://www.osti.gov/biblio/4421057-medical-effects-atomic-bombs-report-joint-commission-investigation-effects-atomic-bomb-japan-volume, last accessed 5 March 2022.

23. M. Susan Lindee, *Suffering Made Real: American Science and the Survivors at Hiroshima* (Chicago: University of Chicago Press, 1994); Frank W. Putnam, 'The Atomic Bomb Casualty Commission in Retrospect', *Proceedings of the National Academy of Sciences* 95 (1998), 5426–38.

24. Janet Farrell Brodie, 'Radiation Secrecy and Censorship after Hiroshima and Nagasaki', *Journal of Social History* 48:4 (2015), 842–64.

25. Angela N. H. Creager, 'Nuclear Energy in the Service of Biomedicine: The US Atomic Energy Commission's Radioisotope Program, 1946–1950', *Journal of the History of Biology* 39 (2006), 649–84.

26. University of Chicago Library, Atomic Scientists' Printed and Near-Print Material Records, 1945–1959, Box 2, Folder 9, Federation of American Scientists, Constitution, Press Releases, Information Papers, Memoranda, etc., January–April 1946. See also Donald A. Strickland, *Scientists in Politics: The Atomic Scientists Movement, 1945–46* (Lafayette, LA: Purdue University Studies, 1968).
27. Morton Grodzins and Eugene Rabinowitch (eds), *The Atomic Age: Scientists in National and World Affairs* (New York: Basic Books, 1963), 17–21.
28. Farrington Daniels, 'Atomic Power Production', *Bulletin of the Atomic Scientists* 1:7 (1956), 13.
29. Charles Krauthammer, 'A Man for All Seasons', *Washington Post*, 25 August 2000.
30. Louis H. Hempelmann, Hermann Lisco and Joseph G. Hoffmann, 'The Acute Radiation Syndrome: A Study of Nine Cases and a Review of the Problem', *Annals of Internal Medicine* 36:2 (1952), Pt 1, 279–510.
31. Austin M. Brues, Hermann Lisco and Miriam Posner Finkel, *Biological Hazards and Toxicity of Radioactive Isotopes*, US Atomic Energy Commission, Argonne National Laboratory, 13 May 1949.
32. Hermann Lisco, 'Radiation Hazards and Radiation Sickness', *Bulletin of the Atomic Scientists* 2:9/10 (1946), 26–7.
33. Statement of Dr John Von Neumann, 31 January 1946, Atomic Energy Act of 1946: Hearings Before the Special Committee on Atomic Energy, United States Senate, 79th Congress, 2nd session, on S. 1717, a Bill for the Development and Control of Atomic Energy, Part 2 (Washington, DC: US Government Printing Office, 1946), 205–18.
34. David Bradley, *No Place to Hide* (Boston, MA: Little Brown, 1948). See also B. C. Hacker, *The Dragon's Tail*, 31; Allan M. Winkler, *Life Under a Cloud: American Anxiety about the Atom* (Urbana: University of Illinois Press, 1993), 252.
35. United States Atomic Energy Commission, Report of the Medical Board of Review, Washington, DC, 20 June 1947, available at: https://nsarchive2.gwu.edu/radiation/dir/mstreet/commeet/meet9/brief9/tab_i/br9i2q.txt, last accessed 17 October 2022.
36. 'Medical Board of Review Reports to U.S.A.E.C.', *Bulletin of the Atomic Scientists* 3:9 (1947), 271–4.
37. David E. Lilienthal, Robert F. Bacher, Sumner T. Pike, Lewis L. Strauss and William W. Waymack, 'Third Semiannual Report to the Congress by the United States Atomic Energy Commission, February 2, 1948', in US Department of Energy, Office of Scientific and Technical Information (OSTI), available at: https://doi.org/10.2172/1362098, last accessed 6 March 2022.
38. Ibid. See also Guzman Barrow, 'The Nation's Medical Research', *Bulletin of the Atomic Scientists* 4:2 (1948), 59–60; US Department of Energy, Advisory Committee on Human Radiation Experiments – Final Report, Part I, The Atomic Energy Commission and Postwar Biomedical Radiation

Research, available at: https://ehss.energy.gov/ohre/roadmap/achre/intro_4.html, last accessed 6 March 2022.

39. William Bloom (ed.), *Histopathology of Irradiation from External and Internal Sources* (New York: McGraw-Hill, 1948).

40. Carl Voegtlin and Herold Hodge (eds), *Pharmacology and Toxicology of Uranium Compounds* (New York: McGraw-Hill, 1949), vols 1, 2.

41. David E. Lilienthal, Robert F. Bacher, Sumner T. Pike and Lewis L. Strauss, 'Fifth Semiannual Report of the Commission to the Congress: Atomic Energy Development, 1947–1948, 1 January 1949', in OSTI, available at: https://www.osti.gov/biblio/1362100-fifth-semiannual-report-commission-congress-atomic-energy-development, last accessed 6 March 2022.

42. David E. Lilienthal, Robert F. Bacher, Sumner T. Pike and Lewis L. Strauss, 'Sixth Semiannual Report of the Commission to the Congress: Atomic Energy and the Life Sciences, July 1949', in OSTI, availableathttps://www.osti.gov/biblio/1362103-sixth-semiannual-report-commission-congress-atomic-energy-life-sciences-july, last accessed 6 March 2022.

43. McGeorge Bundy, *Danger and Survival: Choices About the Bomb in the First Fifty Years* (New York: Random House, 1988); Gregg Herken, *The Winning Weapon: The Atomic Bomb in the Cold War, 1945–1950* (Princeton, NJ: Princeton University Press, 1988); Memorandum by the Counselor (Kennan), Top Secret, [Washington], 20 January 1950, in Neal H. Petersen, John P. Glennon, David W. Mabon, Ralph R. Goodwin and William Z. Slany (eds), *Foreign Relations of the United States, 1950, National Security Affairs; Foreign Economic Policy, Volume I* (Washington, DC: United States Government Printing Office, 1977), Document 7, available at: https://history.state.gov/historicaldocuments/frus1950v01/d7, last accessed 17 October 2022.

44. Holloway, 'Nuclear Weapons and the Escalation of the Cold War, 1945–1962', 376–97.

45. A Report to the National Security Council by the Executive Secretary on United States Objectives and Programs for National Security, 11 April 1950, Harry S. Truman Presidential Library, President's Secretary's Files, Ideological Foundations of the Cold War, available at: https://www.trumanlibrary.gov/library/research-files/report-national-security-council-nsc-68?documentid=NA&pagenumber=1, last accessed 6 March 2022. See also John L. Gaddis, *Strategies of Containment: A Critical Appraisal of American National Security Policy during the Cold War* (New York: Oxford University Press, 1982), 87–124.

46. John Krige, 'Atoms for Peace, Scientific Internationalism, and Scientific Intelligence', *Osiris*, 21:1 (2006), 161–81.

47. David E. Lilienthal, 'Atomic Energy Is Your Business', *New York Times*, 11 January 1948.

48. Richard G. Hewlett and Francis Duncan, *Atomic Shield: A History of the United States Atomic Energy Commission, Vol. 2: 1947–1952* (University Park: Pennsylvania State University Press, 1969), 386.

49. Lewis L. Strauss, 'The Medical Profession and Atomic Energy', *Journal of the American Medical Association* 138:17 (1948), 1225–27.
50. Paul Boyer, 'Physicians Confront the Apocalypse: The American Medical Profession and the Threat of Nuclear War', *Journal of the American Medical Association* 254:5 (1985), 633–43.
51. Edward Teller's interview at 'US Strategic Nuclear Policy: A Video History, 1995–2004. Sandia Labs Historical Video Documents History of U.S. Strategic Nuclear Policy', available at: www.gwu.edu/~nsarchiv/nukevault/ebb361/index.htm, last accessed 6 March 2022.
52. 'Science and the Citizen', *Scientific American* 181:1 (1949), 26–29.
53. Angela N. H. Creager, 'Radioisotopes as Political Instruments, 1946–1953', *Dynamis* 29 (2009), 219–39.
54. Thomas R. Rochon, *Mobilizing for Peace: The Antinuclear Movements in Western Europe* (Princeton, NJ: Princeton University Press, 1988), 55. See AEC General Advisory Committee's Majority and Minority Reports on Building the H-Bomb, 30 October 1949, available at: http://www.shoppbs.pbs.org/wgbh/amex/bomb/filmmore/reference/primary/extractsofgeneral.html, last accessed 6 March 2022.
55. Paul Boyer, *By the Bomb's Early Light: American Thought and Culture at the Dawn of the Atomic Age* (Chapel Hill: University of North Carolina Press, 1985), 103; Lawrence S. Wittner, *Rebels against War: The American Peace Movement, 1933–1983* (Philadelphia, PA: Temple University Press, 1984), 200.
56. 'Statement by the American Institute of Physics', *Bulletin of the Atomic Scientists* 5:6/7 (1949), 176.
57. 'The Fellowship Program: Testimony before the Joint Committee', *Bulletin of the Atomic Scientists Bulletin of the Atomic Scientists* 5:6/7 (1949), 174–6.
58. On the Libby–Pauling controversy, see Linda Marie Richards, 'Rocks and Reactors: An Atomic Interpretation of Human Rights, 1941–1979', PhD dissertation, Oregon State University, 2014, available at: http://hdl.handle.net/1957/48695, last accessed 6 March 2022, 90–141.
59. William L. Lawrence, *Men and Atoms: The Discovery, the Uses and the Future of Atomic Energy* (New York: Simon & Schuster, 1959), 243.
60. Linda Richards, 'Fallout Suits and Human Rights: Disrupting the Technocratic Narrative', *Peace and Change* 38:1 (2013), 56–82.
61. On the debate about nuclear radioactivity's safe threshold, see Barton C. Hacker, 'Radiation Safety, the AEC, and Nuclear Weapons Testing', *Public Historian* 14:1 (1992), 31–53; J. Samuel Walker, *Permissible Dose: History of Radiation Protection*; (Berkeley: University of California Press, 2000).
62. Linus Pauling, 'Genetic Effects of Weapons Tests', *Bulletin of the Atomic Scientists* 18:10 (1962), 16–18.
63. Gerald Kutcher, *Contested Medicine: Cancer Research and the Military* (Chicago: University of Chicago Press, 2009); James L. Nolan Jr., *Atomic Doctors: Conscience and Complicity at the Dawn of the Nuclear Age* (Cambridge, MA: Harvard University Press, 2020).

64. Jacob Darwin Hamblin, *The Wretched Atom: America's Global Gamble with Peaceful Nuclear Technology* (New York: Oxford University Press, 2021).
65. Ryan Edgington, 'Fragmented Histories: Science, Environment and Monument Building at the Trinity Site, 1945–1995', in Chris Pearson, Peter Coates and Tim Cole (eds), *Militarized Landscapes: From Gettysburg to Salisbury Plain* (London: Continuum, 2010); Traci Brynne Voyles, *Wastelanding: Legacies of Uranium Mining in Navajo Country* (Minneapolis: University of Minnesota Press, 2015); Andrew G. Kirk and Kristian Purcell, *Doom Towns: The People and Landscapes of Atomic Testing, A Graphic History* (New York: Oxford University Press, 2016); Jon Mitchell, *Poisoning the Pacific: The US Military's Secret Dumping of Plutonium, Chemical Weapons, and Agent Orange* (Lanham, MD: Rowman & Littlefield, 2020).
66. Lawrence S. Wittner, *Confronting the Bomb: A Short History of the World Nuclear Disarmament Movement* (Stanford: Stanford University Press, 2009).

8

Fighting the Cold War and *Variola*: The American Commitment to Smallpox Eradication

Bob H. Reinhardt

On 18 May 1965, US President Lyndon B. Johnson announced his administration's decision to support the international effort to eradicate smallpox, signalling a shift in the US approach to smallpox and international health.[1] In his announcement, Johnson warned that 'for as long smallpox exists anywhere in the world, no country is safe from it. This dread disease spreads so rapidly, that even a single case creates the threat of epidemic.'[2] Although smallpox had effectively disappeared from the United States by the beginning of the twentieth century, outbreaks due to importations were possible (as demonstrated in a 1947 outbreak in New York that left five people dead), and the 'dread disease' continued to maim and kill elsewhere in the world, with more than 50,000 cases and 9,000 deaths reported in 1965.[3] Against such a fearsome killer in a global disease environment, the United States shared the fate of the rest of the world, said Johnson: 'It is clear that every nation of the world, whether or not it has experienced smallpox in recent years, has a major stake in a worldwide eradication program.' Americans would proudly join their fellow world citizens against a common enemy, with Johnson promising that, 'this Government is ready to work with other interested countries to see to it that smallpox is a thing of the past by 1975'.

Johnson's announcement came as part of a flurry of American anti-smallpox initiatives during 1965. Marking World Health Day in March, Johnson noted the continued danger of smallpox and anticipated that the disease 'will one day be only a memory and that ours will be a healthier and happier world'.[4] The US announcement at the World Health Assembly (WHA) came two months later. And most importantly, in November 1965, the United States announced a smallpox eradication and measles control campaign for eighteen (later, nineteen) countries in West and Central Africa, led by the Communicable Disease Center (CDC, now the Centers for Disease

Control and Prevention). This represented a significant shift in the American position on smallpox eradication. Prior to 1965, the United States had offered general but abstract support for global smallpox eradication, and certainly without significant investment of American dollars. After 1965, the United States sought to take the lead in global smallpox eradication. Why the change?

Many of those who participated in smallpox eradication attribute the shift in American policy to good timing and smart efforts on the part of the CDC – there was an opportunity for the CDC to get involved, and the agency jumped at the chance, proposed a relatively inexpensive programme, and made it happen.[5] Scholarly accounts see a little less coincidence and a little more historical contingency. For example, Erez Manela explains that the CDC's smallpox eradication plans came to the Johnson administration at a moment when that administration wanted to show international good will, make a public demonstration of international cooperation and exercise its internationalist approach.[6] Some of the most interesting and invigorating recent scholarship in the field, especially that from Sanjoy Bhattacharya and colleagues, deliberately turns away from the United States, looking instead to the decisions and actions of nations and individuals in the developing (or Third) world that pushed for and shaped smallpox eradication, pointing to the limits of US hegemony during the 'American Century'.[7]

This chapter contributes to our understanding of the origins of global smallpox eradication by exploring how the Johnson administration's smallpox policy represented a step towards a Global Great Society within the context of the Cold War: an effort to engage with (and win over) the decolonising world through the enthusiasm of American liberalism and the power of the American government.[8] Smallpox eradication was one of a variety of projects in American liberalism that embodied a deep conviction that the power of the modern liberal state could solve the health challenges facing all of humanity, from disease to malnourishment to over-population.[9] Freed from the burden of disease, the people of the developing world could become more economically productive and thereby fend off the looming threat of communism – or so hoped the many advocates of modernisation and economic development, which influenced the evolving American approach to the post-colonial Cold War world of the 1950s and 1960s.[10] International health programmes like smallpox eradication represented an ambitious expansion of that general approach as it developed under the Johnson administration. The Global Great Society would ensure universal access to the universal rights to peace, prosperity and freedom, and it would begin with an international programme to destroy a universally hated scourge. The Johnson administration's pursuit of smallpox eradication, then, manifested a particular strategy in pursuit of the American Century: leveraging an international health programme to both demonstrate benevolent US global leadership and protect against perceived threats to American interests abroad.

As it happened, this expansive vision of a Global Great Society failed to materialise. Budget hawks attacked international health programmes for costing too much, and liberals found themselves torn between advocating for wars on disease that would ostensibly help prevent communism and fighting actual wars against real communists, as in Vietnam. The American smallpox programme reflected the fate of the Global Great Society. Both driven and constrained by the American approach to the Cold War, the American approach to international smallpox eradication narrowed and its meaning and purpose became uncertain – an uncertainty that is clear in the reminiscences and reflections of Americans who participated in the campaign.

Like those American public health workers, this chapter both recognises the limits of the American approach and also acknowledges (and praises) the successes of that approach and those public health workers. In less than five years – and within the budget, as many participants eagerly remind us – the CDC and its partners in West and Central Africa eliminated smallpox. That effort contributed to (and inspired, in many ways) the global programme coordinated by the WHO, which isolated the last naturally occurring case of *variola major* in Bangladesh in 1975, and the last case of *variola minor* in Somalia in 1977. From the official origins of the global smallpox eradication campaign in 1965, it took just over ten years to eliminate a disease that had plagued humanity for millennia. That is an impressive, unprecedented and as-yet unrepeated public health victory, but a victory that was complicated by the Cold War from beginning to end.

Cold War barriers to smallpox eradication

Although Johnson's 1965 announcement boasted of American leadership in international smallpox eradication, the programme had its official origins in a Soviet proposal, which the United States had conspicuously ignored for seven years. At the 1958 WHA, held in Minneapolis, Soviet delegate and minister of health Dr Viktor Zhdanov called for a global campaign against smallpox.[11] Zhdanov began by quoting Thomas Jefferson's 1806 prediction that 'future nations will know by history only that the loathsome smallpox has existed' – a thinly veiled jab at the failure of the United States to fulfil the prophecy of one of its Founders. After noting that the Soviet Union had eradicated endemic smallpox within its enormous borders twenty years previously, Zhdanov made a scientific argument for the eradicability of smallpox, noting advances in the 'modern status of medical science and health protection', especially the 'high grade smallpox vaccine' produced by the Soviet industrial machine. With an effective vaccine, scientific knowledge of the virus and historically proven vaccination programmes like the Soviet Union's, 'there can be no doubt', argued Zhdanov, 'that if our proposals are accepted . . . smallpox, which has been a scourge of mankind for centuries, will be practically eradicated within five years'. Zhdanov's enthusiasm was not universally shared among his fellow WHA delegates, who noted the desirability of smallpox eradication, but asked for further study of the matter.[12] The next year, the WHA discussed the study, which estimated that eradication would cost nearly $98 million; the delegates passed another resolution that gestured to the 'urgency of achieving world-wide eradication', but that 'urgency' was belied by the WHO budget, which allocated only $55,568 for smallpox control.[13]

Meanwhile, the WHO's malaria eradication programme, launched in 1955, consumed its attention and ever more resources: total WHO expenditures on the initiative increased from $2.4 million in 1955 to more than $13 million in 1958.[14] There was, of course, a good reason to prioritise malaria over smallpox eradication: the WHO estimated that malaria killed 1.5 million people per year, compared with the 39,889 deaths attributed to smallpox in 1955.[15] But malaria was initially more 'suitable for eradication' (in the language used by global health authorities at the time) than smallpox for reasons that had very little to do with the diseases themselves. A central factor, as explained in more detail elsewhere, was the diseases' different relationships to their environments, and ideas about science, technology and the non-human natural world.[16] Additionally, the Cold War played an important role in prioritising malaria eradication over smallpox eradication. Political and institutional contingencies in the early 1950s gave the United States a dominant role in the WHO. When the Soviet Union (and the rest of the Eastern Bloc) stayed out of the WHO from 1949 to 1956, citing its 'inflated administrative machinery' that failed to deliver on its constitutional promises to improve health, the United States gained remarkable influence in the organisation.[17] Acting as the sole superpower in the WHO, the United States threw its support behind global malaria eradication, which, as other historians have explained, offered potential foreign policy gains – specifically, turning poorer countries away from communism and towards American-style democracy and free-market capitalism – that could be won without direct, potentially redistributionist (that is, socialist or communist) anti-poverty efforts.[18]

As the Cold War continued, malaria eradication became more explicitly and unapologetically linked with American interests. Congress made malaria eradication a part of the nation's Cold War soft power campaigns when it amended the Mutual Security Act in 1957 to 'declare it the policy of the United States . . . to assist other peoples in their efforts to eradicate malaria'.[19] And in his State of the Union address the next year, President Eisenhower lauded the global malaria eradication campaign and challenged the Soviet Union 'to join with us in this great work of humanity'.[20] Instead, the USSR called for a new eradication programme against smallpox, offering a competitor for the budget and attention allocated to the WHO's three-year-old malaria eradication programme.[21] Zhdanov's proposal came just a few months after a State Department report warned of a broader 'Sino-Soviet economic offensive' that was using communist foreign aid to appeal to less-developed countries, a prospect that alarmed both President Eisenhower and the US Congress.[22] From this perspective, the Soviet's smallpox eradication programme represented a potential threat to American foreign policy interests. In short, malaria became the first candidate for global eradication because, in part, the disease suited the US approach to a globalising world in the Cold War of the 1950s.

The global effort to eradicate smallpox languished into the next decade. In the two years following the Soviet proposal and a large donation of smallpox vaccine, the WHO distributed only 500,000 doses, and the USSR complained that the programme had stalled.[23] The United States, uninterested in debates about the smallpox eradication programme, deserved much of the blame. The United States essentially ignored smallpox eradication while continuing to direct significant funds to the WHO for malaria eradication. By 1960, the United States had contributed $11 million to the WHO's Malaria Eradication Special Account – representing nearly 90 per cent of all donations to the fund ($12,422,038) – while making no contributions to the WHO Special Account for Smallpox Eradication (established following the Soviet proposal in 1958).[24] The WHO's malaria programme monopolised the organisation's attention and resources, with thousands of staff members and millions of dollars dedicated to it. In 1965 alone, the WHO spent more than $12.6 million on malaria eradication, while spending just $233,000 on smallpox.[25] Observing this disparity in the WHO's approach to the two diseases, the USSR delegation to the WHA complained that 'malaria eradication seemed to have been the favoured daughter of WHO, whereas smallpox eradication seemed to have been treated rather as a foster child'.[26] Meanwhile, the Americans kept their mouths and wallets shut, never explicitly opposing the programme, but never providing critical support either.

Such practical obstructionism reflected the opinion of American policymakers that the Soviet Union could not be trusted, even in matters of international health. In December 1960, an interdepartmental health policy advisory group made up of representatives from the Public Health Service, the US Information Agency, the International Cooperation Administration, and the departments of State and Health, Education and Welfare concluded that, 'it will be necessary to make careful judgments between actions of the Soviets that are to be resisted as political and those that are to be accepted and supported as legitimate contributions to world health and to international action under the UN system'.[27] From this perspective of suspicion, the Soviet proposal for global smallpox eradication threatened American foreign policy interests as represented in the malaria eradication programme (which the advisory group lauded as the perfect expression of the correct approach to international health, while saying nothing about smallpox eradication). And without American political, personnel and financial support, the WHO smallpox eradication programme would go nowhere.

Cold War visions of a Global Great Society

That approach began to change under the administration of Lyndon Johnson, which tentatively deployed an integrated approach to foreign diseases and foreign policy that would lead to increased American investment in international health, including smallpox eradication. At home, the Great Society that Johnson introduced in 1964 proposed a broad set of universal rights: housing, education, freedom from poverty and peace, among others.[28] Johnson believed that he could expand the Great Society to the rest of the world; 'My foreign policy', Johnson said, 'is the Great Society.'[29] Speaking to Holy Cross' graduating class in 1964, Johnson explained the need and justification for expanded investment in international health. 'Man's struggle against diseases' like tuberculosis, dysentery, leprosy and measles represented 'the focal point in his war to control the destructive forces of nature', Johnson said. And the United States could, and should, lead the fight in that war. 'We have the knowledge to reduce the toll of these diseases,' Johnson observed. Americans should be using their resources and scientific knowledge 'to avert millions of separate tragedies of needless death and suffering' caused by disease.

Although Johnson claimed that such plans 'do not spring from the Cold War or even from the ambitions of our adversaries', the economic development theories popular among American liberals linked international health programmes to capitalistic economic development and the confrontation with communism. That logic was exemplified in a 1964 speech by Dr Philip Lee, then the Director of Health Services for the State Department's US Agency for International Development (USAID), in which Lee clarified the connection between disease and development.[30] 'The diseases which cause the premature death of large numbers of people result in the loss of human capital,' Lee explained, drawing a direct line between poor health and poor economies. Measles, smallpox and other endemic diseases stunted the growth of the qualities necessary for full participation in the global capitalist economy. Disease also 'decreased initiative and energy', leaving less-developed populations vulnerable to the wiles of communism, and might even reinforce biological inferiority, through 'stunted physical growth and possible mental retardation'. In short, diseases halted a country's progress towards economic development and provided fertile ground for the growth of communism. If the United States wished to encourage economic development and democracy, it must begin by attacking disease.

The occasion of World Health Day in March 1965 gave Johnson the opportunity to announce American support for smallpox eradication, manifesting the broader ideological and political combination of the Cold War and the Global Great Society that had been percolating within his administration. Presented with the idea of global smallpox eradication, Johnson 'loved it', according to Joseph Califano, Special Assistant to the President, with whom Philip Lee discussed smallpox eradication as part of larger effort to expand American leadership in international health programmes.[31] Johnson's message in celebration of World Health Day in March 1965 focused on the importance of smallpox eradication, claiming a long-standing American commitment to 'assisting the World Health Organization in its drive to eradicate smallpox from the face of the globe'.[32] The message said nothing of the Soviet Union's interest in smallpox eradication, instead noting a vague 'spirit of international cooperation and concern'. Two months later, the United States positioned itself as a leader in the campaign by introducing the WHA resolution that would kick-start the stalled global smallpox eradication programme. Explaining his government's position in a speech to the WHA, US Surgeon General Luther Terry cited Johnson's 1964 speech at Holy Cross and the American commitment to 'find new techniques for making man's knowledge serve man's welfare'. Technology and scientific expertise offered both the opportunity and the duty for the world to come together and defeat smallpox, as Terry challenged his colleagues at the WHA: 'Knowledge represents responsibility . . . Each of us individually, and all of us together in WHO, must call on resources available to control disease in every continent . . . and elevate the well-being of mankind.'[33] These were the lofty aims embodied in the resolution backed by President Johnson on 18 May and passed by the WHA the next day. The ideas of the Global Great Society had found their expression in smallpox eradication.

The initial implementation of the American commitment to smallpox eradication would come through a bilateral programme in West and Central Africa, a programme that had been years in the making by health professionals at the CDC and a number of African health ministries. By the early 1960s, the CDC had already begun an assault on diseases around the globe. In 1963 alone, CDC epidemiologists responded to distress calls from the South Pacific to the northern Atlantic, confronting epidemics of polio, cholera, rabies and malaria.[34] In 1964, the CDC agreed to take over the expansion of a measles vaccination programme initiated three years earlier by the National Institutes of Health (NIH), which had been skilfully courted by African health professionals like Paul Lambin, Upper Volta's health minister. Using the public platform of the WHA and his contacts with USAID, Lambin pushed the United States (and the WHO) to go beyond measles and to attack other diseases, including onchocerciasis, malaria, meningitis and smallpox.[35] The CDC was particularly intrigued by smallpox eradication, a topic which it had studied through its Smallpox Unit (created in 1961) and which it had explored specifically in Togo after taking over the NIH's measles vaccination programme. Johnson's May 1965 announcement of support for smallpox eradication gave the CDC and health professionals in West Africa another card to play. Lambin specifically noted the president's announcement in a meeting with USAID officials in Upper Volta, and a month later, USAID received from the CDC a draft plan to couple smallpox eradication to the measles campaign: five years, eighteen countries, 130 million vaccinations, $36.5 million.[36]

The CDC official who developed the plan, D. A. Henderson (who would go on to direct the WHO's eradication programme), said that he was 'convinced that the proposal would be rejected'.[37] Instead, on 23 November 1965, President Johnson announced the new US measles and smallpox vaccination campaign in West and Central Africa. Henderson remembers being 'totally surprised' by the approval of the programme. He perhaps should not have been, considering how well the West and Central Africa programme suited the foreign policy and foreign health objectives and methods of the Johnson administration. The programme promised to improve African health, which would, in turn, develop African economies and stave off the expansion of communism. USAID liked the idea; the agency's director, David Bell, highly recommended the programme to the president, noting that the CDC programmes 'have received exceptional response from governments throughout Africa'.[38] The State Department appreciated the political payoff for a limited investment, and Bell pointedly noted that the programme's 'impact on our balance of payments will be slight'.

The US commitment to smallpox eradication in late 1965 prompted ambitious – but brief – discussions about even more expansive US programmes in international health. For example, in 1966, the House considered H.R. 12453, the International Health Act (IHA), which would have increased funding for the eradication of smallpox and other diseases, invested in Head Start nutrition programmes in the developing world, doubled grants for health training abroad, created family planning programmes, and built an International Career Service in Health to send American doctors out into the world. In his message accompanying the bill, Johnson urged Congress to 'add a world dimension' to the progress it was making on the Great Society at home, for it would be 'shortsighted to confine our vision to this Nation's shorelines'.[39] But those ambitious plans quickly ran into the reality of an expensive war in Vietnam and resistance to spending more American time and talent on the rest of the world's problems. At a time when the United States was on its way to spending nearly $1.5 billion in Vietnam in 1966 alone, the IHA's $54 million price tag seemed unjustifiable.[40] Before Johnson had even introduced the IHA, Assistant Secretary of State Joseph Sisco questioned 'the desirability of such an initiative at this time', particularly in 'view of the overall budgetary stringency which the US is facing owing to the Vietnam situation'.[41] Representative Howard Smith, chairman of the House Rules Committee, lambasted the cost and underlying philosophy of the IHA: 'How are we going to finance the $60 million for [the International Health Act] when Viet Nam is costing so much? Are we going to have a war on poverty for the world? Where are we going to stop?'[42] In this view, the United States should focus on taking care of its own at home and taking care of business in Vietnam, rather than exporting the Great Society to the rest of the world.

The IHA died in committee, presenting an early sign that the Great Society might, in fact, remain bound to American soil. Instead, smallpox eradication became the Global Great Society's last best hope, thanks to its promise of an extraordinary accomplishment at very little cost. The CDC proposed a relatively small budget for the joint measles–smallpox programme in West and Central Africa: just $36 million for five years, compared with $54 million for the IHA in the first year alone. The programme required West and Central African governments to pay for all local costs, including fuel and maintenance for automobiles, which would be made in the United States, per USAID regulations. Bell emphasised these points in his recommendation to the president, as did the White House's announcement of the West and Central Africa programme in November.[43] In this way, the United States could engage with the globalising, post-colonial world, while retaining important control over the specific means of that engagement and simultaneously boosting the American economy. Perhaps most importantly, the West and Central African programme had a finite goal: total and permanent elimination of a disease. Johnson's support of the WHO programme called for eradication in ten years, and the CDC promised to be out of West and Central Africa in five. With a definite end point, a small budget, and a programme already in place, the West and Central Africa programme continued, even as broader visions of a Global Great Society slipped away.

Assessing the complex legacy of smallpox eradication

The smallpox eradication efforts in West and Central Africa generated remarkably fast results: 25 million vaccinations in less than two years; a 50 per cent decrease in smallpox incidence between 1968 and 1969 alone, and effective nil incidence by mid-1969, just three years after the programme started. That success contributed to the WHO's global smallpox eradication programme, which in the eyes of participants and some historians became one of the greatest examples of international cooperation during the Cold War.[44] Although the Soviet Union complained about not receiving enough credit for initiating eradication – at a WHA meeting in 1975, a Soviet delegate noted that it was the USSR, after all, that initially proposed smallpox eradication in 1958, and he 'regretted that a number of articles recently published had given the impression that the programme had not really started until 1967' – doctors and health professionals from the USSR, the United States and dozens of other countries worked side-by-side in the WHO campaign, which isolated the last naturally occurring case of smallpox in 1977.[45] The WHO declared total victory over smallpox in 1980, certifying the first (and, to date, only) deliberate eradication of a human disease. CDC staff from the West and Central Africa programme were and are rightly proud of their success against smallpox. Tony Masso, who worked for the programme in Niger, compared smallpox eradication with another remarkable US achievement inspired in part by the Cold War: landing on the moon in 1969. 'The American space program was going up there', Masso remembers thinking, 'and here we are, and we're going to do something just as important. We're going to wipe a disease off the face of the earth . . . That was tremendously rewarding to be able to say that to those people, to believe it, and then to leave when it was all done.'[46] As Don Moore, who also served in Niger, later put it, the programme showed that, 'one man, or a team of a couple of men, with the backing of a strong government, like the United States, with the Public Health Service behind them, can make a fantastic impact on a large population of people. A country can make a major world health impact.'[47]

Other staff questioned the significance of that accomplishment. Bill White, the operations officer in Upper Volta, says that 'from a philosophical point of view, one of the questions we asked ourselves in late-night conversations with wine and cheese was basically: What were we accomplishing?'[48] He understood the contributions to epidemiology in West and Central Africa, and that 'we accomplished something for the United States in that it took away an infectious disease that could have come here'. 'But the real question', asked White, was 'What was the real benefit in the areas in Africa that we were working in?' In the context of the great needs and demands for healthcare in Africa, the eradication of smallpox seemed somehow insufficient, its legacy somehow ambiguous. Yes, the United States had helped to eradicate a deadly disease. But why? White's comments note the American public health self-interest served by smallpox eradication – the programme 'took away an infectious disease that could have come here'. And, as this chapter argues, American participation in smallpox eradication had been justified in part by American foreign policy interests. White's comments point to the ways in which American self-interest compromised or limited the potential of American involvement in smallpox eradication and global public health efforts more broadly.

As it had complicated the origins of smallpox eradication, so did the Cold War muddle the legacy of smallpox eradication. Initially, American suspicions of the Soviet Union stymied global smallpox eradication, but then the Johnson administration decided to support the programme, in part because of its potential foreign policy gains and the extension of American influence during the American Century. Likewise, the Cold War shaped the conclusion of the global eradication programme. When the WHA officially certified the eradication of smallpox in 1980, some delegates called for the destruction of all remaining stocks of smallpox in scientific laboratories. But US delegate Donald Hopkins, who oversaw the CDC's eradication programme in Sierra Leone, said that it was 'unwise at the present time' to destroy smallpox stocks, citing 'very incomplete' knowledge of other ortho-poxviruses. Soviet delegate V. K. Tatochenko also said there was need for 'considerable scientific research'. And, as it happened, only two laboratories would retain their smallpox stocks: the CDC in Atlanta and the Research Institute of Viral Preparations (RIVP) in Moscow. That reality represents well the extent and limits of this particular effort to leverage a global public health campaign to help build the American Century: a terrible disease eliminated, but a virus left to live on in part due to American foreign policy interests. This complicated legacy of the American Century is equally deserving of both celebration and criticism.

Notes

1. Portions of this chapter were published in *The End of a Global Pox: America and the Eradication of Smallpox in the Cold War Era* (University of North Carolina Press, © 2015). Used by permission of the publisher. For more information visit www.uncpress.org.
2. Lyndon B. Johnson, 'Statements by the President on Announcing US Support for an International Program To Eradicate Smallpox', available at: http://www.presidency.ucsb.edu/ws/index.php?pid=26977.
3. World Health Organization, 'Smallpox: Cases and Deaths in 1965', *Weekly Epidemiological Record* 41:21 (1966), 283–7.
4. Lyndon B. Johnson, 'Statement on World Health Day', 14 March 1965, Ex HE/MC, Box 6, White House Central Files (hereafter, WHCF), Lyndon B. Johnson Library, Austin, TX (hereafter, LBJ Library).
5. See, for example, D. A. Henderson, *Smallpox: The Death of a Disease* (New York: Prometheus Books, 2009); William Foege, *House on Fire: The Fight to Eradicate Smallpox* (Berkeley: University of California Press, 2011).
6. Erez Manela, 'A Pox on Your Narrative: Writing Disease Control into Cold War History', *Diplomatic History* 34:2 (2010), 299–323; Erez Manela, 'Globalizing the Great Society: Lyndon Johnson and the Pursuit of Smallpox Eradication', in Francis J. Gavin and Mark Atwood Lawrence (eds), *Beyond the Cold War: Lyndon Johnson and the New Global Challenges of the 1960s* (New York: Oxford University Press, 2014), 165–81; Erez Manela, 'Smallpox Eradication and the Rise of Global Governance', *The Shock of the Global: The 1970s in Perspective* (Cambridge, MA: Belknap Press of Harvard University, 2010).
7. Sanjoy Bhattacharya, *Expunging Variola: The Control and Eradication of Smallpox in India, 1947–1977* (Hyderabad: Orient Longman, 2006);

Sanjoy Bhattacharya, 'Global and Local Histories of Medicine: Interpretative Challenges and Future Possibilities', in Mark Jackson (ed.), *The Oxford Handbook of the History of Medicine* (Oxford: Oxford University Press, 2011), 135–49; Sanjoy Bhattacharya, 'Reflections on the Eradication of Smallpox', *The Lancet* 375:9726 (2010), 1602–3; Sanjoy Bhattacharya, 'Struggle to a Monumental Triumph: Re-Assessing the Final Phases of the Smallpox Eradication Program in India, 1960–1980', *Historia, Ciencias, Saude Manguinhos* 14:4 (2007), 1113–29; Sanjoy Bhattacharya and Niels Brimnes. 'Introduction: Simultaneously Global and Local: Reassessing Smallpox Vaccination and Its Spread, 1789–1900', *Bulletin of the History of Medicine* 83: 1 (2009), 1–16; Sanjoy Bhattacharya and Rajib Dasgupta, 'A Tale of Two Global Health Programs: Smallpox Eradication's Lessons for the Antipolio Campaign in India', *American Journal of Public Health* 99: 7 (2009), 1176–84; Sanjoy Bhattacharya and Sharon Messenger (eds), *The Global Eradication of Smallpox* (Hyderabad: Orient Longman, 2010); Sanjoy Bhattacharya and Carlos Eduardo D'Avila Pereira Campani, 'Re-Assessing the Foundations: Worldwide Smallpox Eradication, 1957–67', *Medical History* 64:1 (2020), 71–93.

8. A growing body of literature has examined efforts to 'internationalise' or 'globalise' the Great Society. See Ahlberg, Kristin, *Transplanting the Great Society: Lyndon Johnson and Food for Peace* (Columbia: University of Missouri Press, 2008); Francis J. Gavin and Mark Atwood Lawrence (eds), *Beyond the Cold War: Lyndon Johnson and the New Global Challenges of the 1960s* (New York: Oxford University Press, 2014), esp. chapters by Patrick Cohrs, Nick Cullather, Sheyda Jahanbani and Erez Manela; Bob H. Reinhardt, 'The Global Great Society and the US Commitment to Smallpox Eradication', *Endeavour* 34:4 (2010): 164–72.

9. The story of smallpox eradication represents one of the triumphs, albeit complex and limited in many ways, of liberalism and the Great Society, whereas most accounts of that era focus on frustrations and failures. See John Andrew, *Lyndon Johnson and the Great Society* (Chicago, IL: I. R. Dee, 1998); H. W. Brands, *The Strange Death of American Liberalism* (New Haven, CT: Yale University Press, 2001); Gareth Davies, *From Opportunity to Entitlement: The Transformation and Decline of Great Society Liberalism* (Lawrence: University Press of Kansas, 1996); Doris Kearns Goodwin, *Lyndon Johnson and the American Dream* (New York: Harper & Row, 1976); Alonzo L Hamby, *Liberalism and Its Challengers: From F.D.R. to Bush*, 2nd edn (New York: Oxford University Press, 1992); Theodore J. Lowi, *The End of Liberalism: The Second Republic of the United States*, 40th anniversary edn (New York: W. W. Norton, 2009); G. Calvin Mackenzie and Robert Weisbrot, *The Liberal Hour: Washington and the Politics of Change in the 1960s* (New York: Penguin, 2008); Sidney Milkis and Jerome Mileur (eds), *The Great Society and the High Tide of Liberalism* (Amherst,

MA: University of Massachusetts Press, 2005); Irwin Unger, *The Best of Intentions: The Triumphs and Failures of the Great Society Under Kennedy, Johnson, and Nixon* (New York: Doubleday, 1996).

10. For histories of development and modernisation theory and its influence in American foreign policy, see David Ekbladh, *The Great American Mission: Modernization and the Construction of an American World Order* (Princeton, NJ: Princeton University Press, 2010); Nils Gilman, *Mandarins of the Future: Modernization Theory in Cold War America*, New Studies in American Intellectual and Cultural History (Baltimore, MD: Johns Hopkins University Press, 2003); Michael Latham, *Modernization as Ideology: American Social Science and 'Nation Building' in the Kennedy Era* (Chapel Hill: University of North Carolina Press, 2000); Michael Latham, *The Right Kind of Revolution* (Ithaca, NY: Cornell University Press, 2011); Kimber Charles Pearce, *Rostow, Kennedy, and the Rhetoric of Foreign Aid* (East Lancing: Michigan State University Press, 2001).

11. 'Eradication of Smallpox (Draft Resolution Proposed by the Government of the USSR)', 6 March 1958, A11/P&B/1, WHO Library.

12. F. Fenner, D. A. Henderson, I. Arita, Z. Ježek and I. D. Ladnyi, *Smallpox and Its Eradication* (Geneva: World Health Organization, 1988), 369–71.

13. World Health Assembly, Resolution WHA12.54; Fenner et al., *Smallpox and its Eradication*, 369–70.

14. Fenner et al., *Smallpox and its Eradication*, 383.

15. WHO, *Official Records of the World Health Organization: First Report on the World Health Situation*, 20; Cyril William Dixon, *Smallpox* (Lodon: J. A. Churchill, 1962), app. III.

16. Bob H. Reinhardt, 'Smallpox Denaturalized, Demonized, and Eradicable', *Environmental History* 20:4 (2015), 700–9; Bob H. Reinhardt, *The End of a Global Pox: America and the Eradication of Smallpox in the Cold War Era* (Chapel Hill: University of North Carolina Press, 2015).

17. For departure of the USSR and influence of the US in the WHO, see Theodore M. Brown, Marcos Cueto and Elizabeth Fee, 'The World Health Organization and the Transition From "International" to "Global" Public Health', *American Journal of Public Health* 96:1 (2006), 62–72; Marcos Cueto, 'International Health, The Early Cold War and Latin America', *Canadian Bulletin of Medical History/Bulletin Canadien d'histoire de La Médecine* 25:1 (2008), 17–41; Christopher Osakwe, *The Participation of the Soviet Union in Universal International Organizations: A Political and Legal Analysis of Soviet Strategies and Aspirations inside ILO, UNESCO and WHO* (Leiden: Sijthoff, 1972); Javed Siddiqi, *World Health and World Politics: The World Health Organization and the UN System* (Columbia: University of South Carolina Press, 1995). For contemporary reactions at the US Department of State, see 'Associate Membership in WHO', 1948, Box 2, 63D220, Records Pertaining to the World Health Organization

and the Committee on International Health Policy, 1945–1962, RG 59, National Archives and Records Administration, College Park, MD (hereafter cited as NARA).

18. See Marcos Cueto, *Cold War, Deadly Fevers: Malaria Eradication in Mexico, 1955–1975* (Washington, DC: Woodrow Wilson Center Press, 2007); Harry Cleaver, 'Malaria and the Political Economy of Public Health', *International Journal of Health Services* 7:4 (1977), 557–79; DavidKinkela, *DDT and the American Century: Global Health, Environmental Politics, and the Pesticide that Changed the World* (Chapel Hill: University of North Carolina Press, 2011), ch. 2; Amy L. S. Staples, *The Birth of Development: How the World Bank, Food and Agriculture Organization, and World Health Organization Changed the World, 1945–1965* (Kent, OH: Kent State University Press, 2006), 170–1; 'Malaria and Development', SI *Medical Anthropology* (1997), ed. Randall Packard, esp. Litsios, 'Malaria Control, the Cold War, and the Postwar Reorganization of International Assistance', 255–78; Packard, 'Malaria Dreams', 279–94; Packard and Brown, 'Rethinking Health, Development, and Malaria'.

19. 'Disease Eradication', January 1966, Folder 'Diseases: Disease Eradication', Committees-Diseases, Correspondence 1949–1969, Box 40, Office of International Health, RG 90, NARA.

20. President Eisenhower, 'Annual Message to the Congress on the State of the Union', available at: http://www.presidency.ucsb.edu/ws/index. php?pid=11162; Kelley Lee notes that 'In 1956, US President Dwight Eisenhower decided to provide substantial funds for malaria eradication on both humanitarian and foreign policy ground', see Lee, *The World Health Organization*, 39.

21. In a March 1959 meeting, Dr H. van Zile Hyde, the assistant to the Surgeon General for International Health and a US delegate to the World Health Assembly, made a direct comparison between the Soviet (and Cuban) contributions to smallpox eradication and US contributions to malaria eradication. See 'Memorandum of Meeting re: Establishment of an Interdepartmental Committee on International Health Policy and World Health Organization Fund for Conquest of Disease', 13 March 1959, Folder: 'Health: Interdepartmental Committee on International Health Policy – Memoranda (Miscellaneous)', Box 4, Records Pertaining to the World Health Organization and the Committee on International Health Policy, 1945–1962, RG 59, NARA.

22. Department of State, *The Sino-Soviet Economic Offensive in the Less Developed Countries*, US Government Printing Office, 1958. For Eisenhower and Congress' anxiety about Soviet foreign aid and how that anxiety shaped American foreign aid policy in the 1950s, see Burton Ira Kaufman, *Trade and Aid: Eisenhower's Foreign Economic Policy, 1953–1961* (Baltimore, MD: Johns Hopkins University Press, 1982).

23. 'Committee on Programme and Budget, Provisional Minutes of the Thirteenth Meeting', 21 February 1961, A14/PB/Min/13, WHO Library.

24. 'Malaria Eradication Special Account: Report by the Director-General', 21 October 1960, A11/AFL/8, WHO Library; Fenner et al., *Smallpox and Its Eradication*, 401.

25. Fenner et al., *Smallpox and its Eradication*, 384.

26. 'Committee on Programme and Budget, Provisional Minutes of the Twelfth Meeting, Eleventh World Health Assembly', 17 May 1965, A18/P&B/Min/12, WHO Library. For Soviet frustration, see Manela, 'Globalizing the Great Society', 167.

27. Henry Gelfand, 'E-1 Statement for Measles Control and Smallpox Eradication, Mauritania', 29 April 1966, Folder '20 B.4 IHP-61', Box 4, Bureau of International Organization Affairs, Office of International and Economic and Social Affairs, Records Pertaining to the World Health Organization and the Committee on International Health Policy, 1945–1962, RG 59, NARA.

28. Lyndon B. Johnson, 'Remarks at the University of Michigan', American Presidency Project, 22 May 1964, available at: http://www.presidency. ucsb.edu/ws/index.php?pid=26262.

29. Quoted in Ahlberg, *Transplanting the Great Society*, 44.

30. Philip Lee, 'International Health Programs: The Role of the United States Government', 13 October 1964, Folder 'Foreign Relations, International Cooperation Year Reports, Int. Health Activities', Box 42, Correspondence 1949–1969, Education & Training: Foreign Relations, 1966–1967, Office of International Health, RG 90, NARA.

31. Philip Lee, 18 January 1969, Oral History Collection, LBJ Library; Philip Lee, interview by author, telephone, 18 February 2011; Joseph Califano, interview by author, 29 November 2012.

32. Johnson, 'Statement on World Health Day'.

33. 'World Health Assembly, Provisional Minutes of the Eighteenth Meeting', 19 May 1965, A18/VR/7, WHO Library.

34. Etheridge, *Sentinel for Health*, 179.

35. World Health Organization, *Official Records of the World Health Organization, No. 128: Sixteenth World Health Assembly, Geneva, 7–23 May 1963, Part II, Plenary Meetings Verbatim Records, Committees Minutes and Reports*, 1963, World Health Organization Library & Information Networks for Knowledge Database; Walter Sherwin, 'Memorandum of Conversation, Paul Lambin and Walter Sherwin', 22 July 1965, Agency AID, Accession No. 71A3860, Carton 27, Box 1, National Archives and Records Administration (College Park, MD).

36. Walter Sherwin, 'Memorandum of Conversation, Paul Lambin and Walter Sherwin', 22 July 1965, Folder 'HLS Health', Carton 27, Agency AID, Accession No. 71A3860, RG 286, NARA.

37. Henderson, *Smallpox: The Death of a Disease,* 72–3.

38. Quoted in Charles Schultze, 'Memorandum for the President, Subject: Expanded West African Measles/Smallpox Program', 23 November, 1965, Ex HE/MC, Box 6, WHCF, LBJ Library; Telegram from US Embassy, Ougadougou, to Secretary of State, 26 November 1965,

Folder 'PASA–OCCGE Measles Program (Altman)', Box 36, Correspondence 1949–1969, Agreements-Associations, 1966–1967, Office of International Health, RG 90, NARA.

39. Lyndon B. Johnson, 'Special Message to the Congress Proposing International Education and Health Programs', 2 February 1966, Statements of Lyndon B. Johnson, 27 January1966–3 February 1966, Box 175, LBJ Library.

40. Vernon W. Ruttan, *United States Development Assistance Policy: The Domestic Politics of Foreign Economic Aid* (Baltimore, MD: Johns Hopkins University Press, 1996), 495.

41. Joseph Sisco, 'Memo for Douglass Cater', 16 December 1965, Ex HE, Box 1, WHCF, LBJ Library.

42. Ralph Huitt, 'Memorandum for Henry Hall Wilson, Jr.', 17 March 1966, Ex LE/FO 4-2, Box 58, WHCF, LBJ Library.

43. Horace Ogden, *CDC and the Smallpox Crusade* (Atlanta, GA: US Dept. of Health and Human Services, 1987), 24; Schultze, 'Memorandum for the President'.

44. For participant accounts emphasising cooperation, see, for example, Henderson, *Smallpox: The Death of a Disease*; Foege, *House on Fire*. Among historians, Erez Manela has made the argument for cooperation most effectively.

45. For Soviet delegate quote, see World Health Organization, *Official Records of the World Health Organization, No. 227: Twenty-Eighth World Health Assembly, Geneva, 13–30 May 1975, Part II, Verbatim Records of Plenary Meetings, Summary Records and Reports of Committees* (Geneva, 1975), 9.

46. Tony Masso, Interview by Kata Chillag, 14 July 2006, Global Health Chronicle, Centers for Disease Control, Atlanta, Georgia.

47. Don Moore, Interview by Diane Drew, 14 July 2006, Global Health Chronicle, Centers for Disease Control, Atlanta, Georgia.

48. Bill White, Interview by Kata Chillag, 14 July 2006, Global Health Chronicles, Centers for Disease Control, Atlanta, Georgia.

9

Brother's Brother Foundation in Costa Rica: A Case Study in Public–Private Partnerships and Global Health in the American Century

Sarah B. Snyder

The chapter analyses a 1967 immunisation campaign led by Dr Robert Hingson and the non-governmental organisation (NGO) he founded, Brother's Brother Foundation, that was aided by key logistical support from the US government. This collaborative effort to promote public health and eradicate disease reveals one of the diverse ways the US government improved public health and fought disease in the American Century. This programme achieved a degree of 'soft power' for the United States, and it intersects with broader narratives about the role of the United States, American NGOs and US citizens in advancing international health.[1] Examining the episode illuminates American approaches to development in the 1960s, and it highlights an understudied bilateral relationship – that between the United States and Costa Rica, or the hawk and the sparrow, as one author has termed it.[2] Finally, the campaign offers us a means of analysing public–private global health collaboration in foreign countries.

Before the Brother's Brother Foundation campaign in Costa Rica, the United States had a record of cooperating with Latin American governments, at least since the 1940s, on sanitation, medical care and public health.[3] These efforts could also be framed in terms of the potential positive economic benefits – enhanced productivity, increased life expectancy and greater development.[4] In the view of Representative Hugh L. Carey (Democrat, NY), we should see these health interventions as 'effective instrument[s] of foreign policy'.[5] He wrote, 'Historically, American medical help has been used to open new frontiers in our hemisphere and around the world.'[6] Such drives were justified in economic, humane and security terms, and facilitated the expansion and protection of US interests in the Western Hemisphere.[7] As other scholars have shown, the spread of disease in Central America and elsewhere in the developing world posed potential threats to development and therefore US strategic and economic interests.[8] This unchecked transmission of infection therefore represented threats to the ideals, values and capacities of the American Century.

Whereas there is a rich historiography on American corporations and foundations in Costa Rica in the late nineteenth century and first half of the twentieth century, the literature on US–Costa Rican relations in the 1960s is more limited.[9] As US interests shifted during the Cold War, Costa Rica's history as a peaceful country meant that it was not central to US foreign policy and therefore the history of US foreign relations.[10] Yet the United States, in the wake of the 1959 Cuban Revolution, paid heightened attention to the Caribbean region, including Central America. John F. Kennedy travelled to Costa Rica in 1963, and while there he delivered an address that touched on the significance of 'political liberty' and 'social justice'.[11]

One of Brother's Brother Foundation's first missions was a campaign to vaccinate Liberians against smallpox in 1962.[12] Although State Department telegrams characterised the trip as 'strictly private', the organisation coordinated with the Liberian government and US Agency for International Development (USAID) representatives in Monrovia.[13] The US navy also aided the mission by transporting personnel and 200 tons of material to Liberia.[14] Several years later Brother's Brother Foundation's undertook a campaign in Costa Rica in which it secured support from a different branch of the US government – the Pentagon, which loaned the group sixteen jet injectors. Examining Hingson's vaccination campaigns demonstrates the secularisation of development, US government partnerships with non-state actors and a deeper degree of military–private partnerships than the existing literature suggests.[15]

Pistolas de la paz

At the end of August 1967, Costa Rican Minister of Health Alvaro Aguilar wrote to President Lyndon B. Johnson thanking the US Defense Department for loaning sixteen jet injectors, which he termed '*pistolas de la paz*', for a vaccination campaign.[16] The campaign enabled the inoculation of 840,000 Costa Ricans against smallpox and the immunisation of around 210,000 Costa Ricans, primarily babies, against measles. These records, filed under the White House Central Files subject category 'Peace', signalled that the Johnson administration sought to build upon its predecessors' efforts to wage the Cold War by other means and via non-governmental actors. Correspondence in the Lyndon B. Johnson Library reveals that Johnson's intrigue with the minister's language, which transformed vaccine delivery vehicles into transmitters of peace. A 6 September 1967 note records, 'Find out what this is and have Covey Oliver develop a program. "Pistols for Peace" – that sounds pretty good.'[17] Despite the notation, I could find no evidence that replication was pursued elsewhere (Figure 9.1).

The immunisation programme in Costa Rica involved collaboration among the United States, the Costa Rican government, and Brother's Brother Foundation. The foundation provided US medical professionals and utilised resources such as the Pentagon's loan of the jet injectors, which were termed peace guns in Spanish due to their gun-like appearance and painless effects.[18] At a time when US guns were being deployed overseas increasingly to wage war in Vietnam, the US military continued collaborating with humanitarian organisations towards peaceful ends. As with Hingson's other missions, the civilian nature of these efforts was key. They also fit within Vice President Hubert Humphrey's concept of a 'shirtsleeve war' – efforts by civilians to improve health and education.[19]

The Brother's Brother Foundation initiative in Costa Rica built upon earlier undertakings by the Rockefeller Foundation in the region, which began working in Central America and the Caribbean in 1914 and made early efforts regarding international health focused on hookworm, malaria and yellow fever.[20] According to some scholars, the Rockefeller Foundation's efforts, like those of Brother's Brother

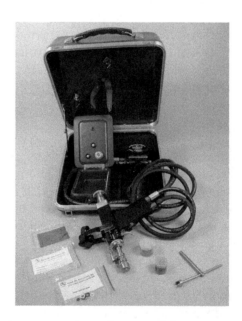

Figure 9.1 A jet injector in the collection of the Division of Medicine and Science, National Museum of American History, Smithsonian Institution

Foundation, were driven by a 'missionary impulse'.[21] Whereas other observers have asserted Rockefeller's international health initiatives and potentially the efforts of Brother's Brother in Liberia sought to aid economic growth.[22]

The literature on US policy towards Latin America has often contrasted the commitment to development and democracy ostensibly embedded in Kennedy's Alliance for Progress programme with the Mann Doctrine of the Johnson years, which in R. D. Johnson's telling privileged 'stability and restraint of Communism'.[23] Despite this shift in emphasis, it is significant that Johnson kept aid to Central America consistent with Kennedy's commitments, especially given that Congress sought diminished foreign assistance considering the costs of the war in Vietnam.[24]

The Johnson administration's support for Brother's Brother Foundation's Costa Rican campaign complemented the president's rhetoric about the interconnections between national and international health. In 1965 remarks announcing more funding for biomedical research facilities, Johnson repeatedly shifted between his and the country's commitment to domestic and international health. For example, he said, 'Malaria and cholera were conquered in America a long time ago . . . The American goal is the complete eradication of malaria and cholera from the entire world.' He argued that the United States was leading 'a worldwide war on disease'.[25]

The Johnson administration's support for Hingson's efforts in Costa Rica also fit with its international health programme, which Johnson proposed in February 1966, saying that the United States should participate in an international effort 'to rid mankind of the slavery of ignorance and the scourge of disease'.[26] Among other objectives articulated by Johnson in this speech was the creation of a civil service devoted to global health. Speaking in 1964, Johnson had said, 'Those who live in the emerging community of nations will ignore the problems of their neighbours at the risk of their own prosperity.'[27] The International Health Act of 1966 sought to ensure that prosperity. The legislation proclaimed: 'It is in the interest of this Government to develop and strengthen the capability of the United States to provide assistance to those countries who are working to help themselves develop needed health services; and that, therefore, it is both necessary and desirable for this Government to assist in providing our share of the health workers needed to man the posts of the health battle throughout the world.'[28]

The International Health Education Act ultimately failed, and Peter J. Hoetz argues that in the aftermath, the United States pulled back from medical missions abroad. Nonetheless the proposed legislation should be seen as an expression of the administration's wish to expand its engagement internationally, including in matters of health.[29]

In addition to supporting Brother's Brother Foundation and Hingson's efforts, the United States also benefited from the good-will and spirit of cooperation such humanitarian missions engendered. Writing to Johnson, the Costa Rican health minister said, 'We believe our governments should unite in the use of the pistolas of peace in preference wherever possible to the use of the guns of war.'[30] Johnson responded to the minister of health and congratulated him in the vaccination campaign.[31] Earlier that year, Johnson had indicated to several Central American presidents, including José Trejos of Costa Rica, that he wanted to expand the fight to eradicate screwworm to that region, demonstrating that the American commitment to improving Central American health went beyond facilitating the loan of *pistolas de la paz*.[32]

United States' support for global health projects in the 1960s also represented a potential counterpoint to its most significant interaction in the world in these years – the war in Vietnam. Hingson explicitly connected the two agendas, contrasting his budgets to vaccinate people in Central American countries to US military spending for Vietnam. Hingson claimed that he could immunise the world's population with 'one-tenth of the military personnel and one-fourth of the budget of the United States' expenditure for the war in Vietnam'.[33]

Hingson: the man and his jet injector

Robert Hingson served in the US Public Health Service before working in medical schools in Colombia and Venezuela in the 1950s.[34] An anaesthesiologist, he was focused on diminishing patients' pain. To that end he worked to develop a medical device, the jet injector, which would innovate vaccination efforts in subsequent years. As part of his studies, Hingson practised on cadavers and himself.[35] The multiple-dose jet injector enabled the vaccination of 1,000 people per hour, a dramatic increase over earlier delivery methods.[36] In addition to enabling increased numbers of patients reached, the innovation of the jet injector, or hypospray, offered other advantages over using a needle and a syringe. Most notably, the jet injector was less painful; half of patients reported a 'complete absence of pain'. In addition, the jet injector did not require sterilisation with each use.[37] The name, 'peace gun', came from a Burmese child – who remarked after receiving a typhoid inoculation, that 'it's not a bad gun; it's a peace gun'.[38]

Among Hingson's motivations for his humanitarian work were religious ones – a professed desire to follow the commandment to love one's neighbour as oneself, as well as potentially a belief in the gospel of public health or the compulsion to protect human life.[39] As one fellow Baptist put it, Hingson felt 'very strongly the commission as expressed in Luke 4:18 that in addition to preaching the gospel to the poor we are to heal the broken hearted'.[40] In 1958, Hingson led the first inter-racial, interfaith and interdisciplinary team of medical professionals to undertake a mission internationally by embarking on an around-the-world-trip to assess medical needs.[41] Funded by the Baptist World Alliance, the team travelled to Japan, the Philippines, Burma, South Korea, India, Hong Kong, Egypt, Kenya, Iran, Tanganyika, Southern Rhodesia, the Belgian Congo, French Equatorial Africa, Nigeria and Liberia. During its journey, the group visited hospitals, performed operations, administered vaccines and delivered medical supplies, among other activities.[42]

Brother's Brother Foundation

After their trip, those involved created a committee to try to address the medical needs they catalogued on their journey.[43] Supported by the Baptist World Alliance, Hingson established Brother's Brother Foundation in Pittsburgh. The organisation took its name from a Nigerian medical student who told Hingson, 'We don't need a keeper; we need a brother'.[44] The organisation's objective was to utilise US medical resources in global health challenges given the overwhelming need its organisers identified in the world. It raised money from wealthy individuals such as Baptist Maxey Jarman and sought and received in-kind donations from pharmaceutical companies. The group also made direct appeals to donors via talks to religious and civic organisations in their community and across the country.

One way to conceive of Hingson and his interdenominational medical colleagues is as medical missionaries. There are examples of Americans serving as medical missionaries as early as 1834, such as Peter Parker in China, but the phenomenon became more prevalent later.[45] The 1932 'Hocking Report' urged American missionaries to move away from their long-standing focus on conversion to prioritise social services such as medical care.[46] Thereafter, American missionary activity evolved away from the 'Christian imperialism' that Emily Conroy-Krutz and others have documented.[47]

Brother's Brother Foundation's immunisation campaign in Costa Rica built upon and was facilitated by its earlier work, especially in Liberia and Honduras.[48] The campaign in Liberia demonstrated that mass vaccination against smallpox was possible. In subsequent years as the World Health Organization (WHO) focused its attention on smallpox eradication in Africa and then Asia, the Americas received less attention. Given that gap, Dr Donald Henderson, who worked for the US Communicable Disease Center and then led the WHO's smallpox campaign, urged Hingson and the foundation to undertake immunisation efforts in the Americas like those they had pursued earlier in Liberia.[49] Hingson emphasised the complementary nature of their efforts in a letter to Johnson in January 1966.[50] Hingson and his fellow medical professionals all held full-time positions and devoted themselves to intensive, international medical missions only occasionally. After Liberia, the next significant Brother's Brother Foundation initiative was a joint effort in 1965 with *Amigos de Honduras*, a group of Texan doctors and volunteers affiliated with the River Oaks Baptist Church in Houston.[51] The group benefited from financial and in-kind donations in its efforts to vaccinate Hondurans against diseases including polio, tuberculosis, smallpox and diphtheria, among others. The team dispensed hundreds of thousands of shots.[52]

Medical intervention in Costa Rica

Brother's Brother Foundation reached out to Latin American governments in 1967 offering medical missions to immunise against polio, tuberculosis, leprosy, smallpox and measles.[53] By responding to requests from health ministers and other government officials, Brother's Brother Foundation worked to avoid 'volunteer colonialism', when locals are not adequately involved in developing and implementing projects.[54] Hingson reported that Brother's Brother Foundation, a small and highly founder-driven NGO, was concentrating its work in Central America because the region was in 'our own backyard'.[55]

Aguilar, the health minister of Costa Rica, responded in early June asking for help in combating a measles epidemic in the country.[56] Health ministry officials estimated that 10,000 Costa Rican children had measles, and one in eleven Costa Rican children with measles were dying.[57] In response, Hingson and Brother's Brother Foundation organised a complex operation that vaccinated 846,000 Costa Ricans against smallpox and immunised them against measles and polio.[58] Hingson pledged that the volunteers would 'be traveling by truck, jeep, plane, boat, horse, donkey, and afoot' to reach 50,000 Costa Ricans a day.[59] At the time, only 60 per cent of Costa Ricans regularly received medical attention.[60]

United States government officials in San José and reporters in the United States tracked the effort. Before the mission commenced, US embassy reporting predicted 9,000 Costa Ricans under the age of ten would be inoculated against measles and smallpox by Brother's Brother Foundation. It also noted that the organisation planned to immunise as many as 1 million Costa Ricans against leprosy, polio and tuberculosis.[61] The *New York Times* covered the eighty-four volunteers, which included members of the Hingson family, as they travelled to Costa Rica for a month-long campaign. Potentially minimising the skills and commitment of the Brother's Brother Foundation participants, the *New York Times* characterised them as 'U.S. medical vacationers', rather than as medical practitioners or missionaries.[62] Local reports revealed that the volunteers would 'eat and sleep wherever they find themselves'.[63]

The team worked together with the Costa Rican public health department as well as the Pan American Health Organization (PAHO), a regional office of the WHO.[64] When Brother's Brother Foundation faced challenges in securing sufficient doses of the measles vaccine, the PAHO was able to provide some doses of the vaccine.[65] The health department of New York City contributed from its stockpile as well.[66] Brother's Brother Foundation also turned to the US ambassador to Costa Rica Clarence S. Boonstra for assistance.[67] Given the scope and urgency of the epidemic, Brother's Brother Foundation ultimately bought vaccine doses beyond its available funds.[68] The Costa Rica mission left Brother's Brother Foundation $101,000 in debt, an amount it tried to reduce through subsequent fundraising activities.[69]

Beyond vaccines, Brother's Brother Foundation also needed jet injectors to deliver the doses. Significantly, the US Department of Defense lent sixteen injectors, which fit into the evolution of the role of the US military in those years.[70] The 1959 US Mutual Security Act had emphasised a shift to focus on 'socio-economic improvement'.[71] Civic action was the component of military assistance that addressed development needs, including medicine and health. This element made up 15.8 per cent of US military assistance to Latin America in 1966.[72] The medical department of the US military services participated in the delivery of medical services and therefore facilitated development efforts. An army report noted, 'Civic action has, therefore, become a strategic concept rather than a military tactic.'[73] Intriguingly, Hingson framed his work in terms of a 'war' against death in which the 'enemy' was disease. The 'army', his band of medical professionals, confronted these challenges with 'weapons' such as vaccine and 'artillery' like the jet injector, making explicit connections with more conventional battles at the time.[74]

The measles immunisations had dramatic effects with total measles cases and deaths decreasing significantly. In contrast to the 3,811

Costa Ricans who were hospitalised with measles in 1967, that number dropped to 97 in 1968.[75] In a sign of the significance with which the Costa Rican government treated the mission, Hingson and Brother's Brother Foundation team members met with the Costa Rican president José Joaquín Trejos to discuss their campaign.[76] Reporting on the endeavour, the US embassy characterised the efforts a 'success' and pointed specifically to the benefits of the jet injector method as easing the process.[77] Boonstra wrote later to Hingson, 'There is no question but that your program was indeed successful.' The ambassador added, 'The campaign has immeasurably strengthened the bonds of friendship and goodwill between Costa Rica and our country,' suggesting it enhanced American soft power in the country.[78]

Conclusion

Historians of development and modernisation have shown that NGOs and non-state actors such as missionaries have long aided the US government in achieving such goals.[79] Historian Amanda McVety has shown a recognition, dating back at least to the 1920s, that security could be facilitated through 'the expansion of human welfare'.[80] Dispensing vaccinations and medicine produced an immediate improvement in health and development as opposed to other types of development that might take much longer to reveal their benefits.[81] A number of voluntary associations, including the health organisations Project Hope and MEDICO were founded after Hingson's medical survey trip. In the view of one observer, these organisations, as well as the Peace Corps, were inspired by similar humanitarian impulses.[82] They also reveal non-governmental responses to the expansion of US power internationally.

Efforts relating to international health in the Johnson years, such as lending the jet injectors, were also part of a broader pursuit of modernisation and economic development at this time. Missionaries, foundations and other groups increased their modernisation efforts in the early years of the Cold War.[83] Historian Amy Staples writes about the years after the Second World War as 'the birth of development' or when the idea began 'that development was an international obligation'.[84] But rather than an obligation, other scholars have argued the United States often saw overseas assistance, including in health, as a 'tool' of its Cold War foreign policy.[85]

United States' support for Brother's Brother Foundation in Costa Rica fit into attempts to internationalise Johnson's domestic vision of a Great Society.[86] United States' efforts regarding disease were driven, in part, by a conviction that many tropical diseases were not necessarily linked to their geography but rather to 'poverty, social deprivation, malnutrition and insanitary conditions'.[87] These factors might also leave a country vulnerable to communist influence, a development of grave concern to US Cold War era leaders. Matthew Connelly argues that defence officials in the Johnson administration saw national and social security as two elements in a 'continuum'.[88] Brother's Brother Foundation's campaign therefore should be considered in the context of the Cold War consensus shaping Americans' conceptions of their individual and collective positions in the world. Support for discrete efforts to eradicate disease and therefore economic under-development and political instability fit into broader reconfigurations of the role of the United States internationally within the American Century.

Notes

1. The author expresses her appreciation to Lauren Carruth, Daniel Fine, Julia Irwin, Jennifer Johnson, Amanda McVety, Amanda Moniz, Inderjeet Parmar, Andrew Preston and Giles Scott-Smith for their feedback and suggestions; to Jaclyn Fox, Matthew Hartwell, Patrick Kendall and Ingrid Korsgard for research assistance; and to American University's School of International Service for research support. Joseph S. Nye Jr, *Soft Power: The Means to Success in World Politics* (New York: Public Affairs, 2004). Like the United States, Cuba has also sought 'symbolic capital' through health diplomacy. Julie M. Feinsilver, 'Cuba as a "World Medical Power": The Politics of Symbolism', *Latin American Research Review* 24:2 (1989), 18.
2. Kyle Longley, *Sparrow and the Hawk: Costa Rica and the United States during the Rise of Jose Figueres* (Tuscaloosa: University of Alabama Press, 1997).
3. Luther L. Terry, 'The Appeal Abroad of American Medicine and Public Health', *Annals of the American Academy of Political and Social Science* 366:1 (1966), 80.
4. Some members of Congress were cautious about disease eradication efforts, fearing that, say the end of malaria, might lead to an explosion in world population. Marcos Cueto, *Cold War, Deadly Fevers: Malaria Eradication in Mexico, 1955–1975* (Washington, DC: Woodrow Wilson Center Press, 2007), 57, 59.
5. Hugh L. Carey, 'A War We Can Win: Health as a Vector of Foreign Policy', *Bulletin of the New York Academy of Medicine* 46:5 (1970), 339.
6. Ibid., 335.
7. Sunil S. Amrith, 'Internationalising Health in the Twentieth Century', in Glenda Sluga and Patricia Clavin (eds), *Internationalisms: A Twentieth-Century History* (New York: Cambridge University Press, 2017), 263–4.
8. Cueto, *Cold War, Deadly Fevers*, 5, 7, 57–61; Randall Packard, 'Visions of Postwar Health and Development and Their Impact on Public

Health Interventions in the Developing World', in Frederick Cooper and Randall Packard (eds), *International Development and the Social Sciences: Essays on the History and Politics of Knowledge* (Berkeley: University of California Press, 1997), 98; Amrith, 'Internationalising Health in the Twentieth Century', 263–4; Bob H. Reinhardt, *The End of a Global Pox: America and the Eradication of Smallpox in the Cold War Era* (Chapel Hill: University of North Carolina Press, 2015), 65; A. E. Brin, 'Backstage: The Relationship between the Rockefeller Foundation and the World Health Organization, Part I: 1940s–1960s', *Public Health* 128 (2014), 130; Amanda Kay McVety, *The Rinderpest Campaigns: A Virus, Its Vaccines, and Global Development in the Twentieth Century* (New York: Cambridge University Press, 2018), 45; Christina Klein, *Cold War Orientalism: Asia in the Middlebrow Imagination, 1945–1961* (Berkeley: University of California Press, 2003), 9; Erez Manela, 'Smallpox and the Globalization of Development', in Stephen J. Macekura and Erez Manela (eds), *The Development Century: A Global History* (New York: Cambridge University Press, 2018), 97–8.

9. See, for example, Steve Marquardt, 'Pesticides, Parakeets, and Unions in the Costa Rican Banana Industry, 1938–1962', *Latin American Research Review* 37:2 (2001), 3–36; Lara Putnam, *The Company They Kept: Migrants and the Politics of Gender in the Caribbean Costa Rica, 1870–1960* (Chapel Hill: University of North Carolina Press, 2002); Steve Marquardt '"Green Havoc": Panama Disease, Environmental Change, and Labor Process in the Central American Banana Industry', *American Historical Review* (2001), 49–80; Kirk S. Bowman, '¿Fue el Compromiso y Consenso de las Élites lo qu Llevó a la Consolidación Democrática en Costa Rica?: Evidencias de la Década de 1950', *Revista De Historia* 41 (2000), 91–127; Steven Palmer, 'Central American Encounters with Rockefeller Public Health, 1914–1921', in Gilbert M. Joseph, Catherine C. LeGrand and Ricardo D. Salvatore (eds), *Close Encounters of Empire: Writing the Cultural History of US–Latin American Relations* (Durham, NC: Duke University Press, 1998), 311–32.

10. Rodolfo Cerdas Cruz, 'Costa Rica since 1930', in Leslie Bethell (ed.), *Central America since Independence* (Cambridge: Cambridge University Press, 1991), 299; Jon Hurwitz, Mark Peffley and Mitchell A. Seligson, 'Foreign Policy Belief Systems in Comparative Perspective: The United States and Costa Rica', *International Studies Quarterly* 37:3 (1993), 248. Through the 1960s, Costa Rica had a Guardia Civil, whose members numbered around 1,200. Graeme S. Mount, 'Costa Rica and the Cold War, 1948–1990', *Canadian Journal of History* 50:2 (2015), 296; Juan Carlos Zarate, *Forging Democracy: A Comparative Study of the Effects of US Foreign Policy on Central American Democratization* (New York: University Press of America, 1994), 29.

11. John F. Kennedy, 'Remarks at the University of Costa Rica in San Jose', 20 March 1963, American Presidency Project, available at:

https://www.presidency.ucsb.edu/documents/remarks-the-university-costa-rica-san-jose, last accessed 21 September 2016.

12. For more on Brother's Brother Foundation's origins and initial mission to Liberia, see Sarah B. Snyder, 'Guns of Peace and an Early Campaign Against Smallpox', *Historical Journal* 65:2 (2022), 462–81.

13. Monrovia to Secretary of State, 12 January 1962, 876.55/1-1262, Box 2769, Central Decimal File, 1960–1963, Record Group 59 General Records of the Department of State, National Archives and Records Administration, College Park, MD (hereafter RG 59 and NARA); Department of State to Monrovia, 19 January 1962, ibid.; Orr to Adler, 12 January 1962, Brother's Brother, Container 2, Entry #P616, Subject Files, 1961–1969, Record Group 286 Records of the Agency for International Development, NARA (hereafter RG 286); Orr to McConnell, 16 January 1962, ibid.

14. USS *Diamond Head* (AE-19) Ship's History, Naval History and Heritage Command, Washington, DC.

15. This literature will be enhanced by Julia Irwin, *Catastrophic Diplomacy: US Foreign Disaster Assistance in the American Century* (Chapel Hill, University of North Carolina Press, forthcoming).

16. Telegram 15167, 30 August 1967, PC 3, Confidential File Box 75, White House Central Files, Lyndon B. Johnson Library, Austin Texas (hereafter LBJL).

17. Note, 6 September 1967, PC 3, Confidential File Box 75, White House Central Files, LBJL.

18. Rostow to Johnson, 5 September 1967, PC 3, Confidential File Box 75, White House Central Files, LBJL; '"Peace Gun" Kills Inoculation Pains: Jet Injector can Administer Vaccines without Needle', *New York Times*, 5 October 1968, 58. Hingson asserted that the Pentagon's contribution 'made the difference between success and failure' given problems with Brother's Brother Foundation's injectors. Hingson to President, 30 August 1967, Hingson, Robert Name File, White House Central Files, LBJL.

19. Scott Felipse, 'The Latest Casualty of War: Catholic Relief Services, Humanitarianism, and the War in Vietnam, 1967–1968', *Peace and Change* 27:2 (2002), 251.

20. Alison Bashford, 'Global Biopolitics and the History of World Health', *History of the Human Sciences* 19:1 (2006), 71; James L. A. Webb Jr, *Humanity's Burden: A Global History of Malaria* (New York: Cambridge University Press, 2009), 146; Palmer, 'Central American Encounters with Rockefeller Public Health, 1914–1921', 311.

21. Marcos Cueto and Steven Palmer, *Medicine and Public Health in Latin America: A History* (New York: Cambridge University Press, 2015), 109.

22. Brin, 'Backstage', 130.

23. Robert David Johnson, 'Constitutionalism Abroad and at Home: The United States Senate and the Alliance for Progress, 1961–1967', *International History Review* 21:2 (1999), 434; Robert A. Packenham,

Liberal America and the Third World: Political Development Ideas in Foreign Aid and Social Science (Princeton, NJ: Princeton University Press, 2016), 95.

24. John H. Coatsworth, *Central America and the United States: The Clients and the Colossus* (New York: Twayne Publishers, 1994), 111; Thomas M. Leonard, *Central America and the United States: The Search for Stability* (Athens: University of Georgia Press, 1991), 153.

25. Lyndon B. Johnson, 'Remarks at the Signing of the Health Research Facilities Amendments of 1965', 9 August 1965, American Presidency Project, available at: https://www.presidency.ucsb.edu/documents/remarks-the-signing-the-community-mental-health-centers-act-amendments-1965, last accessed 21 March 2023; Elena Conis, *Vaccine Nation: America's Changing Relationship with Immunization* (Chicago: University of Chicago Press, 2015), 53.

26. Lyndon B. Johnson, 'Special Message to the Congress Proposing International Education and Health Programs', 2 February 1966, American Presidency Project, available at: https://www.presidency.ucsb.edu/documents/special-message-the-congress-proposing-international-education-and-health-programs, last accessed 2 April 2018.

27. Francis J. Gavin and Mark Atwood Lawrence, 'Introduction', Francis J. Gavin and Mark A. Lawrence (eds), *Beyond the Cold War: Lyndon Johnson and the New Global Challenges of the 1960s* (New York: Oxford University Press, 2014), 1.

28. H.S. 12453 [Report No. 1317], 11 March 1966.

29. Peter J. Hoetz, 'Vaccines as Instruments of Foreign Policy', *EMBO Reports* 21:101 (2001), 864; Bob H. Reinhardt, 'The Global Great Society and the US Commitment to Smallpox Eradication', *Endeavour* 34:4 (2010), 169.

30. Telegram 15167, 30 August 1967, PC 3, Confidential File Box 75, White House Central Files, LBJL.

31. American Embassy San Jose, 1 September 1967, PC 3, Confidential File Box 75, White House Central Files, LBJL.

32. Memorandum of Conversation, 11 April 1967, Costa Rica, vol. I 4/64-10/68, Box 15, National Security File, LBJL.

33. Cyril E. Bryant, *Operation Brother's Brother* (Old Tappan, NJ: Fleming H. Revell, 1968), 32. For more on the intersection of peace, the Vietnam War, and the Cold War, see Petra Goedde, *The Politics of Peace: A Global Cold War History* (New York, Oxford University Press, 2019). For more on the intersection of the war in Vietnam and smallpox eradication, see Reinhardt, *The End of a Global Pox*, 91, 101.

34. Abram to Moyers, 7 September 1965, Hingson, Dr Robert, Box 263, Office Files of John Mach, LBJL; Biographic Data, Hingson, Dr Robert, Box 263, Office Files of John Macy, LBJL.

35. Bryant, *Operation Brother's Brother*, 37.

36. 'Robert Hingson, Founder Of Brother's Brother Foundation', Brother's Brother Foundation, available at: http://www.brothersbrother.org/bbfs-founder, last accessed 23 June 2017; Robert A. Hingson, Hamilton S.

Davis and Michael Rosen, 'The Historical Development of Jet Injection and Envisioned Uses in Mass Immunization and Mass Therapy Based upon Two Decades of Experience', *Military Medicine* 128:6 (1963), 516–524. Aaron Ismach also played a role in developing jet injectors. Erez Manela, 'Globalizing the Great Society: Lyndon Johnson and the Pursuit of Small-pox Eradication,' in Francis J. Gavin and Mark Atwood Lawrence (eds), *Beyond the Cold War: Lyndon Johnson and the New Global Challenges of the 1960s* (New York: Oxford University Press, 2014), 170.

37. Robert A. Hingson, 'The Development of the Hypospray for Parenteral Therapy by Jet Injection', *Anesthesiology* 10:1 (1949), 66–75; Robert A. Hingson, 'America's Challenge in the Field of Public Health', *Journal of the National Medical Association* 50:2 (1958), 114–16; Robert A. Hingson, Hamilton S. Davis and Michael Rosen, 'Clinical Experience with One and a Half Million Jet Injections in Parenteral Therapy and in Preventive Medicine', *Military Medicine* 128:6 (1963), 525–8; Hingson, Davis and Rosen, 'The Historical Development of Jet Injection and Envisioned Uses in Mass Immunization and Mass Therapy Based Upon Two Decades of Experience', 516–24.

38. Bryant, *Operation Brother's Brother*, 39, 63.

39. Ibid., 22; Charles E. Rosenberg, *The Cholera Years: The United States in 1832, 1849, and 1866* (Chicago: University of Chicago Press, 1987), 213.

40. Robert S. Denny, 'Dr. Hingson's Magnificent Obsession', *Baptist World* (1965), 16.

41. Hingson and Brother's Brother Foundation repeatedly demonstrated a commitment to religious and racial inclusion in the composition of their missions. Bryant, *Operation Brother's Brother*, 56–7.

42. Ibid., 62–7; 'Bishop to Preach on Vietnam War', *Washington Post*, 15 April 1967, E13.

43. Bryant, *Operation Brother's Brother*, 70.

44. 'Robert Hingson, Founder of Brother's Brother Foundation', Brother's Brother Foundation, available at: http://www.brothersbrother.org/bbfs-founder, last accessed 23 June 2017.

45. John R. Haddad, *America's First Adventure in China: Trade, Treaties, Opium, and Salvation* (Philadelphia, PA: Temple University Press, 2013), 100–8.

46. Melani McAlister, *The Kingdom of God Has No Borders: A Global History of American Evangelicals* (New York: Oxford University Press, 2018), 21.

47. Emily Conroy-Krutz, *Christian Imperialism: Converting the World in the Early American Republic* (Ithaca, NY: Cornell University Press, 2015), 52.

48. The focus on Brother's Brother Foundation in this chapter is not intended to neglect the role of non-American actors in smallpox eradication. For a call to foreground those contributors, see Sanjoy Bhattacharya and Carlos Eduardo D'Avila Pereira Campani, 'Re-assessing the Foundations: Worldwide Smallpox Eradication, 1957–67', *Medical History* 64:1 (2020), 71–93.

49. Bryant, *Operation Brother's Brother*, 100–1.
50. Hingson to Johnson, 15 January 1966, Hingson, Robert Name File, WHCF, LBJL.
51. Cleland to Johnson, 25 September 1965, Hingson, Robert Name File, WHCF, LBJL.
52. Gainer F. Bryan Jr, 'Doctor Gives Honduras Shot in the Arm', *Plain Dealer Sunday Magazine*, 12 August 1965.
53. In these years, the Bacille Calmette-Guérin (BCG) vaccine was utilised in many cases against tuberculosis and leprosy.
54. Joseph H. Blatchford, 'The Peace Corps: Making It in the Seventies', *Foreign Affairs* 49:1 (1970), 129.
55. '"Peace Gun" Kills Inoculation Pains: Jet Injector Can Administer Vaccines Without Needle', *New York Times*, 5 October 1968, 58.
56. Robert J. Holmes, 'Costa Rican Plea for Aid Answered', *Cleveland Plain Dealer*, 28 July 1967, 1; Bryant, *Operation Brother's Brother*, 119–20. Such steps were necessary because as historian Steve Marquardt argues, the Costa Rican government historically 'legitimized its rule through a paternalistic hygienicist stance'. Marquardt, 'Pesticides, Parakeets, and Unions in the Costa Rican Banana Industry, 1938–1962', 30.
57. Bryant, *Operation Brother's Brother*, 122, 153. Costa Rican President Jose Trejos was also concerned about outbreaks of smallpox cases in Colombia and Peru, as well as polio in Nicaragua and Panama. Holmes, 'Costa Rican Plea for Aid Answered'.
58. Wolfgang Saxon, 'Robert Andrew Hingson, 83, A Pioneer in Public Health', *New York Times*, 12 October 1996.
59. Holmes, 'Costa Rican Plea for Aid Answered'. Hingson also pulled a team together to combat a polio epidemic in Nicaragua at the same time. 'Nicaragua Polio Aid is Organized', *Cleveland Plain Dealer*, 5 July 1967, 29; Jon Bixler, 'Westlake Firm Helps Fight Nicaragua Polio', *Cleveland Plain Dealer* 11 July 1967, 27. See also Bryant, *Operation Brother's Brother*, 112–18.
60. American Embassy San Jose to Department of State, 7 April 1967, POL 2-1 Costa Rica 1/1/67, Box 2004, Central Foreign Policy Files, 1967–1969, RG 59, NARA. The population of Costa Rica in 1967 was 1.695 million. 'Costa Rica', available at: http://data.worldbank.org/country/costa-rica, last accessed 29 June 2017.
61. American Embassy San Jose to Department of State, 24 June 1967, POL 2-1 Costa Rica 1/1/67, Box 2004, Central Foreign Policy Files, 1967–1969, RG 59, NARA.
62. 'US Medical Vacationers to Immunize Costa Ricans', *New York Times*, 29 July 1967, 25; Bryant, *Operation Brother's Brother*, 127; and Interview with Ralph Hingson, 29 May 2018.
63. Mary Hirschfeld, '85 Ohio Nurses, Doctors Pack for Antimeasles War', *Cleveland Plain Dealer*, 18 July 1967, 13.
64. Interview with Ralph Hingson, 29 May 2018.
65. Bryant, *Operation Brother's Brother*, 124.

66. Holmes, 'Costa Rican Plea for Aid Answered'. Unfortunately, the records of New York City Health Commissioner Edward O'Rourke did not reveal the genesis of this donation.
67. Bryant, *Operation Brother's Brother*, 123.
68. In a letter 'to Americans', Hingson expressed some frustration that the US government or USAID would not support this effort through allocation of funding for vaccine doses. 'A Plan to Save 1500 Costa Rican Children from Death and Eliminate Measles and Smallpox', Hingson, Robert Name File, White House Central Files, LBJL. Later correspondence shows support from Catholic charities, the First Baptist Church of Cleveland, and the American Baptist Convention. Hingson to President, 30 August 1967, Hingson, Robert Name File, White House Central Files, LBJL.
69. Bryant to Denny, 16 September 1967, Folder 5.6D, Box 57, Baptist World Alliance Archives, American Baptist Historical Society, Atlanta, Georgia (hereafter BWA Archives); Bryant, *Operation Brother's Brother*, 126, 147.
70. Although documentary evidence to support such a claim does not exist, Hingson's brother James worked in the Pentagon and perhaps marshalled its resources to support Brother's Brother Foundation's work. Hingson to Tolbert and Tolbert, 10 May 1965, Folder 5.6C, Box 57, BWA Archives. The PAHO also provided one jet injector gun. Bryant, *Operation Brother's Brother*, 124.
71. US Army Civic Action Report, LATAM vol. V 1963–1967, Box 7, Accession Number 338-99, Record Group 530 US Southern Command, NARA (hereafter RG 530).
72. Leonard, *Central America and the United States*, 165–6.
73. US Army Civic Action Report, LATAM vol. V 1963–1967, Box 7, Accession Number 338-99, RG 530, NARA.
74. Robert A. Hingson, 'Amigos de Honduras Fight War with "Peace Guns"', *Medical Tribune*, 16–17 October 1965, 6.
75. Bryant, *Operation Brother's Brother*, 162.
76. Ibid., 125.
77. American Embassy San Jose to Department of State, 8 September 1967, POL 2-1 Costa Rica 1/1/67, Box 2004, Central Foreign Policy Files, 1967–1969, RG 59, NARA.
78. Bryant, *Operation Brother's Brother*, 135.
79. David Ekbladh, *The Great American Mission: Modernization and the Construction of an American World Order* (Princeton, NJ: Princeton University Press, 2010), 23.
80. McVety, *The Rinderpest Campaigns*, 45.
81. Manela, 'Smallpox and the Globalization of Development', 85.
82. Bryant, *Operation Brother's Brother*, 146.
83. Ibid., 154.
84. Amy L. S. Staples, *The Birth of Development: How the World Bank, Food and Agriculture Organization, and World Health Organization*

Changed the World, 1945–1965 (Kent, OH: The Kent State University Press, 2006), 2.

85. Julia F. Irwin, *Making the World Safe: The American Red Cross and a Nation's Humanitarian Awakening* (New York: Oxford University Press, 2013), 2. Some sceptics suggest these Cold War era efforts were often driven by political motivations. Gavin and Lawrence, 'Introduction', 7.

86. See, for example, Sheyda Jahanbani, 'One Global War on Poverty: The Johnson Administration Fights Poverty at Home and Abroad, 1964–1968', in Francis J. Gavin and Mark Atwood Lawrence (eds), *Beyond the Cold War: Lyndon Johnson and the New Global Challenges of the 1960s* (New York: Oxford University Press, 2014), 97–117; Nick Cullather, 'LBJ's Third War: The War on Hunger', in Francis J. Gavin and Mark Atwood Lawrence (eds), *Beyond the Cold War: Lyndon Johnson and the New Global Challenges of the 1960s* (New York: Oxford University Press, 2014), 118–40.

87. David Arnold, 'Introduction', in D. Arnold (ed.), *Warm Climates and Western Medicine: The Emergence of Tropical Medicine, 1500–1900* (Atlanta, GA: Rodopi, 1996), 4. Historian David Engerman has emphasised that development aid 'helped shape new patterns of relations between nations'. David C. Engerman, 'Development Politics and the Cold War', *Diplomatic History* 1:1 (2017), 1. But, due to lack of Costa Rican records from the Trejos years, we cannot see to what extent Costa Rica made claims utilising Cold War or development rhetoric with Hingson and the US government.

88. Matthew Connelly, 'LBJ and World Population: Planning the Greater Society One Family at a Time', Francis J. Gavin and Mark Atwood Lawrence (eds), *Beyond the Cold War: Lyndon Johnson and the New Global Challenges of the 1960s* (New York: Oxford University Press, 2014), 145.

10

AIDS and Reproductive Rights in the American Century

Emma Day

'If a pregnant woman tested positive for the AIDS virus, would you recommend an abortion?' one reporter asked Surgeon General Charles Everett Koop as he stood among a crowd of journalists and twenty-two television cameras at the National Press Club on 24 March 1987. All of those present anticipated that the surgeon general's words – the answer from a self-proclaimed evangelical Christian, nominated by the avowed anti-abortion President Ronald Reagan – would be headlined on the evening news and next day's papers.[1] 'If you wanted to give her all the possibilities that were available to her, you would have to mention abortion,' Koop replied.[2] While Koop later reassured reporters that his personal opposition to abortion had not changed, his conservative advocates viewed his pronouncement as an evidence of his 're-thinking' on the subject.[3] Although Koop's commitment to public health compelled him to confirm that abortion was legal and possible in 1987, he was never motivated by a duty to affirm women's reproductive rights. Instead, like many other government officials, he wanted to protect children from HIV.

'One of the things I think is most important about this,' he continued, 'is my great concern for the babies who are born to positive mothers. I think no woman should contemplate a pregnancy without voluntarily wanting to be tested for the AIDS virus.'[4] In September 1982, after receiving reports of immunodeficiency disorders in young, White men, the Centers for Disease Control and Prevention (CDC) defined a new disease, AIDS (acquired immunodeficiency syndrome), as the presence of Kaposi sarcoma, *Pneumocystis carinii* pneumonia, and a series of other opportunistic infections that suggested the failure of an otherwise healthy person's immune system.[5] The CDC reported its first notices on AIDS in infants three months later.[6] In 1985, the Food Drug Administration (FDA) approved ELISA, the first commercial test to screen human blood for HIV. By the end of the year, they confirmed that women could transmit HIV during pregnancy, childbirth and breastfeeding.[7] The news that infants became infected primarily through mother-to-child transmission, that rates of transmission varied from 30 to 70 per cent, that infants born with HIV would likely become seriously ill and cripple the state financially in the process, and that rates of AIDS in women and children were rising – 3,601 and 737, respectively in 1987 – political and public health figures like Koop called for testing to identify HIV-positive women and advise those who tested positive to not have children in the 1980s.[8]

Deep-seated cultural anxieties over infant mortality and disability in children informed Koop's advice. In the early to mid-twentieth century, lawmakers seeking to limit births among those deemed 'unfit' to promote Anglo-American dominance and avoid the expense of caring for disabled and unwell children in a for-profit health system in which care is considered a privilege and not a right introduced policies that restricted women's reproductive freedoms in the name of public health. This eugenicist thinking also informed the political response to AIDS in the 1980s, as conservative lawmakers and political commentators who expressed concern about the financial and moral cost of caring for HIV-positive children worked to limit the reproductive freedoms of multiply marginalised women with HIV – those whose identities and social status placed them at the intersection of more than one vector of discrimination and limited their access to elite power structures. Using AIDS as a wedge to expand power over women's bodies, the official response to AIDS in women violated the values of freedom, equality and cooperation in the American Century. This power manifested in increasingly coercive and punitive ways as public health became more privatised and politicised over the course of the century.

The AIDS epidemic emerged at a moment of conservative backlash against women's reproductive rights, including the right to plan for, terminate or bring a pregnancy to term. After the Supreme Court upheld a woman's constitutional right to abortion in the 1973 case *Roe* v. *Wade*,[9] conservatives mobilised to overturn the decision. Establishing that a foetus is a person with moral and legal rights equal to a woman's was central to their strategy. Immediately after *Roe*, conservative members of Congress began introducing statutes and amendments to the constitution declaring that life began at conception, thereby equating abortion and murder.[10] As attempts to ban abortion nationally floundered, anti-abortion activists pursued other options, passing the Hyde amendment which banned the use of Medicaid to fund abortions in 1976.[11] As Congress succeeded in making abortion less accessible to low-income women, the language of foetal rights informed abortion restrictions at the state level.[12] The fight to establish foetal personhood also advanced with the 'war' on drug use against communities of colour in the 1980s, as medics began testing and disproportionately reporting to law enforcement pregnant Black and Native American women suspected of using substances that allegedly harmed their foetuses.[13] The same logic that the state should intervene to protect foetuses from the behaviours of supposedly 'irresponsible' women, and society from the financial and emotional cost of caring for sick and apparently 'undesirable' children, similarly underwrote the testing, reporting and punishment of HIV-positive women in connection with their pregnancies.

The assault on reproductive rights since *Roe* symbolised the punitive turn that accompanied the advance of neoliberalism in American politics at the end of the twentieth century. In the 1970s, lawmakers proposed competing visions of the causes of and solutions to the challenges facing the country following the social, economic and political upheavals of the previous decades. Those calling for cuts in welfare support for the supposedly 'non-working' poor tapped into entrenched racial and gender prejudices that attributed the presence of poverty and social unrest in certain racial communities to their perceived pathology, and especially the apparent shortcomings of single, non-White women. Instead of addressing the inequalities that underpinned social disparities by, for example, investing in public healthcare, conservative policymakers shifted the responsibility of supporting marginalised communities from state agencies to private organisations and the White, heterosexual, middle-class, male-headed nuclear family whom they framed the regulator of acceptable private behaviour. The shrinking of the welfare state, and emphasis on the family and private sector as the guarantors of public order, did not signal a reduction in government size, capacity or will. Instead, the state 'redeployed' its administrative power, increasing funding to law enforcement departments and building new prisons to punish those seen to have violated the strict standards of normative behaviour that the rising 'family values politics' of this period prescribed.[14] With this retrenchment of the welfare state and the expansion of the carceral state that underpinned the development of neoliberalism in the late twentieth century, conservative lawmakers framed the state as the 'protector' of 'innocent' citizens from the supposedly 'immoral' lifestyles of those who fell beyond the boundaries of normative society, including – from the 1980s onwards – multiply marginalised women with HIV and their children.

In line with the gutting of social welfare programmes and the move towards a neoliberal social agenda that dovetailed with the expansion of the carceral state in the 1980s, the official response to AIDS in women shifted the responsibility for dealing with the social issues related to illness away from the government and onto people with the fewest resources. Reflecting the historical expectation of women to put the symbolic needs of children before their own, the state placed this burden on women. But government figures tended not match their rhetorical concern for foetuses and infants with structural support to help HIV-positive women get tested and, if positive, navigate their illness, their reproductive wishes or the illness of their child. Instead, they restricted their access to the abortion care and the other family planning services that enabled them to control their reproductive health and passed legislation criminalising the pregnancies of women who failed to prevent conception. These measures did not help infants or women. Rather, they advanced the family values agenda of promoting sex and pregnancy in marriage, relying on the nuclear family to provide support for vulnerable groups in the absence of a social safety net, and punishing those who suffered from a lack of state support. Political figures vilified multiply marginalised HIV-positive women to justify the use of criminal penalties, seeking to absolve the government of the responsibility of investing in what Steven W. Thrasher has termed the 'conceptual prophylaxis' of housing, education and freedom from incarceration that protects people from disease and supports them caring for their children.[15] Koop's speech at the Press Club therefore illustrates how HIV testing became interwoven with structural inequalities beyond homophobia and racist xenophobia, including the underacknowledged struggle over reproductive justice.[16]

In the context of the anti-abortion, anti-welfare and tough-on-crime politics of the 1980s, the alarm that some government officials expressed over the cost and care of HIV-positive children therefore resulted in increased efforts to control women's reproductive health choices. Initially, these concerns drove some physicians to pressure HIV-positive women to end their pregnancies. They did not, however, result in a widening of abortion access, as the government figures who called for prevention framed their arguments not in terms of women's reproductive health rights but foetal rights. The same currents of thought informing advice for women to abort underwrote abortion restrictions, and the surveillance of women. The case study of AIDS and reproductive rights is an example of the government using disease outbreaks not as an opportunity to expand access to affordable and effective healthcare, but to reinscribe the hierarchies of sex, gender, race and class fuelling socio-economic inequality.

Testing women

On 14 November 1988, thirty-eight-year-old Carol Doe, a five-month pregnant Haitian woman living in New York, visited Jamaica

Hospital in New York City for a routine prenatal check-up. During the visit, Doe received a test for HIV as part of her prenatal care which came back positive. Three days later, Doe met Dr Maurice Abitbol, chief of obstetrics and gynaecology at Jamaica Hospital. Since learning her test result, Doe had decided that she wanted to carry her pregnancy to term. A nurse recommended that she have an abortion, claiming that Doe was likely to pass HIV to her baby. Dr Abitbol agreed that Doe should terminate the pregnancy, adding that HIV-positive children placed a heavy burden on society. Doe was already a mother to a daughter born with spina bifida and Abitbol claimed that giving birth to a HIV-positive child was worse. After pleading with Abitbol and other practitioners to allow her to continue her prenatal care with Jamaica Hospital's high-risk programme, Abitbol referred Doe to King County Hospital, claiming that it provided superior care for HIV-positive women. Three weeks later, Doe received a second-trimester abortion at King County Hospital. The following year, the Center for Constitutional Rights (CCR) – a New York-based legal advocacy organisation founded in 1966 to advance civil rights legislation that in the 1980s helped people with HIV/AIDS facing discrimination in areas of employment, housing and reproductive rights – filed a suit on Doe's behalf against Jamaica Hospital, Kings County Hospital and the staff that treated her at both institutions, alleging that they breached their duties to provide appropriate care and obtain her informed consent.[17] Moreover, Doe claimed that the conduct of the staff violated her rights as a person with a disability as protected by section 504 of the Federal Rehabilitation Act 1973.[18] Although Justice Scholnick of the New York Supreme Court found that the requirements of section 504 did not apply, he ruled that Doe provided sufficient evidence to create an issue of fact as to whether Dr Abitbol negligently offered inaccurate advice upon which she acted in deciding to have an abortion.[19] Doe represented the many women who early in the epidemic saw the desire on the part of medical professionals and federal agencies to control their reproductive decisions as undermining their right to become pregnant or to carry a pregnancy to term.

Throughout the twentieth century, the outbreak of diseases that caused congenital disorders raised questions over who had the authority to determine whether a woman could plan for, terminate or continue a pregnancy. The political responses to these diseases had different implications for women's rights, especially along the lines of race, class, health and ability. During the Progressive Era, as reformers feared that increased immigration threatened Anglo-American dominance in US society and physicians warned that venereal disease increased sterility and harmed developing foetuses, several states – illustrative of their role in intermingling with reproductive rights – passed laws mandating premarital testing for venereal diseases, hoping to increase birth rates among White, married, 'respectable' and 'healthy' couples.[20] Driven by the same desire to decrease birth rates among the seemingly 'unfit', namely, recent immigrants, Black Americans, poor people, people with physical and intellectual disabilities and 'promiscuous' women, numerous states also legalised sterilisation and banned inter-racial marriage.[21] Scientists also routinely experimented on the bodies of Black, Latina, Native American and Puerto Rican women to develop new reproductive tools designed to tackle issues such as poverty, over-population and alcohol use.[22] The eugenicist thinking that informed these policies also shaped the state response to other genetic disease outbreaks, including Huntington's chorea in the early twentieth century.[23] In the 1960s, following an outbreak of German measles, a movement of doctors, religious leaders and lawmakers presented abortion as a necessary procedure that protected both women from giving birth to children with physical and intellectual disabilities and society from having to pay for their care. The fact that society perceived German measles as mostly afflicting White, heterosexual, middle-class women deemed responsible and respectable helped to liberalise attitudes to abortion.[24] In the presence of foetal defects, many perceived abortions for family and eugenicist reasons as acceptable.

Whether or not doctors like Abitbol provided substandard care, their view that HIV-positive women should end their pregnancies aligned with prevailing medical opinion. In December 1985, the CDC published guidelines urging 'at risk' women considering pregnancy – a designation that implied HIV impacted only certain women to the detriment of public health – to get tested and advised those who tested positive to 'delay' pregnancy 'until more is known about perinatal transmission of the virus'.[25] All states bar New Jersey followed the CDC in advising HIV-positive women to avoid pregnancy.[26] Physicians published articles in prominent medical journals such as the *Journal of the American Medical Association* supporting this position, citing the possibility women passing HIV on to their infants and the chance that pregnancy might accelerate their illness.[27] The advice mirrored that given to women in the context of Huntington disease and German measles in previous decades whom physicians and social workers told to delay or end pregnancy either through abortion, celibacy or sterilisation.[28] Although the CDC did not offer suggestions for how a woman might 'delay' pregnancy, women's health advocates such as Carola Marte and Kathryn Anastos expressed concern that without the prospect of scientists discovering a vaccine or cure soon and, in light of the increasing limits placed on abortion access in the form of public funding restrictions and physical harassment, doctors might pressure women to make unwanted decisions about their pregnancies.[29] As Jennifer Nelson noted, the threat of involuntary sterilisation increased in the absence of legal abortion.[30] In urging all 'at risk' women to get tested and advising that those who tested positive not to have children, the government's response to HIV drew on the same tactics used to tackle congenital diseases in the past.

Physicians spoke more candidly of their conviction that HIV-positive women should not have children beyond the pages of academic journals. At a 1988 conference on AIDS in the workplace, director of the CDC's AIDS programme, James Curran, described undetected cases of AIDS in pregnancy as 'a national tragedy' and asserted that the imperative to test pregnant women for HIV exceeded that of rubella or syphilis because AIDS 'is much, much, much, much worse. With AIDS, the baby will die and the mother will die'. Curran not only raised the alarm about AIDS mortality. Dovetailing with federal efforts to reduce healthcare spending under Reagan, he also raised concerns about the costs that HIV-positive children posed to the state. Through the 1981 Omnibus Budget Reconciliation Act (OBRA), Reagan introduced block grants that gave states less money for health and welfare programes but greater discretion over how to spend it, enabling them to reduce the number of people eligible for support. Vilifying people reliant on state aid, Reagan's policy proposals shaped a political discourse hostile to welfare which crystalised a decade later in the major welfare reform of President Bill Clinton.[31] As Congress worked to shrink the federal contribution to Medicaid, Curran also argued that HIV-positive women should avoid pregnancy to reduce healthcare costs. The 'small state' rhetoric of the Reagan administration that exploited deep-seated racist and gendered stereotypes about who is deserving of support informed Curran. Arguing that, as the expense of paediatric AIDS exceeded that of adults, and that 'Babies with AIDS have no parents' – a sweeping statement that lacked qualification – Curran protested that the burden of care would fall to the state. Although Curran's concerns over AIDS mortality were not unfounded – in 1988, AIDS was listed as the underlying cause of death for 249 children aged under fifteen and 1,430 for women aged 15–44 – calling HIV-positive women who wanted to become pregnant illogical betrayed his disregard for the multifaceted reasons informing a woman's wish to have a child.[32] Such inflammatory comments, reprinted in mainstream media outlets like the *Washington Post*, contributed to the presentation of HIV-positive women who became pregnant or continued a pregnancy as selfish and created a perception of 'crisis' in which coercive testing policies and advice appeared more acceptable.[33] Some male journalists agreed on the necessity of abortion in the presence of diseases, callously noting that 'any pregnant woman who has the lethal AIDS virus' or whose newborn 'will have a non-fatal affliction such as spina bifida or Down's syndrome . . . won't find me barring the door to the abortion clinic'.[34] These comments reveal assumptions about who should decide whether and when pregnancies continue or end and when it should be appropriate. Here, male journalists echoed the view of leading male physicians that the social cost of caring for sick infants outweighed the rights of HIV-positive women and their prospective children. This view reflected the conservative context committed to withdrawing state support in which they operated as well as the deep cultural anxiety about infant mortality and disability in children as seen throughout the American Century.

Punishing pregnancy

The historical association between genetic testing, the eugenics movement, and racist, classist and ableist reproductive control informed women's health advocates and activists' concerns over federal and state efforts to test HIV-positive pregnant women and infants.[35]

States responded differently to the CDC's 1985 guidance on perinatal HIV testing and lacked uniformity in the application of this public health measure. In Oregon, authorities mandated that medics report the names of infants who tested positive at anonymous testing sites, and, in 1987, New York mandated that doctors offer counselling and voluntary HIV testing to all pregnant women. As infants receive antibodies against different infections from women during pregnancy which they retain for several months after birth, testing infants for HIV antibodies only revealed the HIV status of the woman, not the baby.[36] Women's health advocates criticised the strategy of using an infant's test results as a 'proxy' for a woman's status, and called for voluntary testing, counselling, and follow-up treatment to all women considering pregnancy and all pregnant women giving birth. Moreover, widespread cuts to prenatal care and family planning services and abortion restrictions that limited women's ability to translate knowledge of their status into action raised concerns that health authorities might use the test results against women.[37]

The concurrent efforts of lawmakers to criminalise HIV transmission raised the stakes of state-wide initiatives to identify people with HIV. Driven by what Trevor Hoppe described as the combined impetus to control disease through coercion and punishment and regulate sex and gender norms in the post-war period, eight states – Florida, Georgia, Idaho, Michigan, Missouri, Oklahoma, South Carolina and Washington – enacted HIV exposure or non-disclosure laws in the 1980s. Implemented in mostly Republican states, the geographic sweep of these laws reflected the reach of the political agenda to 'criminalise sickness'. Lawmakers initially utilised the media panic over sex workers 'carrying' AIDS to the 'general' population to pass HIV-specific felony penalties targeting sex workers that they then applied to all people living with HIV.[38] The punishment of HIV-positive sex workers mirrored previous initiatives to police women's sexual behaviour in the name of public health, as well as the growing contemporary impetus to penalise those who engaged in non-normative and anti-normative sexual and gender behaviour during the era of advancing family values and tough-on-crime politics.[39]

The notion that the state should protect 'innocent' citizens from the supposedly 'immoral' behaviour of those seen as threatening public order also mirrored contemporary efforts to punish women for using substances that allegedly harmed foetuses during pregnancy. In 1985, the publication of a dubious medical study claiming that crack cocaine use during pregnancy harmed foetuses dovetailed with a moral panic about rising rates of drug use in Black communities and the supposed decline of Black families, both of which lawmakers in a political backlash against women's and civil rights blamed on Black single mothers.[40] The report sparked a public outcry that empowered law enforcement to target drug users as well as drug dealers, including pregnant women.[41] The focus on crack cocaine revealed the racism underlying these initiatives, just as the disproportionate targeting of women in public hospitals exposed class biases. Although White women used cocaine at a similar level to Black women, Black communities tended to smoke it in crack form.[42] Moreover, medical professionals tested the urine of Black pregnant patients without their consent more regularly, reporting those who tested positive to the police and child welfare authorities.[43] Judges also tended to prosecute the Black women whose cases came before them at higher rates.[44] The media representation of crack babies as Black solidified the association between the new so-called 'underclass' of infants supposedly destined to grow into 'troublesome' children, just as the media discussion of foetal alcohol spectrum disorders (FASDs) framed it as an 'Indian problem' for which judges sent Native women to prison and removed children from their care.[45]

In 1990, the federal government reinforced efforts to criminalise sickness through federal law, passing the Ryan White Care Act that provided funding for states AIDS services. The Act made receipt of federal funding dependent on a state's willingness to use criminal laws to prosecute any HIV-positive person who knowingly exposed a non-consenting adult to HIV.[46] A total of forty-five states enacted measures that made possible the criminalisation of HIV exposure and transmission, and this legislation continues today in thirty-five of them. The broad wording of these laws enabled the prosecution of HIV-positive women in relation to their pregnancies in most states.[47] The fact that some pregnant women who were tested for drugs were also tested for HIV underscores how the war on crack cocaine overlapped with the AIDS epidemic to put multiply marginalised women who wanted to have children at risk from punitive state intervention.[48]

As Carol Mason argued, abortion opponents' calls for 'foetal protection' took on a new meaning in the context of state efforts to regulate the pregnancies of women of colour. While anti-abortion advocates pushed for restrictions like the partial-birth abortion ban to stop White women ending their pregnancies, the threat of punishment disproportionately levelled against Black and Native American women encouraged them to end their pregnancies, suggesting that a racist desire not only to protect foetuses from the actions of women, but society from the social and financial costs of supporting supposedly 'undesirable' children drove these measures.[49] State and federal legislation that criminalised HIV transmission and exposure, coupled with the vilification of women wanting to continue their pregnancies, surely encouraged abortion in general. As Koop noted in 1987, 'in major obstetrical clinics on the East Coast, where the population has a high incidence of AIDS virus . . . women who are pregnant under 13 weeks are being advised to have abortions and about 50 percent of those, I understand, are indeed having abortions'.[50] Criminal legislation encouraged abortion without lawmakers endorsing the procedure out loud.

Nonetheless, the sentiment that HIV-positive women should not have children did not result in a widening of abortion access in the first decade of the epidemic. Rather, as officials like Koop advanced the notion that a foetus is an 'unborn child' requiring protection from women's bodies framed as harmful hosts and that abortion, while medically viable, constituted the 'slaughter of the unborn', the arguments informing the pressure for HIV-positive pregnant women to abort morphed into arguments underwriting abortion restrictions.[51]

In July 1989, the Supreme Court, in *Webster* v. *Reproductive Health Services,* upheld the right of states to deny women access to abortion counselling and procedures in publicly funded facilities and to require testing for viability if a woman was twenty or more weeks pregnant. The preamble to *Webster* drew on Koop's language of foetal rights, stating that 'the life of each human being begins at conception' and 'unborn children have protectable interests in life, health, and wellbeing'.[52] *Webster* set a precedent for further state-wide restrictions, including restrictions during the first trimester of pregnancy, mandated counselling before an abortion, wait times and warnings about the procedure's psychological risks.[53] These restrictions made abortion less accessible for all women, and especially low-income and young women, and women of colour with restricted access to healthcare.

The deep investment of women in the health of their pregnancies, future children and newborns cast a very different light on the rhetoric that identified them as a health threat to their children. In 1991, the AIDS Clinical Trials Group (ACTG), an organisation established in 1987 to develop AIDS research at the National Institute of Allergy and Infectious Diseases (NIAID), began recruiting women for a new treatment protocol, 076. This HIV trial was the first to include women in a major way as researchers initially excluded women from trials, fearing that women may become pregnant during the trials and the treatment might harm the pregnancy. Funded through the Department of Health and Human Services (HHS), National Institutes of Health (NIH) and NIAID, researchers designed the trial to establish whether azidothymidine (AZT) could prevent perinatal transmission of HIV if given to women during pregnancy and to infants after birth.[54] The trial began in 1993 and involved over 700 pregnant women.[55] As activists from ACT UP, African American Women United Against AIDS, and women doctors such as Janet Mitchell, a Black physician based at Harlem Hospital debated the ethics of enrolling women of colour given the toxicity of AZT and the long history of racialised medical abuse suffered in the name of objective science, many women expressed their desire for the trial to take place, eager to find a treatment that would stop them transmitting HIV during or after pregnancy.[56]

The trial went ahead as planned and had ground-breaking results, finding that AZT effectively reduced the risk for perinatal transmission from 25 per cent to less than 8 per cent. The US Public Health Service (PHS) recommended that doctors give pregnant women AZT to reduce the risk of perinatal transmission of HIV in 1994, leading to a sharp drop-off in paediatric AIDS cases from the mid-1990s onwards.[57]

The approval of the use of AZT in pregnancy in 1994 ended many of the political debates over prevention, abortion and motherhood and at least gave women who could access the drugs the possibility of reducing perinatal transmission without undermining their right to choose when and whether to have a child. The introduction of effective medicine nevertheless put women at increased risk of coercive HIV testing, as the CDC began recommending that states test women unless they specifically declined it (the opt-out approach), a measure that relies on physicians giving women clear information about the test to ensure informed consent. Several states, including North Carolina, Alabama and Arkansas, ignored this recommendation, either requiring or allowing physicians to test pregnant women without their consent.[58]

Moreover, the notion that women posed a threat to their pregnancies continued to contribute to the erosion of women's reproductive rights in the following decades. Since the 1980s, medical professionals and law enforcement officials have tested, arrested and detained several hundreds of mostly low-income and non-White women for actions taken during their pregnancies that allegedly harm their foetuses. Law enforcers have also punished women, mostly those believed to have used illegal drugs, on account of their HIV-positive status. Moreover, the testing of newborns and infants for HIV set a precedent for testing newborns and pregnant women without their consent, resulting in charges for drug delivery, manslaughter, homicide and other crimes.[59] Women have also continued to live with the legal consequences of the earlier moral panic over pregnant women infecting their children with HIV.

Conclusion

In January 2008, police arrested thirty-seven-year-old Cecelia Ann Sliker, a White woman, in her home in Bradenton, Florida, on a felony child neglect charge. Authorities charged Sliker for failing to seek treatment to prevent perinatal transmission of HIV when she became pregnant in 2004, as improvements in treatment options for children apparently left no excuse for her not to have pursued care. Sliker pleaded guilty to the charge at the trial where Circuit Judge Debra Johnes Riva sentenced her to fifteen years in prison. As part of a plea deal, Judge Riva reduced Sliker's sentence to two years' probation in Port Manatee jail. In the thirty-five states where HIV criminalisation laws are still active, pregnant women are legally obliged to disclose their HIV status to a partner and seek medical treatment on behalf of their pregnancies.[60]

Sliker is one of many women who has carried the burden of the earlier moral panic over pregnant women infecting their children with HIV. In 2009, the US District Judge for Maine, John Woodcock, doubled the sentence of QLT, a twenty-eight-year-old, HIV-positive, five-month pregnant woman from Cameroon originally arrested for falsifying immigration documents. Woodcock explained that he detained QLT until she gave birth to ensure that she took her anti-retroviral medication and stop her from 'assault(ing)' her 'unborn child' through HIV transmission, despite her having already arranged medical care in the United States.[61]

Woodcock's ruling perpetuated several harmful mis-assumptions that have informed the mistreatment of HIV-positive women wishing to become pregnant and bring a pregnancy to term in medicine, policy and law since the 1980s. These include the idea that women are the containers for foetuses who are already children with rights; secondly, that foetal health is distinct from women's health, and that women's bodies are harmful to developing pregnancies; thirdly, that women, and, especially those deemed unworthy of the privileges of citizenship on account of their immigration or legal status, are incapable of making rational judgements about their medical needs; and, fourthly, that the state is obliged to intervene in a woman's reproductive life to not only 'protect' a foetus from the apparently harmful actions of its mother, but society from the moral and financial costs of caring for the sick infant. These assumptions have become more institutionally entrenched since the 1980s, as medical advances have empowered hostile law enforcement and judges to exercise their biases, challenging historians to resist neat endings following scientific discoveries. It also reflects how far coercion and punishment have come to shape the political approach to women's health since the Reagan era.

Ronald Reagan came to office in 1981 as policymakers calling to 'get tough' on groups requiring government support began winning the argument about what the state should prioritise in preserving public order. Reagan advanced this emerging 'law and order' agenda, promising to roll-back recent advances in civil rights in part through the re-establishment of prescriptive normative sex and gender roles in what became known as the 'family values politics' of the 1980s. Public figures leading the early AIDS response operated within a political context committed to upholding White, middle-class heteronormativity in ways that blunted effective, systematic measures to curb the epidemic. In the following decades, subsequent administrations continued to channel administrative energy and resources away from social welfare and towards law enforcement programmes, pursuing increasingly punitive policy objectives that harmed women as well as other vulnerable populations, including the obliteration of welfare, the expansion of prisons and the failure to implement universal health reform. The extreme anti-gay, anti-woman, anti-immigrant and anti-welfare agenda of the Trump administration marked the culmination of a forty-year campaign on the part of conservative lawmakers and activists to restore White, heteronormative 'traditional values' and punish those seen to exist in opposition to them.

The HIV/AIDS epidemic illuminates the struggle between the US government and society over who is considered deserving and undeserving of state support and included or excluded from the idea of 'the public'. As with other health crises in the American Century that called into question the responsibility of the state to citizens and citizens to one another to advance public health, officials responding to HIV/AIDS expected women to put the symbolic needs of children before their own. This expectation manifested in increasingly coercive and punitive ways as public health became more politicised and privatised over the course of the century. The coercive and punitive response to AIDS has done nothing to help women or children. Instead, the spectre of punishment, and the fear, stigma and shame that it engenders, deters women from seeking HIV testing, treatment and prenatal care, and therefore fails as a public health measure. The official response to HIV/AIDS contributed to the devaluation of women's right to motherhood and undermined reproductive justice, thus presenting a threat to the ideals, values, and capacities of the American Century.

Notes

1. Memorandum from Donald A. Clarey to Nancy J. Risque, 'Dr. Koop's Speech at the Press Club', 24 March 1987, Box 1, fol. 'AIDS – HHS/Koop' (1 of 2), T. Kenneth Cribb files, Ronald Reagan Presidential Library, Simi Valley, California (hereafter, RRPL).
2. 'Pre-Pregnancy AIDS Test Urged', *AP-NY*, 25 March 1987, 1, Box 1, fol. 'AIDS – HHS/Koop' (1 of 2), Cribb files, RRPL.
3. Jack Fowler, 'Koop Report to Find No Proof of Abort Damage to Women', *Lifeletter* 4 (1988), 2, Box 14, series II, Nancy Risque files, RRPL.
4. 'Pre-Pregnancy AIDS Test Urged,' 1.
5. CDC, 'Current Trends Update on Acquired Immune Deficiency Syndrome (AIDS) – United States', *Morbidity and Mortality Weekly Report* 31:37 (1982), 507–8, 513–14.
6. CDC, 'Epidemiological Notes and Reports Possible Transfusion-Associated Acquired Immune Deficiency Syndrome (AIDS) – California', *Morbidity and Mortality Weekly Report* 31:48 (1982), 652–4;

CDC, 'Unexplained Immunodeficiency and Opportunistic Infections in Infants – New York, New Jersey, California', *Morbidity and Mortality Weekly Report* 31:49 (1982), 665–7.

7. CDC, 'Current Trends Recommendations for Assisting in the Prevention of Perinatal Transmission of Human T-Lymphotropic Virus Type III/ Lymphadenopathy-Associated Virus and Acquired Immunodeficiency Syndrome', *Morbidity and Mortality Weekly Report* 34:48 (1985), 721–6, 731–2.

8. Margaret Engel, 'An AIDS "Epidemic" in Babies', *Washington Post*, 27 May 1985; 'High Costs Cited for AIDS Boarder Babies', *New York Times*, 9 October 1988, 34; Peri Klass, 'AIDS', *New York Times*, 18 June 1989; CDC, 'AIDS Weekly Surveillance Report', *HIV/AIDS Weekly Surveillance Report*, 28 December 1987, 1.

9. *Roe* v. *Wade* 410 US 113 (1973). The decision was eventually overturned in 2022. *Dobbs* v. *Jackson Women's Health Organization*, No. 19-1392, 597 U.S. ___ (2022).

10. Neil Young, *We Gather Together: The Religious Right and the Problem of Interfaith Politics* (New York: Oxford University Press, 2016), 212.

11. Mary Ziegler, *Abortion and the Law in America: Roe v. Wade to the Present* (Cambridge: Cambridge University Press, 2020), 28–9.

12. See, for example, *Webster* v. *Reproductive Health Services* 492 US 490 (1989).

13. Janet Golden, '"An Argument that Goes Back to the Womb": The Demedicalization of Fetal Alcohol Syndrome, 1973–1992', *Journal of Social History* 33:2 (1999), 269–98; Rachel Roth, *Making Women Pay: The Hidden Costs of Fetal Rights* (Ithaca, NY: Cornell University Press, 2000); Carol Mason, *Killing for Life: The Apocalyptic Narrative of Pro-Life Politics* (Ithaca, NY: Cornell University Press 2018); Laura Briggs, *Taking Children: A History of American Terror* (Oakland: California University Press, 2020).

14. Julilly Kohler-Hausmann, *Getting Tough: Welfare and Imprisonment in 1970s* (Princeton, NJ: Princeton University Press, 2017), 7; Nicholas F. Jacobs, Desmond King and Sidney M. Milkis, 'Building a Conservative State: Partisan Polarization and the Redeployment of Administrative Power', *American Political Science Association* 17:2 (2019), 453.

15. Steven W. Thrasher, *The Viral Underclass: The Human Toll When Inequality and Disease Collide* (New York: Celadon Books, 2022), 182.

16. Jennifer Brier, *Infectious Ideas: US Political Responses to the AIDS Crisis* (Chapel Hill: University of North Carolina Press, 2009); Trevor Hoppe, *Punishing Disease: HIV and the Criminalization of Sickness* (Oakland: University of California Press, 2018); Karma R. Chávez, *The Borders of AIDS: Race, Quarantine, and Resistance* (Seattle, WA: University of Washington Press, 2021).

17. Ellen Bilofsky, 'The Coercion of Carol Doe', *Health/PAC Bulletin* (1990), 16, Box 139, fol. 14, Boston Women's Health Book Collective (BWHBC).

18. Maxwell Gregg Bloche, 'Beyond Autonomy: Coercion and Morality in Clinical Relationships', *Health Matrix* 6:229 (1996), 231–2.
19. *Doe v. Jamaica Hospital* 608 NYS.2d 518 (NY App.Div. 1994).
20. Allan Brandt, *No Magic Bullet: A Social History of Venereal Disease in the United States since 1880* (New York, 1987), 19; Harriet Washington, *Medical Apartheid: The Dark History of the Medical Experimentation on Black Americans from Colonial Times to the Present* (New York: Oxford University Press, 2006), 191.
21. Beth Widmaier Capo, *Textual Contraception: Birth Control and Modern American Fiction* (Columbus: Ohio State University Press, 2021), 111.
22. Washington, *Medical Apartheid*, 192, 202–3.
23. Alice Wexler, *The Woman Who Walked into the Sea: Huntington's and the Making of a Genetic Disease* (New Haven, CT: Yale University Press, 2008).
24. Leslie J. Reagan, *Dangerous Pregnancies: Mothers, Disabilities, and Abortion in Modern America* (Berkeley: University of California Press, 2010), 6.
25. CDC, 'Current Trends Recommendations for Assisting in the Prevention of Perinatal Transmission of Human T-Lymphotropic Virus Type III/Lymphadenopathy-Associated Virus and Acquired Immunodeficiency Syndrome'.
26 , Bloche, 'Coercion and Morality in Clinical Relationships', 232.
27. See, for example, Anthony J. Pinching and Donald J. Jeffries, 'AIDS and HTLV-III/LAV Infection: Consequences for Obstetrics and Perinatal Medicine', *Obstetrical and Gynecological Survey* 92:1211 (1985), 569–70; Howard L. Minkoff and Richard H. Schwarz, 'AIDS: Time for Obstetricians to Get Involved', *Obstetrics and Gynecology* 68:2 (1986), 267; Donald P. Francis and James Chin, 'The Prevention of Acquired Immunodeficiency Syndrome in the United States: An Objective Strategy for Medicine, Public Health, Business, and the Community', *Journal of the American Medical Association* 257:10 (1987), 1361.
28. Wexler, *The Woman Who Walked Into the Sea*, 162–3; Reagan, *Dangerous Pregnancies*.
29. C. Marte and K. Anastos, 'Women: The Missing Persons in the AIDS Epidemic, Part II', *Health PAC Bull.* 20:1 (1990), 11–18. PMID: 10104816.
30. Jennifer Nelson, *Women of Color and the Reproductive Rights Movement* (New York: New York University Press, 2003), 65.
31. Jacobs, King and Milkis, 'Building a Conservative State', 456–61; Beatrix Hoffman, *Healthcare for Some: Rights and Rationing in the United States Since 1930* (Chicago: University of Chicago Press, 2012), 170–1.
32. Fern Schumer Chapman, 'Official Advocates AIDS Testing of Pregnant Women', *Washington Post*, 20 September 1988; Susan Y. Chu et al., 'Impact of the Human Immunodeficiency Virus Epidemic on Mortality in Women of Reproductive Age, United States', *Journal of the American*

Medical Association 264:2 (1990), 225–6; Susan Y. Chu et al., 'Impact of the Human Immunodeficiency Virus Epidemic on Mortality in Children, United States', *Pediatrics* 87:6 (1991), 807.

33. Carl T. Rowan, 'Children with AIDS', *Washington Post*, 10 September 1988.

34. Douglas Pike, 'In Search of Answers on the Abortion Issue', *Philadelphia Inquirer*, 8 August 1988.

35. Wendy Chavkin, 'Preventing AIDS, Targeting Women', *Health/PAC Bulletin* (1990), 22.

36. Jeffrey L. Reynolds, 'Keep Policy on Newborns' HIV Test', *Viewpoints*, 2 June 1994, 105, Box, 5, fol. AIDS 1992, Women's Action Coalition Records (WAC), NYPL Manuscripts and Archives Division.

37. Marte and Anastos, 'Women: The Missing Persons in the AIDS Epidemic Part II', 11–13; Chavkin, 'Preventing AIDS, Targeting Women', 20.

38. Hoppe, *Punishing Disease*, 4–5, 116.

39. Brandt, *No Magic Bullet*, 21, 31–2, 94.

40. Enid Logan, 'The Wrong Race, Committing Crime, Doing Drugs, and Maladjusted for Motherhood: The Nation's Fury over "Crack Babies"', *Social Justice* 26:1 (1999), 134–5; Dorothy E. Roberts, *Killing the Black Body: Race, Reproduction, and the Meaning of Liberty* (New York: Vintage, 1999), 3.

41. Briggs, *Taking Children*, 12.

42. Washington, *Medical Apartheid*, 212, 215.

43. Logan, 'The Wrong Race', 124.

44. Roth, *Making Women Pay*, 146–7.

45. Washington, *Medical Apartheid*, 212; Golden, '"An Argument that Goes Back to the Womb"', 281.

46. 'Text – S. 2240, 101st Congress (1989–1990): Ryan White Comprehensive AIDS Resources Emergency Act of 1990', 18 August 1990, 603, available at: https://www.congress.gov/101/statute/STATUTE-104/STATUTE-104-Pg576.pdf.

47. Gena Corea, *The Invisible Epidemic: The Story of Women and AIDS* (New York: HarperCollins, 1992), 48; Aziza Ahmed, 'HIV and Women: Incongruent Policies, Criminal Consequences', *Yale Journal of International Affairs* 6:1 (2011), 32–42, 37.

48. Timothy Ross and Anne Lifflander, 'The Experiences of New York City Foster Children in HIV/AIDS Clinical Trials', Vera Institute of Justice, January 2009, 65.

49. Mason, *Killing for Life*, 94, 91, 97; Roth, *Making Women Pay*, 21.

50. Martha F. Rogers, MD, 'Transmission of Human Immunodeficiency Virus Infection in the United States', in Benjamin K. Silverman and Anthony Waddell (eds), 'The Surgeon General's Workshop on Children with HIV Infection and their Families', 18; Clarey to Risque, 'Dr. Koop's Speech at the Press Club'.

51. C. Everett Koop, *Koop: The Memoirs of America's Family Doctor* (New York: Random House, 1991), 334, 348.

52. *Webster* v. *Reproductive Health Services* 492 US 490 (1989).
53. Rachel Louise Moran, 'A Women's Health Issue?: Framing Post-Abortion Syndrome in the 1980s', *Gender & History* 33:3 (SI Health, Healing and Caring) (2021), 790–804, 800–1.
54. Marion Banzhaf, interview by Sarah Shulman, 18 April 2007, interview 070, transcript, 56–7, *ACT UP Oral History Project*.
55. Carrie Wofford, 'Sitting at the Table', *Outweek*, 2 April 1991, 22.
56. Banzhaf, interview by Sarah Shulman, 56–63.
57. CDC, 'Recommendations of the Public Health Service Task Force on Use of Zidovudine to Reduce Perinatal Transmission of Human Immunodeficiency Virus', *Morbidity and Mortality Weekly Report* 43:RR-11 (1994), 1–20; CDC 'Achievements in Public Health: Reduction in Perinatal Transmission of HIV Infection: United States, 1985–2005', *Morbidity and Mortality Weekly Report* 55:21 (2006), 592–7.
58. Catherine Hanssens, Alison Mehlman and Margo Kaplan, 'Pregnancy and HIV: Medical and Legal Considerations for Women and their Advocates', *Center for HIV Law and Policy* (2009), 12–13.
59. Lynn M. Paltrow and Jeanne Flavin, 'Arrests of and Forced Interventions on Pregnant Women in the United States, 1973–2005: Implications for Women's Legal Status and Public Health', *Journal of Health Politics, Policy and Law* 38:2 (2013), 315, 316; Michele Goodwin, 'How the Criminalization of Pregnancy Robs Women of Reproductive Autonomy', *Hastings Center Report* 47:S3 (2017), S19, S24.
60. Michael A. Scarcella, 'Woman with HIV Didn't Seek Care for Baby', *Herald Tribune*, 11 January 2008; HIV Justice Network, 'US: Florida Woman Guilty of Mother-to-Child HIV Transmission', available at: https://www.hivjustice.net/cases/us-florida-woman-guilty-of-mother-to-child-hiv-transmission; Centre for HIV Law Policy, 'What HIV Criminalization Means to Women in the US', undated, 3, available at: https://www.hivlawandpolicy.org/sites/default/files/Women%20and%20HIV%20Criminalization.pdf.
61. Margo Kaplan, 'Behind Bars for Being Pregnant and HIV-Positive', 8 June 2009, available at: https://www.hivlawandpolicy.org/fine-print-blog/behind-bars-being-pregnant-and-hiv-positive; Ahmed, 'HIV and Women', 39.

11

The Making of Entitled Consumers: Neoliberal Ideas in the Medicare Modernization Act of 2003

Yifei Li

On 16 August 2022, President Joe Biden signed into law the Inflation Reduction Act (IRA) to provide a $70 billion subsidy for those who enrol in Medicare,[1] the federal health insurance programme for American seniors and some younger people with disabilities. Roughly 13 million Medicare beneficiaries will be spared from big increases in their out-of-pocket expenses during a year beset by record-high inflation.[2] However, for those who have faith in Biden's commitment to build on Obamacare – a major achievement in the progressive dream for American universal healthcare long deferred – the IRA has largely failed their expectations. Neither has it removed the incentive of Medicare-approved private plans to limit the amount of medical care for more profits, nor significantly reduced the number of the uninsured or the 'underinsured', a well-captured and well-researched phenomenon in which the health insurance owned by individuals and families still falls short when illness strikes.[3] From another perspective, an even more concerning narrative emerges when we consider the distinct feature about American healthcare: the unreasonably high cost and low coverage, a narrative that says less about the triumph of entitlement programmes and more about the dismantling of New Deal liberalism. In fact, the IRA has left intact a Medicare system predicated on what Gary Gerstle called 'the neoliberal order': the primacy of health consumerism, the emphasis on individual risk management, and the unbridled faith in the private sector as the first and the best means of tackling problems of all kinds.[4]

Traditional Medicare was not built on neoliberal principles. The original legislation of 1965 was strong on a philosophy of entitlement: Part A (hospital insurance) was financed through payroll taxes and Part B (for outpatient services) through general federal revenues. An important reason for associating the programme with payroll was to enhance a sense of entitlement and distance Medicare from the welfare tradition of charity.[5] Ever since, the debate on Medicare has been centred around cost control and expansion of benefits, but the principle of social insurance was sustained until Medicare's surging expenditure and the prevailing cultural ethos of market-driven healthcare urged the federal government to reorganise the programme. The 1980s saw a change in the way Medicare paid hospitals. Instead of paying retrospectively, the new system paid hospitals a fixed price based on estimated per capita costs, a so-called prospective payment mechanism. At the same time, there has been a rise in what was labelled as managed care, which generally took three forms: health maintenance organisations (HMOs); preferred provider organisations (PPOs); and point-of-service (POS) plans. These managed care plans sprang from the concept of 'consumer-directed Medicare', which involved high-deductible coverage and personal medical accounts for out-of-pocket spending. The Balanced Budget Act (BBA) of 1997 further enhanced this notion by introducing the Medicare+Choice programme.[6] Allowing additional managed care plans to participate in Medicare, the Act was intended to expand enrolment in private plans and incentivise Medicare beneficiaries to 'get more skin in the game'.[7]

Over the years, as we shall see, there has been a revealing change in how Medicare and the healthcare industry as a whole are understood to function: from an emphasis on shared risk, with Medicare and non-profit insurers never charging higher rates to less healthy enrolees, to a powerful discourse on individual risk management, with for-profit private insurers setting rates according to each enrolee's medical experience and expected medical costs.[8] From a public health perspective, this restructuring is important both because of its potential impact on access to healthcare and its implications on the boundaries of state intervention in promoting a healthy population in a political climate that emphasises individual responsibility and limited government. An analysis on the neoliberal revolution of Medicare as the United States' single largest health insurance programme, therefore, is necessary if we are to understand the broader change in the values and ideals of public health in America.

A landmark of this revolution, this chapter argues, is the Medicare Prescription Drug, Improvement, and Modernization Act (MMA) of 2003. The legislation warrants lengthy analysis for two reasons. First, the MMA diverted from the dominant pattern of Medicare reform since the 1980s to prioritise restructuring of Medicare over cost control as its principal goal. It established a $724 billion prescription drug benefit (also known as Medicare Part D) to allow beneficiaries to pay for their prescription drugs and medications through private health insurance plans, marking the biggest expansion of

Medicare since its creation in 1965. Secondly, the MMA significantly challenged the imagined boundaries between being a 'citizen' and being a 'consumer' by placing its emphasis on consumer choice and empowerment.[9] More broadly, the MMA also marks the entrenchment of neoliberalism in healthcare, because the idea of 'moral hazard' – people would not be cost-conscious about their healthcare if their insurance plans covered all their claims,[10] has been underpinning the reform agenda of the MMA and was championed by a variety of neoliberal think tanks.[11] Neoliberal demands for efficiency and cost reduction served as the larger justification for consumer-driven healthcare, a concept that emerged in the 1980s and gained momentum in the Clinton administration. Together, these features make the MMA a particularly valuable case when understanding the transformation of the American healthcare system since the 1960s.

The following part of this chapter details the guiding principles of the MMA and examines the new benefits and regulations it mandated, based on which I illustrate four major characteristics of the new system of American healthcare. The first is a change of medical service delivery from a right that accompanies citizenship to a commodity to be purchased, with consumer choice being prioritised over access to and quality of healthcare. This brings us to the second point: encouraging more private healthcare insurance plans to participate in such social programmes as Medicare under the banner of managed competition has deeply altered the values, bases of legitimacy and practical actions of medical services, with trust being undermined by competition, caring and compassion being compromised by cost-containment measures, and the professional ethos being replaced by a commercial ethos.[12] In the meantime, the reform agenda of American healthcare increasingly features the celebration of the private sector as a better solution to major risks than the government. The enthusiasm for delegation and deregulation is nothing new,[13] but the power to shape the institutional landscape of American public health and disease has now been consolidated in corporate interests, and enhanced by a belief that the invention of new accountability mechanisms and medical technologies have finally solved the problems of risk management that once bedevilled private healthcare insurers.[14] The third characteristic, therefore, is a revealing shift away from socialised medicine, with the government taking the responsibility for risk management, to a powerful discourse of personal responsibility for health and disease that placed blame on individuals and their families. Taken together, the new healthcare system calls forth a change in people's relationship with the state, and represents a moral crusade for smaller government, economic vitality and self-sufficiency.[15]

Taking a broader view, the MMA also facilitated a new form of governing by changing Medicare's beneficiaries' initiatives when purchasing healthcare. Specifically, the law marks the culmination of the decades-long effort (detailed below) to reorganise healthcare around neoliberal ideas, namely, opening public health insurance to private, for-profit companies, facilitating market competition in areas formerly dominated by the public system, and emphasising the ability of beneficiaries as consumers to choose among various insurance plans.[16] However, while competition is supposed to boost efficiency and make private insurers accountable to a commodified healthcare agenda, mass privatisation may unleash a large number of private schemes and see immediate effects such as disruption of services and rising costs. After all, 'without active collective management on the demand side, the medical plans would be free to pursue profits or survival using numerous competitive strategies that would destroy equality and efficiency and that individual consumers would be powerless to counteract'.[17] Therefore, ironically, reforms intended to scale back the government and empower market forces by contracting out some services sometimes lead to intense government involvement and subsequently a new set of regulations.[18]

Market solutions for a massive social problem: the MMA and consumer-directed healthcare

The passage of the MMA did not fit comfortably into common assumptions for an era with intense partisan competition. This is because, at least at the outset, liberal Democrats opposed providing a new benefit for American seniors and conservative Republicans advocated for an expensive addition to existing Medicare plans, especially in a fiscal context that favoured welfare retrenchment as well as a political context where a Republican president was expected to take advantage of a unified government and significantly scale back the welfare state.[19] However, a closer inspection suggests that the reality was far more nuanced than the assumption. On the one hand, Democrats thought the coverage was inadequate and drafted a much more generous prescription drug plan to 'turn back Medicare' (to its original architecture). On the other hand, except for the expensive addition to Medicare as a strengthening of 'compassionate government',[20] the Bush administration also delegated the management of pharmacy benefits to the private sector as part of the 2003 reform. This allowed conservatives and their allies in the healthcare industry to embrace the expensive new benefits without appearing to be supportive of an expansion of government, and, more importantly, it reflected that the core of the 2003 legislation was not payment issues but the broader transformation of the value and aim of American healthcare.

There had been previous efforts to develop private plans in Medicare, but none of them had a substantial impact.[21] Managed care plans (provided in a variety of settings like HMOs and PPOs) have been available to Medicare beneficiaries as an alternative to traditional fee-for-service (FFS) Medicare since 1973.[22] Yet efforts to boost enrolment in managed care plans between the 1970s and the early 1980s largely failed, primarily because the capitation payment (a flat fee for each patient it covers) was not financially viable for the HMOs or other prepaid plans. The Tax Equality and Fiscal Responsibility Act (TEFRA) of 1982 attempted to address such problems by simplifying the contracting requirements and introducing a new arrangement similar to the processes that managed care organisations used in the private sector.[23] It also entailed a 95 per cent per capita compensation for HMOs with the expectation that they would save the other 5 per cent. Yet a 1991 study found that Medicare actually paid more for clients in HMOs than for those in traditional Medicare with similar benefits.[24] The establishment of the Medicare+Choice programme as part of the Balanced Budget Act of 1997 as well as the increased payments to private plans in areas with low FFS costs provided other evidence that the capitated payment structure, that is, a fixed amount that insurers paid to medical providers, could neither change Medicare to a competitive market nor lead to savings as intended.[25]

The MMA, however, not only banned the government from negotiating with drug companies for lower prescription drug costs as a promise to secure a profitable status quo in the private sector, despite the sizeable bargaining unit Medicare could bring to the table,[26] but also established a regional PPO option to significantly increase payments to private plans by about $60 million over ten years.[27] It was expected that PPOs could serve as an alternative to traditional Medicare and other types of supplemental insurance, such as Medigap, and encourage plans to serve regions (especially rural areas) that had been ignored by private insurance companies with the new regulations and payment incentives, including a regional plan stabilisation fund, a blended payment rate adjusted according to plans' actual bids in the regions, as well as a network adequacy fund to cover payments of regional hospitals outside the plan's network.[28] Policymakers hoped that private plans could offer better services and more benefits than traditional Medicare, with these over-payments, and their decision to delay the enactment of risk adjustment measures to make private plans be 'held harmless' from financial losses further shifted Medicare to the private sector's advantage.

The force to drive patients out of traditional Medicare did not end with PPOs. Enrolment in private fee-for-service plans (PFFS) contracting with Medicare, working as an alternative to traditional Medicare for those beneficiaries in areas with fewer private plan options, was also greatly boosted by the MMA's substantial subsidies. The number of beneficiaries in PFFS grew from 20,000 in 2003 to 800,000 in 2006, accounting for 'about half of the recent growth in Medicare Advantage (MA) plan enrolment'.[29] With such promising prospects of enrolment and profits (they were paid an 11 per cent subsidy on average for each client with the MMA), PFFS plans then moved from the margins to the centre of Medicare sub-programmes.[30] With these options, beneficiaries could enjoy 'one-stop shopping' that included both drug benefits and healthcare insurance coverage after the 2003 bill came into force, while beneficiaries who stayed in traditional Medicare but sought comprehensive coverage had to purchase Medigap or standalone prescription drug plans.[31] This has made traditional Medicare less user-friendly and more costly – another facilitator of privatisation. In this sense, 'The ideological goal of privatizing more of Medicare trumped the stated goal of using "competition" to restrain the rate of growth in Medicare costs.'[32]

The significance of the MMA as a neoliberal reform

The immediate impact of MMA was undoubtedly an expansion of the federal government's role given the new expensive benefit entitlement it introduced, yet in the long run the Act was part and parcel of what Oberlander termed 'the new politics of Medicare',[33] inasmuch as it involved a cluster of neoliberal ideas that sought to transform Medicare's structure and philosophy. First, the MMA took market-oriented reform to a new level. For the first time in Medicare history, a benefit was provided solely by private insurers; beneficiaries could get prescription drug benefits either through stand-alone plans or as part of the Medicare Part C (later known as Medicare Advantage after the inception of the MMA). Even in areas with no such plans, Medicare could not offer prescription drug benefits directly to beneficiaries; it had to be administered by private insurers with Medicare assuming the risk by paying the government's share of the costs.[34] Besides, although the MMA did not herald a switch to a defined-contribution approach,[35] the law mandated a demonstration project in six metropolitan areas, whereby beneficiaries would be given vouchers to buy either FFS Medicare or private plans.[36]

Certainly, Medicare has always been a public–private mixture – the government has relied on the private sector to deliver medical care since the programme's inception, and has symbolised both an expansion of government power into healthcare and a promise to secure profits of the medical industry since its inception. Yet the MMA ceded a whole area of programme benefits to market-oriented private plans that developed at the expense of traditional Medicare. Further eroding Medicare's original principle as a single-payer programme, the MMA significantly boosted consumer-driven healthcare by enshrining a new version of the Medical Savings Account (MSA), created in 1996 to allow self-employed individuals to open accounts where tax-deferred deposits could be used for medical expenses.[37] In a 2001 article for the *Public Interest*, the neoliberal economist Milton Friedman commented quite pessimistically on the developments of healthcare policy in the 1990s, but was excited about one single advancement: the MSA.[38] Being 'minor in current scope' but 'pregnant of possibilities',[39] the MSA was reincarnated in 2003 as the Health Savings Account (HSA). In general, HSAs are tax-favoured accounts that can be used to pay healthcare costs. Anyone who has no plans other than an expensive high-deductible health insurance plan can enjoy both tax-deductible contributions and tax-exempt interest.[40]

What is unique about the HSA, however, is not the benefits it mandates but its expanded scope and accessibility. Before the MMA, Republicans were divided on the approach: the leadership favoured an insurance-based premium support plan to administer managed care plans in Medicare and deliver drug benefits, while a number of conservatives embraced a consumer-directed mechanism and contended that premium support would foster big government. To gain support from both sides, the final legislative package universalised the availability of HSAs, which were previously for self-employed individuals and small businesses with fewer than fifty employees only, so that anyone (both non-elderly and Medicare beneficiaries)[41] who had a high-deductible plan were eligible to open an HSA.[42] This fitted within a neoliberal view of healthcare for two reasons. First, it was a potentially lucrative source of revenue for the finance industry, as these accounts were estimated to hold up to $300 billion a year in 1997, constituted some 20 per cent of all employer-based plans in 2003, and were expected to gain more market share over the next few years.[43] Secondly, and more importantly, requiring HSAs to be attached to high-deductible health insurance plans could greatly advance the 'consumerisation' of healthcare. By letting people spend their own money, HSAs were established with an aim of inducing price-sensitive behaviours so that overall healthcare expenditure could be held down in the long run.[44]

In this vein, the MMA also redefined standards for Medicare's solvency in order to place limits on its expenditure. Shortly after its establishment, policymakers on the Medicare prescription drug bill proposed an additional cost-containment bill to set a policy presumption that general funds would pay no more than 45 per cent of Medicare expenditures. Should the general fund share of Medicare costs exceed the 45 per cent threshold some time in the next seven years,[45] not only would the president be required to come up with a new policy to bring the percentage below 45 per cent, but also a new Senate rule would come into force automatically to prevent any increases in benefits or payments to private insurers and healthcare providers unless extra costs could be fully offset.[46] This surely allowed substantial room for Medicare reformers to manoeuvre, because the extent to which Medicare could be changed if its costs went beyond the limit was not specified. In this regard it was also an overt ideological agenda, as there were a number of less ideologically loaded ways to contain costs, such as increasing payroll taxes or shifting part of the financing for drug benefits or physician and outpatient services from general revenues to payroll taxes. Put another way, the crisis of Medicare financing had become a genuine political crisis, especially as all parts of Medicare except for hospital costs were supposed to be funded by general revenue and premiums. This meant, further, that increases in the regressive payroll tax and Medicare premiums were favoured over progressive revenue-raising measures achieved through higher income tax.[47]

A final change mandated by the MMA was means-testing premiums and insurance benefits. Previously, all beneficiaries paid the same Part B premiums. Yet from 2007 onward premiums would vary according to beneficiaries' ability to pay and need for help. Specifically, Part B premiums for better-off seniors with an annual gross income above $80,000 (single) and $160,000 (household) would be set at a higher rate than the previous (approximate) 25 per cent benchmark, and Part D drug benefits would be more generous for beneficiaries with incomes below 135 per cent of the federal poverty level, with the premium being completely subsidised and cost-sharing limited to less than 5 per cent per prescription.[48] While this seemed fair to some, it was doubted by many. When Senator John Kerry (Democrat, MA) favourably discussed the idea of making the wealthy pay more during his 2004 presidential campaign, opponents also regarded it as fiscally misleading and politically inappropriate. First, premiums for Part B paid for only one-fourth of the programme's cost, and the number of wealthy elderly was seen as too small to make a difference to Medicare's fiscal future.[49] More importantly, proportional or progressive contributions were applicable for mandatory social insurance programmes because they provided income protection that reflected government responsibility regardless of specific characteristics, risks and circumstances of the individual.[50] For voluntary plans, however, introducing a steep income-related mechanism might very likely have prompted the wealthier and healthier to opt out of Part B. This, in turn, would 'undermine the diversified risk pool and widespread popular support that have sustained Medicare since its inception'.[51]

Whatever their merits, these critics illuminated an important issue: Medicare had been greatly diverted from its original architecture in terms of financing and values. It is clear that 'the politics of differentiation', as Oberlander put it, was on the rise in Medicare politics as these income-related premiums prevailed,[52] and was very likely to sustain even if such policies contributed 'no more than a drop in the bucket' to Medicare's overall fiscal stability.[53] Notably, it is not the MMA that initiated debates on income-related premiums; it was first proposed as part of the Medicare Catastrophic Coverage Act of 1988, mentioned in the failed 1994 Clinton Health Care Plan, and seriously considered after the Balance Budget Act of 1997.[54] By 2003, the problem of rising drug costs, the declining ability of beneficiaries to secure supplemental coverage, and the willingness of members of both parties in Congress to compromise on the issue of drug assistance given the increasing public dissatisfaction about managed care, created the circumstances for major reform.[55] The introduction of income-related premiums demonstrated how policies were shaped by a combination of motives as long-term efforts mixed with short-term partisan expediency and ideological principle.

Moreover, the means-testing in Medicare was quite limited in scope. Had policymakers really wanted substantial subsidies to save low-income beneficiaries from potential bankruptcy, Medicare would have included income-related premiums for its mandatory parts. In this vein, the so-called 'doughnut hole' in Medicare co-payments (that is, beneficiaries still needed to pay the full cost of prescription drugs between $2,250 and $5,100 per year) was particularly relevant.[56] The fact that such a large coverage gap was originally designed to motivate people to use generic drugs also showed that the means-testing premium was not an anomaly in neoliberal efforts to privatise Medicare. Similar to the economic incentive offered by the doughnut hole, it was just another modest attempt to secure the stability and competitiveness of the Medicare market. In this sense, almost all parts of the MMA were designed to enhance competition and privatise healthcare. As stated by Oberlander, the MMA 'provide[d] a testing ground for . . . [conservative] belief that competition, consumer choice, and market forces can govern Medicare much better than the federal government can'.[57]

Promises unkept: 'choice' and 'efficiency' in consumer-directed healthcare

Regarding access to healthcare, the impact of the MMA was quite complicated. The guaranteed ability of all seniors to enrol in the revised Medicare Part D was certainly helpful to some, given the government subsidies for 75 per cent of the cost of a benefit which would, in turn, cover nearly 50 per cent of prescription drug costs. Yet since the drug benefit did not entail full reimbursement, how much it improved the situation for seniors varied greatly from one beneficiary to another on the basis of their income and secondary insurance coverage. Three groups of beneficiaries would significantly benefit from the new plan: those who had no private supplemental coverage and thus had high drug costs; Medigap clients, because Medicare Part D provided better coverage than Medigap premiums (50 per cent vs 37 per cent on average); beneficiaries whose income was too high for Medicaid but low enough for low-income subsidies established by the MMA, as in many states Medicaid plans were limited to people with incomes below 74 per cent of the federal poverty level, while the MMA's low-income subsidies were for those with incomes up to 150 per cent of the poverty level.[58]

However, 'sicker' people or those with chronic diseases were particularly disadvantaged by the new arrangements. This is because some plans either charged fees not required of beneficiaries with FFS Medicare or Medigap or excluded coverage for certain medical treatments.[59] Thus, beneficiaries in poor health usually had much greater out-of-pocket costs than they would have in traditional Medicare. For example, enrolees in a plan in Florida were required to pay $325 per day as part of co-payments for hospital stays up to a total of $3,350, yet in traditional Medicare they needed to pay only a flat $1,068 fee for stays up to sixty days.[60] Besides, beneficiaries who enjoyed generous supplemental retiree coverage prior to the MMA had seen a significant reduction of their private drug benefits. It is hard to tell whether such changes resulted from the MMA or the long-standing trends in private retiree plans, because employer-sponsored retiree insurance has been declining since the early 1990s. What is certain, however, is that the number of seniors who completely lost their retiree benefits has increased sharply after the introduction of the Act.[61]

Another major group who was not better off under the MMA, taking a broader view, is those known as dually eligible beneficiaries. That is, Medicare beneficiaries who received prescription drug coverage through Medicaid before 2003. Under the MMA, this group was required to switch from Medicaid to Medicare Part D plans so that their prescription drug benefits would not be interrupted, but many faced decreased benefits and higher payments under the new plan. This is because the MMA explicitly prohibited states from using federal matching payments to supplement Part D coverage for this group of people. The net result, therefore, was a higher co-payment on the new plan than what many Medicaid programmes required them to pay,[62] as well as a significant increase in out-of-pocket drug costs for some 3.9 million dually eligible beneficiaries.[63] Taken together, the MMA had a mixed impact on different groups. As policymakers loaded the dice heavily in favour of private plans, all parts of Medicare were subjected to the market logic, and no beneficiary could distance themselves from its consequences.

This brings us to another set of mixed impacts of the MMA, which concerns the concept of consumer-directed healthcare as its core principle and a focus of the neoliberal reform as a whole. On the one hand, the general public have been wary about the MMA because many people found their private plans covered less but cost more. There is strong evidence that enrolees in consumer-directed health plans felt less satisfied with overall performance and more vulnerable to high medical bills, and were very likely to change health plans if given the opportunity. Ironically, it was the target groups of consumer-directed healthcare – better-off, healthier people – who were most likely to have these reservations.[64] On the other hand, consumer-directed healthcare has attracted support from various groups with different interests. The Health Insurance Association of America strove to eliminate obstacles to its expansion and constantly sent lobbyists to Congress because of their preference for a defined-contribution system.[65] Employers embraced consumer-directed healthcare because a core part of it, HSAs, required lower administrative costs and made the company's health expenditure more predictable. Banks, interestingly, also preferred healthcare consumerism because managing HSAs brought more income for account processing and was therefore very lucrative, so lucrative that some private health insurance companies even started to handle their own banking services.[66]

On the other hand, for Medicare beneficiaries specifically, the concept of consumer-directed healthcare under the MMA was quite deceptive as well. When advertising the new orientation, the Bush administration once hung its pitch primarily on the principle of individual choice. Bush stated his complete faith in the market to yield optimal outcomes in December 2003: 'For the seniors of America more choices and more control will mean better healthcare, we are putting individuals in charge of their healthcare decisions, and as we move to modernize and reform other programs of this government, we will always trust individuals and their decisions and put personal choice at the heart of our efforts.'[67] 'Choice' in this sense was conflated with rights, freedom and consumer empowerment. However, as the rights of the consumer dominated the public discourse, there were surprisingly few appeals to citizenship even from those who positioned themselves as liberal healthcare reformers.

In fact, many beneficiaries have also found their benefits to be lower than under their previous FFS plans after they joined the system of consumer-directed healthcare. This is largely because the concept of choice is somewhat misleading. Some scholars believed efforts to move beneficiaries out of traditional Medicare had been relying more on carrots than sticks,[68] but this is only partly true. 'The strategy of the MMA is to make Medicare Advantage plans so attractive that most beneficiaries will voluntarily switch out of traditional Medicare,' as testified by Joseph Antos of the American Enterprise Institute,[69] a prominent think tank founded to promote neoliberal ideology. Nevertheless, in practice beneficiaries were often compelled (ironically with the rhetoric of choice) to desert the traditional programme. First, the enrolment rule of the prescription drug coverage was a significant departure from conservatives' rhetoric about 'voluntary switch',[70] because beneficiaries had to enrol in a private plan if they were to receive this benefit. Besides, prior to the MMA, most Medicare beneficiaries had been using Medigap or other types of subsidy, such as retiree coverage, to pay for services that FFS Medicare did not cover. Yet after 2003 these supplements had been declining – another implicit form of compulsion.[71]

Additionally, most private healthcare plans restricted beneficiaries to a small network of hospitals and doctors; some plans allowed members to use providers outside the network, but required them to pay extra to do so. This is hardly an expansion of choice compared with Medicare in the past, as less-advantaged patients will simply give up their free choice if the cost is too high. Under the new rules, seniors were not entitled to an out-of-pocket limit if they chose to stay in traditional Medicare. Even if beneficiaries had the opportunity to switch back to traditional Medicare from Medicare Advantage plans during an open enrolment season, it was hard for them to protect themselves from unexpected costs by purchasing supplemental coverage if they had medical problems.[72] This is because the MMA allowed private providers to adjust drug prices and formulas on a weekly basis, while beneficiaries were only permitted to change benefit provider once a year. That is a painfully long period for those who were suddenly caught by serious disease, especially as in managed care plans they also need a referral from a primary care doctor to consult a specialist (in traditional Medicare that is not required). In this sense, the MMA particularly limited the choice of beneficiaries who wanted financial protection yet favoured traditional Medicare due to its greater flexibility of choosing medical providers.

A further critique in this regard concerned the distinctiveness of seniors as a demographic group. While Medicare beneficiaries were expected to be well-informed 'rational consumers' who could always choose the option that had optimal benefits, the choices provided by the MMA seemed to escape this consumer logic. The discount card programme as part of the MMA was both complicated and confusing. While seniors' limited ability to figure out their actual needs and options should be taken into consideration, there is strong evidence that both seniors and their caregivers found the researching process complex and time-consuming.[73] Even if Families USA, a non-profit consumer health advocacy organisation, held a traveling expo and recorded a video to provide guidance for seniors about what benefits were included and which discount card to use, the effect was quite limited because seniors faced a major obstacle when clarifying what their medical problems were to determine which card could best meet their needs.[74] Consequently, although it was speculated that beneficiaries would enrol in private plans due to additional benefits, the complicated directions often confounded seniors.

Lack of information was in general a major concern. Approximately 78 per cent of the participants in a 1998 Princeton Survey Research Associates poll supported the law that required managed care companies to 'provide people with more information about their health plan'.[75] In 2005, just before the MMA's implementation, the Kaiser Foundation also reported that around 46 per cent of respondents chose 'I don't know enough about it', and 37 per cent chose 'its too complicated' when asked about the reason they did not enrol in a Medicare drug plan.[76] This had allowed private plans substantial room to manoeuvre when appealing to clients. In most cases, private insurers claim that their plans provide the 'same' coverage as traditional Medicare; after all, many seniors would be reluctant to abandon their FFS plans without such assurances. Yet the fact is that private plans only provided equal out-of-pocket costs to the public system. This means they could change the type of benefits or structure of cost-sharing quite flexibly to cover different groups of beneficiaries. For instance, including benefits such as discounted fitness club memberships could attract healthier beneficiaries who were less costly to cover.[77]

Not only did insurance companies mislead beneficiaries on their benefits, but they also lied about the reason beneficiaries would have extra benefits or lower premiums. Emphasising their aim to encourage members to have regular physical examinations so that some ailments could be found at an early stage (that is, to be treated at relatively low costs), private plans claimed that extra benefits were made possible by lower overall costs.[78] In fact, however, these extra benefits promised by insurance companies were 'overwhelmingly – not financed out of plan efficiency, but rather by the Medicare program and other beneficiaries', as Medicare Payment Advisory Committee Chairman Glenn Hackbarth noted.[79] This means some beneficiaries got more benefits at the expense of others, and that private plans were taking advantage of the flat fee paid by the government regardless of beneficiaries' actual healthcare costs. Further contributing to this argument, there is strong evidence that insurance companies had exaggerated the health problems of their clients by 'upcoding' them, that is, assigning diagnosis codes for more severe illnesses to beneficiaries, so that government payments to these companies could be inflated.[80] In this sense, the Medicare Advantage option had been diverted away from its alleged aim to rein in costs through competition and act as a vehicle to diversify plan offerings that would cater to beneficiaries' varied needs.[81]

Overall, the MMA has done little to improve the efficiency of the Medicare system. As a matter of fact, 'each dollar's worth of enhanced benefits in private FFS (PFFS) plans costs the Medicare program over three dollars'.[82] Broadly speaking, payments to Medicare Advantage plans have always exceeded what FFS Medicare would have spent for similar beneficiaries, and Medicare Advantage costs per client were roughly 114 per cent of comparable FFS spending.[83] Regarding other aspects on which neoliberals once pinned high hopes, like choice and competition, the MMA was misleading as well. Obviously, the MMA was channelling more federal funds into private companies for doing more, whether or not more meant appropriate. What we observe, at least from a patient experience perspective, is that beneficiaries' 'free choices' were not free at all. Some scholars have regarded this as the 'second face' of neoliberalism, in that constraining choices could change beneficiaries' economic incentives, therefore actually becoming another form of extended governing.[84] The logic was that restraining members to a small network of providers would make beneficiaries more 'cost-conscious' by allowing plans to bargain for better rates *beforehand*, yet it is hard to say whether such 'extended governing' has improved consumers' cost-consciousness or sent more money to private insurers. In this vein, the MMA's impact on fuelling competition is ambiguous as well, as private plans are competitive only because they play on an uneven field.

Conclusion

Few public policy initiatives have been more complicated than the MMA. First, its establishment was remarkable in a political environment where ideological conflict over the role of government created almost insurmountable barriers to Medicare reform – the deliberative, bipartisan process of Medicare policymaking was turned into a highly polarised, deadlocked debate with the ascendancy of a Republican majority in 1994.[85] This was largely because the enormous subsidies the MMA entailed attracted enough supporters from various interest groups: employers, rural healthcare providers, hospitals and managed care plans would get substantial short-term subsidies,[86] and pharmaceutical manufacturers would be spared from the direct administration of benefits by the federal government as well as explicit cost control measures.[87] For some analysts, the law was 'a classic election-year giveaway, a year early'[88] and even some kind of 'corporate welfare'.[89] Secondly, American healthcare has been renowned for its quality – a utopia of cutting-edge research, top medical technologies and effective interventions, on the one hand, and the substantial gap between what is known to work and what patients are actually experiencing, on the other. The implementation of the MMA has demonstrated a substantial disjuncture between the promise to provide Medicare beneficiaries with better care and more medical resources and its actual impact on different beneficiary groups: some beneficiaries enjoyed lower premiums and better medical services under the MMA, while others found their choices being limited, the overall inefficiency of the system was maintained, and their benefits were inadequate and even fewer than under their traditional FFS Medicare. Thus, in terms of the three touchstones to evaluate healthcare systems – cost, quality and access[90] – the MMA has reinforced the notion that access to and affordability of medical care in the United States is subordinated to the profits of giant hospital chains, pharmaceuticals and private insurers.

From a neoliberal perspective, the MMA's impact on American healthcare was also clear. Given the seemingly contradictory fact that the MMA at once emphasised consumer choice and entailed a variety of limitations, it illustrated two distinctive aspects of a consumer-directed system. The first was a reframing of citizens as consumers in the market rather than holders of social rights. This means Medicare beneficiaries had a right to be well informed when 'purchasing' their medical services and the right to complain when services did not fulfil their expectations, but could no longer count on the government to give them particular rights, especially with regard to welfare. The beneficiaries' choices about which medical insurance and services to choose were informed more by financial considerations than under premium support or social insurance systems. Thus, even if opening Medicare to the private sector largely emphasised 'choice' over service quality instead of 'voice' in terms of democratic participation, according to neoliberals, consumerism could enhance citizenship because rising expectations could motivate citizens to challenge perceived inadequacies in service, thus activating the market by fuelling competition. More broadly, as the reform agenda of healthcare becomes increasingly dominated by proposals to enhance competition and develop private plans, one also sees a deep loss of what Putnam called 'social capital', namely, a sense of trust and duty, norms of reciprocity that arise from connections among individuals, and a bond that ensures solidarity in the face of adversity.[91]

The MMA also represented a change of focus from collectivist social rights to individual responsibilities, and inequality and social risk were no longer regarded as a systematic pathology but rather as an individual aberration.[92] Citizenship was redefined as a contract rather than a status, and entitlement became conditional on the fulfilment of certain duties.[93] As a result, personal responsibility became accompanied with personal consequences with regard to health, service quality, access and costs. There is no remedy for poor choices because neither insurers nor the government would be there to provide a safety net. Such a major transition did not happen overnight. The notion of market-oriented systems has been introduced gradually, on the premise of not bringing significant disruptions to coverage for enrolees, and was built through policy layering which led to the programme reconstruction of the MMA. However, as Goldsmith contended, while market logic became a major feature of US healthcare, 'the real task of policymakers is not to supplant, but to leverage those marketplace forces'.[94] The experience of the MMA has already shown that private plans alone cannot sustain the huge and diversified system of Medicare, and for those who think that a well-functioning healthcare system without government involvement would be a workable compromise, the issue of entrenched commercial interests in the medical industry has to be confronted.

Notes

1. A. Beam, 'Biden Bill to Help Millions Escape Higher Health Care Costs', *US News*, 19 August 2022, available at: https://www.usnews.com/news/health-news/articles/2022-08-19/biden-bill-to-help-millions-escape-higher-health-care-costs.

2. Ibid.
3. C. Schoen, M. M. Doty, S. R. Collins and A. L. Holmgren, 'Insured But Not Protected: How Many Adults are Underinsured?' *Health Affairs Web Exclusive*, 14 June 2005
4. G. Gerstle, *The Rise and Fall of the Neoliberal Order: America and the World in the Free Market Era* (Oxford: Oxford University Press, 2022).
5. T. Marmor, *The Politics of Medicare*, 2nd edn (Hawthorne, NY: Aldine de Gruyter, 2000), 16.
6. D. Beland and A. Waddan, *The Politics of Policy Change: Welfare, Medicare, and Social Security Reform in the United States* (Washington, DC: Georgetown University Press, 2003).
7. D. Altman, 'What's Trending in Health Care? Conservative Ideas', *Wall Street Journal*, 14 July 2014.
8. J. Quadagno and J. B. McKelvey, 'The Transformation of American Health Insurance', in J. S. Hacker (ed.), *Health at Risk: America's Ailing Health System – And How to Deal With It* (New York: Columbia University Press, 2008), 10–31.
9. E. West, 'Mediating Citizenship Through the Lens of Consumerism: Frames in the American Medicare Reform Debates of 2003–2004', *Social Semiotics* 16:2 (2006), 243–61.
10. M. Pauly, 'Means-testing in Medicare', *Health Affairs* 23:1 (2004), W4-557.
11. A. Gaffney, 'The Neoliberal Turn in American Health Care', *International Journal of Health Service* 45:1 (2015), 33–52.
12. B. Gray, 'Trust and Trustworthy Care in the Managed Care Era', *Health Affairs* 16:1 (1997), 34–49; D. Mechanic, 'The Functions and Limitations of Trust in the Provision of Medical Care', *Journal of Health Politics, Policy, and Law* 23 (1998), 661–86.
13. A. L. Fairchild, D. Rosner, J. Colgrove, R. Bayer and L. P. Fried, 'The EXODUS of Public Health: What History Can Tell Us About the Future', *American Journal of Public Health* 100:1 (2010), 54–63.
14. This is because private insurance companies often conduct 'risk selection' to attract healthier and younger enrolees and avoid high-cost enrolees based on their anticipated medical expenses. Invention of proper accountability mechanisms and information technology can help to reduce such phenomenon. For detailed analysis, see H. J. Aaron, J. M. Lambrew and P. F. Healy, *Reforming Medicare: Options, Tradeoffs, and Opportunities* (Washington, DC: Brookings Institution Press, 2008).
15. D. Light, 'Comparative Institutional Response to Economic Policy Managed Competition and Governmentality', *Social Science and Medicine* 52 (2001), 1151–66.
16. H. Ratna, 'Medical Neoliberalism and the Decline in US Health Care Quality', *Journal of Hospital Management and Health Policy* 4:7 (2020), 1–9.
17. A. C. Enthoven, *Theory and Practice of Managed Competition in Health Care Finance* (Amsterdam: North Holland, 1988).

18. D. W. Light, 'The Sociological Character of Markets in Health Care', in G. L. Albrecht, R. Fitzpatrick and S. C. Scrimshaw (eds), *Handbook of Social Studies in Health Care and Medicine* (London: Sage, 2000), 394–408.

19. T. R. Marmor and J. S. Hacker, 'Medicare Reform and Social Insurance: The Clashes of 2003 and Their Potential Fallout', *Yale Journal of Health Policy, Law and Ethics* 5 (2005), 479–85.

20. D. Milbank and C. Deane, 'President Signs Medicare Drug Bill', *Washington Post*, 9 December 2003, A1.

21. Century Foundation, *Medicare Reform: A Century Foundation Guide to the Issues* (New York: Century Foundation Press, 2001); N. DeParle, 'As Good As It Gets? The Future of Medicare+Choice', *Health Affairs* 27 (2002), 500.

22. Health maintenance organisations (HMOs), the first form of managed care, was first introduced by the Health Maintenance Organization Act.

23. J. Moore, 'Medicare Managed Care: Current Requirements and Practices to Ensure Accountability', in S. B. Jones and M. Ein Lewin M (eds), *Improving the Medicare Market: Adding Choice and Protections* (Washington, DC: National Academies Press, 1996).

24. K. R. Levit, H. C. Lazenby, C .A. Cowan and S. W. Letsch, 'National Health Expenditures, 1990', *Health Care Financing Review* 13:1 (1991), 29–54.

25. B. Biles, L. H. Nicholas, B. S. Cooper, E. Adrion and S. Guterman, 'The Cost of Privatization: Extra Payments to Medicare Advantage Plans: Updated and Revised'," *Issue Brief (Common Fund)*, 23 (2006), 1–16, available at: https://pubmed.ncbi.nlm.nih.gov/17153271.

26. Kaiser Family Foundation (KFF), 'The Medicare Part D Prescription Drug Benefit Fact Sheet', Kaiser Family Foundation, Medicare, September 2014, aAvailable at: https://files.kff.org/attachment/medicare-prescription-drug-benefit-fact-sheet.

27. CBO, 'A Detailed Description of CBO's Cost Estimate for the Medicare Prescription Drug Benefit', Congressional Budget Office, 2004, available at: https://www.cbo.gov/publication/15841.

28. US GAO, 'Medicare Demonstration PPOs: Financial and Other Advantages for Plans, Few Advantages for Beneficiaries', United States Government Accountability Office, 2004, available at: https://www.gao.gov/products/gao-04-960.

29. The PFFS is one of the most common types of Medicare Advantage plans, the other three are: Health Maintenance Organization (HMO) plans; Preferred Provider Organization (PPO) plans; and Special Needs Plans (SNPs). For detailed analysis on this issue, J. see Zhang and V. Fuhrmans, 'Seniors Flock to Private Fee-for-Service Medicare Plans', *Wall Street Journal*, 29 August 2006.

30. M. Freudenheim, 'Luring Customers from Medicare; Fee-for-Service Health Plans Flourish With Government Help', *New York Times*, 22 September 2006.

31. R. Berenson, 'Medicare Disadvantaged and the Search for the Elusive "Level Playing Field', *Health Affairs* (web exclusive, 15 December 2004), available at: https://www.healthaffairs.org/doi/abs/10.1377/hlthaff.W4.572.

32. K. Patel and M. E. Rushefsky, *Healthcare Politics and Policy in America*, 4th edn (New York: M. E. Sharpe, 2014).

33. J. Oberlander, *The Political Life of Medicare* (Chicago: University of Chicago Press. 2003).

34. J. O'Sullivan, H. Chaikind, S. Tilson, J. Boulanger and P. Morgan, *CRS Report for Congress: Overview of the Medicare Prescription Drug, Improvement, and Modernization Act of 2003* (Washington, DC: Congressional Research Service, 2003).

35. In a speech to an organisation called Coalition for Medicare Choice, President G. W. Bush emphasised the advantage of private plans to provide benefits that were not available in traditional FFS Medicare, and stated 'The defined benefit plan in Medicare limits the capacity of seniors to meet their needs, and that doesn't seem right to me', 2002.

36. T. Rice and K. A. Desmond, 'Distributional Consequences of Premium Support', *Journal of Health Politic, Policy and Law* 29:6 (2004), 1187–226.

37. 'Health Savings Accounts and Other Tax-Favoured Health Plans', *Irs.gov.*, Internal Revenue Service, 2005, available at: https://www.irs.gov/pub/irs-pdf/p969.pdf.

38. M. Friedman, 'How to Cure Health Care', *The Public Interest* (Winter 2001), available at: https://www.hoover.org/research/how-cure-health-care-0.

39. Ibid., 3.

40. P Fronstin, 'The Potential Impact of Consumer Health Savings Accounts as a Market-Based Approach for Improving Quality and Reducing Costs', Wisconsin Family Impact Seminars, 2005, available at: https://www.purdue.edu/hhs/hdfs/fii/wp-content/uploads/2015/07/s_wifis21c02.pdf.

41. Although a person automatically loses HSA eligibility once they enrol in Medicare, they can always contribute to the account before they turn sixty-five, and can still use the money in the HSA to pay for their healthcare after they start to benefit from Medicare. That said, advantages of the HSA are also available to Medicare beneficiaries.

42. A. Minicozzi, 'Medical Savings Accounts: What Story Do the Data Tell?' *Health Affairs* 25 (2006), 256–67.

43. A. W. Gaffney, 'The Neoliberal Turn in American Health Care', *Jacobin*, 15 April 2014.

44. T. Jost, *Health Care At Risk: A Critique of the Consumer-Driven Movement* (Durham, NC: Duke University Press, 2007).

45. Technically, the trigger time is the date on which the Board of Trustees of Federal Hospital Insurance and Federal Supplementary Medical Insurance trust funds both report that the 45 per cent threshold will be

reached seven years from now, including the current year and the six subsequent years.

46. R. Greenstein, J. R. Horney, R. Kogan and E. Park, 'President and Senate Budget Committee Embrace Misguided "45-Percent Trigger"' (Washington, DC: Center on Budget and Policy Priorities, 2006).
47. E. Park, R. Greenstein and R. Kogan, 'Overlooked Element of the Medicare Trustees' Report Could Spell Trouble for Beneficiaries in Future Years' (Washington, DC: Center on Budget and Policy Priorities, 2004).
48. M. V. Pauly, *Means-testing in Medicare*, Project Hope (Washington, DC: People to People Health Foundation, Inc., 2004).
49. H. J. Aaron, 'The Grand Delusion', *Century Issues*, 15 October 2003, available at: http://www.brook.edu/views/op-ed/aaron/20031015.htm.
50. T. R. Marmor, J. L. Marshall and P. L. Harvey, *America's Misunderstood Welfare State: Persistent Myths, Enduring Realities*, reprinted edn (New York: Basic Books, 1992).
51. Marmor and Hacker, 'Medicare Reform and Social Insurance, 479–85.
52. J. Oberlander, 'Through the Looking Glass: The Politics of the Medicare Prescription Drug, Improvement, and Modernization Act', *Journal of Health Politics, Policy and Law* 32:2 (2007), 187–219.
53. L. Bakk, 'Medicare Prescription Drug, Improvement, and Modernization Act of 2003: Implications for the Future of Health Care', *Health & Social Work* 34:1 (2009), 59–63.
54. D. G. Smith, *Entitlement Politics: Medicare and Medicaid 1995–2001* (Hawthorne, NY: Aldine de Gruyter, 2002).
55. T. Oliver, P. R. Lee and H. L. Lipton, 'A Political History of Medicare and Prescription Drug Coverage', *Milbank Quarterly* 82:2 (2004), 283–354.
56. R. Conti, S. B. Dusetzina and R. Sachs, 'How the ACA Reframed the Prescription Drug Market and Set the Stage for Current Reform Effort', *Health Affairs* 39:3 (2020), 445–52.
57. Oberlander, 'Through the Looking Glass', 203.
58. D. Jaenicke and A. Waddan, 'President Bush and Social Policy: The Strange Case of the Medicare Prescription Drug Benefit', *Political Science Quarterly* 121:2 (2006), 217–40.
59. Kaiser Family Foundation (KFF), 'Costs Under Private Medicare Advantage Plans Higher than Traditional Medicare for Some Beneficiaries, GAO Report Finds', *Kaiser Daily Health Policy Report*, 28 February 2008.
60. B. Biles, L .H. Nicholas, B. S. Cooper, E. Adrion and S. Guterman, 'Medicare Beneficiary Out-of-Pocket Costs: Are Medicare Advantage Plans a Better Deal?" *Commonwealth Fund: Issue Brief* 19 (2006), available at: https://www.commonwealthfund.org.
61. J. Gabel, H. Whitmore and J. Pickreign, 'Retiree Health Benefits After Medicare Part D: A Snapshot of Prescription Drug Coverage', *Commonwealth Fund: Issue Brief* 46 (2008).
62. As of 2005, eleven states do not charge co-payments, and thirteen states have co-payments lower than the established Part D levels.

63. J. Angeles and M. Moon, 'The Medicare Prescription Drug Law: Implications for Access to Care', *American Medical Association Journal of Ethics* 7:7 (2005), 493–5.

64. Kaiser Family Foundation (KFF), 'National Survey of Enrollees in Consumer Directed Health Plans', 2006, available at: https://www.kff.org/wp-content/uploads/2013/01/7594.pdf.

65. Health Insurance Association of America, available at: http://www/ahip.org.

66. B. Werner, 'Blue Cross Banks on Health Savings Plans', *The State*, 2 March 2007, available at: http://www.thestate.com/mid/thestate/business/16812989.

67. CNN., 'President Bush Signs Landmark Medicare Bill into Law', CNN live event/special, 2003, available at: https://edition.cnn.com/2003/ALLPOLITICS/12/08/elec04.medicare.

68. Oberlander, 'Through the Looking Glass', 203.

69. J. Antos, 'Will Competition Return to Medicare?' Working Paper No. 125 (Washington, DC: American Enterprise Institute, 2006).

70. R. Berenson, 'Doctoring Health Care, II', *American Prospect* (January/February 2007), 13–14.

71. J. Lambrew and K. Davenport, 'Has Medicare Been Privatized? Implications of the Medicare Modernization Act, Beyond the Drug Benefit', *Center for American Progress*, 2006, aailable at: https://cdn.americanprogress.org/wp-content/uploads/kf/MEDICARE_PRIVATIZATION.PDF.

72. T. Newman, 'Traditional Medicare Disadvantaged?' KFF, 2016, available at: https://www.kff.org/medicare/perspective/traditional-medicare-disadvantaged.

73. K. Lind, 'Medicare Drug Discount Card Program: How Much Does Card Choice Affect Price Paid?' *AARP Bulletin Online*, 1 November 2004, available at: https://www.aarp.org/health/drugs-supplements/info-2004/medicare_drug_discount_card_program_how_much_does.html.

74. Kaiser Family Foundation (KFF) and Harvard University School of Public Health, *The Medicare Drug Benefit: Beneficiary Perspectives Just Before Implementation*, 2005, available at: https://www.kff.org/medicare/poll-finding/the-medicare-drug-benefit-beneficiary-perspectives-just-2.

75. Kaiser Family Foundation (KFF) and Harvard University School of Public Health, *Survey of Americans' Views on the Consumer Protection Debate* (Storrs, CT: Roper Center, 17 September 1998).

76. Kaiser Family Foundation (KFF) and Harvard University School of Public Health, *The Medicare Drug Benefit: Beneficiary Perspectives Just Before Implementation*, 2005, available at: https://www.kff.org/medicare/poll-finding/the-medicare-drug-benefit-beneficiary-perspectives-just-2.

77. MPAC, 'Report to the Congress: Issues in a Modernized Medicare Program', *Chapter 2: Medicare Advantage Payment Areas and Risk Adjustment*, Medicare Payment Advisory Commission, June 2005.

78. M. Morrissey, 'Medicare Privatization: A Cautionary Tale', Economic Policy Institute, 2009, available at: https://www.epi.org/publication/pm142.

79. G. M. Hackbarth, 'Report to the Congress: Medicare Payment Policy', *MedPAC*, 17 March 2009, available at: https://www.medpac.gov/wp-content/uploads/import_data/scrape_files/docs/default-source/congressional-testimony/testimony-report-to-the-congress-medicare-payment-policymar09.pdf, 18.

80. US Congressional Budget Office, *Designing a Premium Support System for Medicare*, December 2006.

81. M. Miller, *Private Fee-For-Service Plans in Medicare Advantage*, written testimony of MedPAC Executive Director Mark E. Miller before the Health Subcommittee of the House Ways and Means Committee, 22 May 2007.

82. Hackbarth, 'Report to the Congress: Medicare Payment Policy', 19.

83. Ibid.

84. L. T. Larsen and D. Stone, 'Governing Health Care Through Free Choice: Neoliberal Reforms in Denmark and the United States', *Journal of Health Politics, Policy and Law* 40:5 (2015), 942–71.

85. Oliver, Lee and Lipton, 'A Political History of Medicare and Prescription Drug Coverage'.

86. A. Goldstein, 'Medicare Bill Would Enrich Companies', *Washington Post*, 24 November 2003, A1.

87. G. Harris, 'Drug Makers Move Closer to Big Victory', *New York Times*, 25 November 2003, A20.

88. R. Abelson and M. Freudenheim, 'Medicare Compromise Plan Won't Cut Costs, Critics Say', *New York Times*, 4 September 2003, C6.

89. C. Tucker, 'Prescription Drug Plan Is Expensive Boondoggle', *Baltimore Sun*, 1 December 2003, 15A.

90. European Economic and Social Committee and the Committee on the Regions, *Modernizing Social Protection for the Development of High-Quality, Accessible and Sustainable Health Care and Long-Term Care: Support for the National Strategies Using the 'Open' Method Of Coordination* (Brussels: European Parliament, 2004).

91. R. D. Putnam, 'The Prosperous Community', *American Prospect* 4:13 (1993), 35–42. For other interpretations of social capital, see P. Bourdieu, 'The Forms of Capital', in J. Richardson (ed.), *Handbook of Theory and Research for the Sociology of Education* (New York: Greenwood, 1986), 241–58; J. S. Coleman, 'Social Capital in the Creation of Human Capital', *American Journal of Sociology* (1988) S95–S120. For a comprehensive literature review of this concept, see A. Portes, 'Social Capital: Its Origins and Applications in Modern Sociology', *Annual Review of Sociology* 24 (1998), 1–24.

92. P. Henman, 'Governing Individuality', in C. Howard (ed.), *Contested Individualization: Debates about Contemporary Personhood* (New York: Palgrave Macmillan, 2007), 171–86.

93. J. Handler, *Social Citizenship and Workfare in the United States and Western Europe: The Paradox of Inclusion* (Cambridge: Cambridge University Press, 2004).

94. J. Goldsmith, 'Death of a Paradigm: The Challenge of Competition', *Health Affairs* 3:3 (1984), 5–19.

12

'Real Men Wear Masks': COVID-19 and the Crisis of American Masculinity

Olga Thierbach-McLean

'I was strongly against getting the vaccine. Just because we're a strong conservative family.'[1] This statement, given by thirty-one-year-old Daryl Barker as he was battling COVID-19 in a Missouri hospital, illustrates a current American impasse. In its enthymematic simplicity, it encapsulates how personal health choices, political attitudes and traditional notions of masculinity have interlocked into a vaguely conceived but all the more viscerally felt causal cluster. Following a pattern familiar from numerous other deathbed pleas – an unsettling news genre that cropped up during the pandemic – Barker expressed a change of heart and spoke out in favour of getting vaccinated, despite the fact that he had himself dismissed similar appeals by other COVID-19 patients as nothing more than a hoax peddled by Democrats for political gain.

Accounts of such hardened ideological fronts usually begin with Donald Trump. By politicising the health crisis and staging himself as a virus-defying strongman, he set up COVID-19 as a highly partisan and gendered issue. However, a narrow focus on his personal influence runs the risk of neglecting the broader cultural context in which the conflict has been amplified and sustained. Counter to a common narrative, Trump's emergence as a conservative leader, male identification figure and poster child of pandemic denialism has not been a *sui generis* phenomenon but rather the continuation of historical antecedents. In many ways, Trump was merely the fuse that lit the fire on a national mentality steeped in anti-statist and individualist ideals which have been customarily framed in gendered terms.

Since the beginning of the COVID-19 pandemic, the interconnections between masculinity, individualism and healthcare have shifted into public attention as US citizens, and particularly men, have turned out to be eminently vulnerable to the virus. 'We live in a culture of rugged individualism run amok,' diagnosed Carolina A.

Miranda in view of the national struggles with the pandemic.[2] Hers is just one among many voices drawing direct connections between America's strong individualist tradition and the depth of its current healthcare crisis. However, the oft-observed dominance of individualist tenets in American public life does not mean that they have remained unchallenged by top-down approaches. Especially 'early American responses to epidemics exerted considerable state authority and substantially limited individual freedoms in order to achieve great public health victories'.[3] More often than not, the frictions arising between the competing claims of individual self-determination and the common good have been tied to cultural narratives of what it means to be a 'real man'. From the antebellum era, when yellow fever outbreaks were construed as 'social panacea because [they] efficiently weeded out lesser men', to the 1918 Spanish influenza pandemic, in which 'masculine resistance to hygiene rules associated with mothers, school marms, and Sunday school teachers [made men] weak links in hygienic discipline', to the HIV/AIDS crisis of the 1980s, which was initially conceived as a condition affecting only homosexual men, US discourses on infectious disease have habitually revolved around notions of rugged, straight masculinity.[4]

In that regard, the precursors of the present cultural moment can be traced back centuries. But at the same time, the COVID-19 pandemic marks a deep caesura in US history. When the Trump administration announced its intention to withdraw from WHO membership in May 2020, it effectively signalled the relinquishment of America's claim to leadership in global health. The country's particularly high rate of morbidity and mortality – with roughly 4 per cent of the global population it currently accounts for 16 per cent of COVID cases and deaths worldwide – has been read as a sign of national decline, a marker of the end of the American Century. 'At the height of the crisis, with more than 2,000 dying each day', wrote cultural anthropologist Wade Davis, 'Americans found themselves members of a failed state, ruled by a dysfunctional and incompetent government largely responsible for death rates that added a tragic coda to America's claim to supremacy in the world'.[5] The nation that had spearheaded medical innovation for many decades, successfully leading the global charge against smallpox, polio and AIDS, was now on the receiving end of medical aid from China and Russia.[6] A survey conducted in 2020 by the Pew Research Center found that the international reputation of the United States dropped to a historic low point during the pandemic.[7] More than just a crisis of US healthcare, the failure to respond effectively to the coronavirus at home and abroad has been interpreted as a failure of core American principles, including its extolling of individual choice, free-market economy and polarisation-prone two-party system.

This chapter looks at how masculinist norms factor into this national downturn. Taking an intersectional approach, it examines the inter-relatedness of masculinity, conservatism and pandemic-related attitudes in the cultural context of the United States. In particular, it lays out how present-day conservative responses to COVID-19 are shaped by a brand of individualism that is oriented at male-connoted traits such as competitiveness, autonomy and personal strength. This not only runs counter to understanding personal restraint as an instrument for positive collective change, but also exacerbates politico-ideological and gender divides in this pandemic.

The focus on male sensitivities and discontents is neither to lay the blame for the ideological turmoil in the United States squarely at the feet of men nor to diminish the challenges faced by other genders. Rather, this chapter seeks to go beyond rigid boundaries of sex and gender to demonstrate how present-day images of American masculinity are informed by broadly embraced cultural tenets generating problematic effects throughout US society. In contextualising American responses to the COVID-19 crisis within the wider framework of a gendered political mindscape, it sheds some light on the cultural reasons why the pandemic has taken a particularly heavy toll on the US population in general and male Americans in particular.

Maleness and conservatism: two compounding risk factors

According to international data, men are at a higher risk for an adverse outcome of COVID-19 than women. Multiple studies have found that male patients are more likely to be hospitalised, more likely to require ICU treatment and more likely to die from the coronavirus. While this is partly attributable to biological differences, these do not fully explain the disproportionately severe impacts the virus has had on men. It has been determined that, alongside other non-medical factors, including such aspects as the structure of the labour market and demographic age distribution, social constructions of gender play a decisive role in this disparity. For instance, a 2020 Promundo study has found that 'masculine norms can encourage many men and boys to take risks and be more individualistic, meaning they may take lockdown and social distancing rules less seriously'.[8] Another survey published by the American Psychological Association in 2021 detected that conformity to traditional masculinity ideology (TMI), which drives behavioural norms such as 'toughness, dominance, risk-taking, [and] self-reliance', is associated

with lower adherence to recommended pandemic mitigation practices.[9] Such cultural codes not only put men at a higher risk of contracting the virus but also make them less likely to seek medical help
once infected.

In the United States, this gender disparity has manifested in several key metrics. Although women contracted the virus at higher
rates, namely, at 53 per cent versus 47 per cent, men accounted for
51 per cent of hospitalisations, 60 per cent of ICU admissions and
55 per cent of COVID-19 fatalities.[10] Adding to the severity of the
situation, these numbers must be read against a troubling new aspect
of American exceptionalism: from March 2020 on, the United States
has consistently been the country with the highest total number of
infections and deaths worldwide, thus finding itself in the company
of nations with far less sophisticated healthcare systems.[11] Being a
US resident and being male have thus emerged as two compounding
risk factors.

Revealingly, this elevated national risk has been distributed
unevenly with regard to political partisanship. In contrast to many
other Western societies where resistance to corona measures spans
the entire political spectrum from the far left to the far right, in the
United States conflicts over how to handle the health crisis – and
whether such a crisis veritably existed – have been fought mainly
along the lines of political affiliation. From the onset of the pandemic, it has been observed that 'the more a county favoured Donald
Trump over Hillary Clinton in the 2016 election, the less that county
exhibited physical distancing'.[12] In a Gallup poll conducted in June
2021, 46 per cent of Republicans said that they had no plans to get
vaccinated as compared with 6 per cent of Democrats.[13] The partisan
standoff continued unabated even after President Biden's repeated
appeals to 'put politics aside and face the pandemic as a nation'.[14]

The gendered dynamic of this political conflict is further evidenced by the fact that public anger over lockdowns, social distancing and mask mandates has been aimed disproportionally at female
elected officials.[15] A particularly stark example is Democrat Michigan
Governor Gretchen Whitmer whose virus containment measures
elicited denouncements of her as 'an overbearing mother, a nanny,
witch, queen and a menopausal teacher punishing her students with
edicts to prevent the spread of COVID-19'.[16] She even became the
target of a politically motivated kidnapping plot for which fourteen
male suspects, seven of them members of a right-wing militia group,
were arrested in October 2020 on charges of domestic terrorism.[17]
Earlier that year, on 30 April 2020, hundreds of mostly White male
protesters, many of them armed, invaded the Michigan State Capitol

demanding an end to Whitmer's stay-at-home orders. In hindsight, this seems like a prelude to the Capitol riots of 6 January 2021. Probably more than any other event, this right-wing insurrection sealed the image of Trumpism as a movement of 'angry White men' as images of the predominantly male, Caucasian – and conspicuously maskless – crowd flooded screens all over the world.

And yet the gendered component to Trump's appeal is not as racially exclusive as is often assumed. After all, as many as a quarter of men of colour voted for Trump in the 2020 election, regardless of his publicly displayed sympathies for White supremacism and his infamous labelling of non-White male immigrants as drug dealers, criminals and rapists.[18] This is not to understate the distinct racial divide in Trump support – by comparison, he secured a substantially larger share, roughly two-thirds, of the White male vote – but rather to highlight that the gendered pull to Trumpism is often strong enough to over-ride pressing racial concerns.

Pertinently, maleness has also shown a strong gravitational effect when it comes to the intersection between gender and race with education. In an election that was held amid a full-blown pandemic and was widely perceived as the make-or-break choice between science and irrational conspiracy theories, masculine identity outweighed educational status, belying the cliché of Trump as the candidate of the educationally disadvantaged. Although it is true that non-college-educated White men were particularly responsive to his messaging with 70 per cent of the ballot, he also secured 51 per cent among college-educated White male voters.[19] This gender-driven margin was even more pronounced in the 2016 election, in which Trump competed against Hillary Clinton as the first female presidential nominee in US history. In that run, he received 71 per cent among working-class and 53 per cent among college-educated White men.[20] Often interpreted as a historical fluke, this gender divide in Trump support is in fact a culmination of a pre-existing tendency of the Republican Party to draw more men than women.

Political partisanship and performative masculinity

This trend first became palpable in the 1980 presidential election, when Ronald Reagan campaigned on the image of rugged manliness against incumbent Jimmy Carter, who projected a more pensive and sensitive persona. Reagan beat Carter to the presidency by almost ten percentage points but led by only one single point, namely, 46 to 45 per cent, among female voters.[21] If the GOP has been under-performing among women and people of colour ever since, it is not

least because it increasingly channelled cultural anxieties over changing social norms into a narrative of American manhood under siege.
Framing liberal support for the burgeoning women's rights, gay
rights and racial justice movements as a corruption of traditional
masculinity has been a staple conservative strategy from the times of
Richard Nixon's 1968 law and order campaign. Ever since, Democrat candidates have been routinely cast as effeminate 'wimps' too
soft to measure up to the role of national protector.

Even if one is prepared to accept the problematic premise that
masculine bravado is a desirable trait in a modern political leader,
it is striking that among those who were derided as effete weak-
lings were decorated war veterans like George McGovern and John
Kerry. By contrast, the Republican candidates that were presented as
rugged alpha males were often mere performers of male mythology,
like Ronald Reagan, or came from sheltered upper-crust circles, like
George W. Bush. Be that as it may, as a result of this reformulation
of political discourses in aggressively gendered terms, the blueprint
of the ideal conservative politician morphed from the earnest gentle-
man of measured temperament into the hardy swashbuckler. And
like many of his predecessors, Trump embraced this model, whether
it be through militarist language ('I will bomb the shit out of [ISIS]'),
crudely misogynist remarks ('Grab 'em by the pussy') or bashing of
cultural elites ('I don't need to be politically correct').

He abided by the same gendered playbook when the pandemic
reached the United States, mocking Biden's social distancing as
cowardly 'hiding in the basement' and hyperbolically referring to
his rival's unremarkable face covering as 'the biggest mask I've ever
seen'. Even after he contracted COVID-19 and was hospitalised in
autumn 2020, Trump continued downplaying the virus by tweeting
that 'I feel better than I did 20 years ago!' His subsequent return
to the White House was a pageant of triumphant masculinity as he
demonstratively removed his mask for the cameras against the backdrop of military insignia. Conservative media outlets even started
portraying his infection as a heroic act of patriotism, claiming that
by virtue of exposing himself to the coronavirus he had proven himself the superior leader. 'He has experience – now – fighting the virus
as an individual,' submitted Erin Perrine, the director of press
communications for the 2020 Trump campaign. 'Those firsthand
experiences – Joe Biden, he doesn't have those.'[22]

The discrepancy between such histrionic renderings of physical
resilience and Trump's well-documented lack of athleticism suggests
that the US public's strong investment in the bodily fitness of sitting presidents may be less about their concrete capability to fulfil

political duties than about the symbolic affirmation of traditional images of masculinity. When Trump encourages violence against his adversaries, tweets video of himself wrestling to the ground a figure representing CNN or assures the world press that he does not have a small penis, he enacts the signifiers of unapologetic machismo which is particularly appealing to men who feel adrift in the tide of rapidly changing social norms. The key role that performative masculinity plays in the polarisation of American politics is not least evidenced by the choice of a song titled 'Macho Man' as the theme music for Trump's 2020 campaign.

In fact, conservative opinion makers have long been explicit about tapping into the political potential of male discontent. For instance, former *Fox News* host Andrea Tantaros declared in 2016 that '[t]he Left has culturally tried to feminize this country in a way that is disgusting. And you see blue-collar voters – men – this is like their last vestige, their last hope is Donald Trump to get their masculinity back.'[23] By the same token, Canadian clinical psychologist Jordan Peterson, who has been catapulted to stardom in US conservative circles on the crest of a predominantly male followership energised by his unapologetic endorsement of patriarchal codes, has attributed Trump's political rise to the fact that men have been 'pushed too hard to feminize'.[24] Hence, the emergence of the pandemic as an arena for the cultural negotiation of masculinity did not come out of nowhere but rather follows an established template of casting the rivalry between the two main parties as a clash between masculinity and femininity.

The pandemic as a challenge to masculinity across class, racial and religious identities

If US conservatives have charged the political Left with disregarding the cultural anxieties of men, especially White working-class men, they do indeed have a point. Against the priority of advancing gender and racial equality, it has become something of a liberal taboo to divert attention to the fact that members of a privileged gender and/or race are facing their own fundamental struggles. In a time when traditional notions of sex and gender are dismantled and taken-for-granted male privileges are dislodged, men are confronted with the profound psychological challenge of radically revising their self-concepts and behavioural habits. At the same time, conventional images of male dominance, stoicism and autonomy are being promoted as vigorously as ever, notably also in the pop–cultural realm. For instance, the US cinematic landscape is more than ever populated by hypermasculine superheroes who face down existential threats through a mix of chivalry and superior physical power. Meanwhile, in the real world, what only recently counted as gracious gestures of men towards women, such as holding open doors and offering to carry heavy bags, is coming under attack as 'benevolent sexism'. This creates a barrage of contradictory and disorienting cultural signals for what it means to be a man.

In addition to the expiration of long-standing cultural norms, the transformation of the labour market as a result of increasing automation and the rise of the service sector has been rendering physical strength increasingly obsolete, thus eroding a traditional wellspring of masculine pride and distinction. The associated psychological pressures have only intensified with the onset of the pandemic given that the skill set required to weather this once-in-a-century calamity – caution, limited physical mobility, collective cooperation – runs diametrically counter to classic masculinist ideals of toughness, competitiveness and risk-taking. Lockdowns and shut-down economies have also reduced many men's concrete financial ability to live up to their archetypal role as providers.[25]

While these changes have unfolded globally, American men arguably had to operate against a particularly challenging cultural baseline. When compared with male members of Western societies with more collective-minded intellectual traditions – and concomitantly more generous social safety nets – they have been under more practical and psychological pressure to prove their 'manliness' by exhibiting resilience, resourcefulness and self-reliance. Kurt Andersen has recently observed that climbing up the economic ladder is now 'lots harder in the United States than it is in other rich countries . . . A 2018 World Bank study ranked each of the world's countries by its fraction of younger citizens . . . born into the economic lower half who made it to the top quarter before they were old. Among the fifty countries at the bottom of the two hundred, those with the least economic mobility, are forty-six developing countries, and, between Indonesia and Brazil, the United States.'[26]

With economic success increasingly difficult to achieve and cultural norms in flux, American lower-class men in particular may feel like their bodies are the only remaining venue for asserting their masculinity. Demonstrating indifference towards the virus thus becomes a mental proxy for coping with more complex and elusive socioeconomic changes. With that in mind, it is not surprising that the MAGA agenda of dismissing the pandemic and taking America back to the allegedly simpler 'good old days' particularly resonates with men, creating a self-reinforcing logic in which masculinist self-images and hostility to anti-contagion legislation enter into an elective ideological affinity.

Having said that, it should be stressed that a different set of factors comes into play for non-White men. The high level of vaccine hesitancy observed among African Americans, for instance, is rooted in a deep-seated distrust of a medical establishment that has a history of treating them not only as second-class patients but even as involuntary test objects in inhumane medical experiments such as the infamous Tuskegee Syphilis Study. Such racial traumas loom large in the collective memory, making many Black Americans loath to follow government-issued health guidelines. Not to mention that particularly for African American men, wearing a face covering often means weighing health concerns against the danger of being racially profiled. Reports about Black men being confronted by armed police during ordinary activities like grocery shopping on the grounds that their surgical masks made them 'look suspicious' is another reminder that men of colour navigate a different social reality than their White counterparts. Their failure to wear a mask may therefore not stem from a desire to project an image of stalwart masculinity but instead from the need to appear as unthreatening as possible.[27]

Besides race, other parameters that impact preventive behaviour include age, disability, place of residence and religion. For instance, older adults have been more prone than younger ones to get inoculated due to a higher sense of personal risk. Meanwhile, people with disabilities have been only half as likely as the general population to be vaccinated, often reporting impeded access to health facilities as a major reason.[28] Since not all available data are gender-disaggregated, it remains for future research to substantiate how far male and female behaviour diverges within particular demographic segments. But even where statistics are not specifically mapped for gender, they sometimes point to a gendered dimension at least indirectly, such as seems to be the case for the rural–urban divide in vaccination rates. Here, lower rates among rural populations have been linked to a combination of properties comprising less developed healthcare infrastructure, a sense of spatial seclusion from the virus, a higher Trump vote share and the dominance of traditionally male-dominated industries, with rates being lowest 'in farming and mining-dependent counties and highest in recreation-dependent counties'.[29]

Gender also plays an inherent role in connection with religion, which turned out to be another strong predictor for pandemic-related attitudes. The correlation between religiousness and 'more distrust in science and being less likely to get vaccinated', which has been detected for various denominations, has been chiefly ascribed to the collision of religious tenets with recommended preventive practices.[30] For instance, Catholic communities have raised ethical objections to the use of foetal cell lines in the production and testing of some COVID-19 vaccines, whereas people of Muslim faith have commonly cited non-halal contents of vaccines as an obstacle to getting inoculated. But even as specific religious customs differ, one feature widely shared across confessions is the notion 'that someone's disease was the will of God and that nothing should go against it, neither a vaccine'.[31]

This belief in divine destiny is also common among evangelical Christians who represent the most politically influential religious group in present-day America, and at the same time the most vociferous in its opposition to COVID-19 containment efforts. Yet tellingly, their dissent has been articulated in the language of political partisanship rather than religious doctrine, being geared more towards supporting Trumpian politics than towards asserting spiritual principles. The fact that a religious movement championing the return to traditional family values has so enthusiastically endorsed as its figurehead a twice-divorced bon vivant known for consorting with nude models and adult film actresses has been widely pointed out as an ideological oxymoron. But what is often perceived as a moral disconnect fully tallies with evangelical convictions regarding God-ordained gender roles. In this context, sociologist of religion Samuel L. Perry has explained that conservative Christians of both sexes subscribe to the belief that 'women are designed to be responders, helpers, and nurturers', while men are seen as 'natural sexual initiators and are understood to "struggle" with issues of lust more than women'. Accordingly, even as men's sexual transgressions are considered sinful, they also serve to affirm their 'God-given masculinity' as well as the notion that '[e]verybody, from presidents to pastors, is in need of grace and forgiveness'.[32]

As so often the case, the willingness to put a positive spin on the breach of moral standards is politically selective. While Democrat president Bill Clinton was condemned by conservative America for his extramarital affairs, Trump is not the first Republican leader to be championed by evangelicals despite his deviation from conservative social norms. After all, when the evangelical movement aligned with the Republican Party in the 1980s, it was under no other than Ronald Reagan, the first ever divorcée president in US history. This bond between politics and religion was forged over the explicit common goal of reversing the tide of cultural liberalism and restoring White male authority. Given this historical connection, the current evangelical push-back against social distancing, masks and vaccines arguably owes more to the secular longing for old-fashioned masculinity than to concerns over the details of theological dogma.

Individualist culture as an amplifier of masculine gender norms

While such intersections between masculinity, conservatism and reticence to health protection have also appeared in other Western societies, generally speaking they have manifested in less dramatic forms than in the United States. Nowhere did anti-restriction emotions run quite as high quite as quickly, with assaults on restaurant staff, retail employees and educators over mask-wearing disputes being reported from across the country already in the early days of the pandemic. The most common reason given for this animosity is 'that these measures represent an undue restriction on individual freedom', indicating that, beyond the immediately polarising effects of Trumpism, it is driven by prevalent assumptions about the priority of individual over collective judgement.[33]

Although the oft-noted national emphasis on personal autonomy, individual initiative and private conscience has also been a source of cultural vitality, critical voices have long cautioned against the problematic effects which all too literal interpretations of individualist principles can have on the social fabric as well as on the individual psyche. To invoke some of these commentators, the seminal book *Habits of the Heart* (1985) by Robert N. Bellah et al. pointed out that US citizens' strong identification with individualist models of personhood makes it hard to mobilise them for collective goals.[34] Along the same lines, Nina Eliasoph observed in her study *Avoiding Politics* (1998) that, as a result of being socialised in an individualistically charged social environment, Americans are susceptible to the notion that 'what is shared is oppressive'.[35] More recently, Kurt Andersen's *Fantasyland* (2017) has traced the ways in which individualist ideas have shaped US culture and politics, stressing that the resulting everyone-for-themselves mentality does not only throw the individual back on themselves materially, but also fosters self-referential modes of truth-finding. Andersen has argued that the national celebration of the unfettered self has normalised subjectivity as a viable epistemological mode, so that 'the principle of absolute tolerance became axiomatic in our culture and internalized as part of our psychology – *What I believe is true because I want and feel it to be true* – individualism turned into rampant solipsism'.[36] Within this cultural matrix, people are encouraged to believe that their spontaneous impressions are as good as empirical facts, and that personal experience is the only relevant source of information. This is precisely the mental predisposition that has posed the main obstacle to creating trust in government, experts and even the accounts of peers, opening the doors to pandemic denialism and the notion that health and sickness ultimately depend on individual self-control. The COVID-19 crisis has thus become a convergence point at which national myths of rugged individualism, conventional images of masculinity and reactionary politics coalesce.

Here it should be clarified that ideals of personal freedom and responsibility are by no means exclusively conservative. In fact, they are widely shared in the United States across boundaries of political affiliation. Nevertheless, important differences have emerged between the two main political camps. To adopt the outline offered by sociologist Robert Wuthnow, American liberals have traditionally phrased their claims 'in the name of diversity and the right to choose', while conservatives 'cast their arguments in terms of freedom from government'.[37] But in the course of this pandemic, we have seen a striking deviation from this pattern, with conservatives appropriating the classic liberal language of individual conscience and personal dignity to make their case against restrictive measures. By now it has become a conservative default to frame collective virus-containment efforts as a violation of fundamental personality rights, whether it be Trump calling on his supporters to 'LIBERATE MINNESOTA!' and 'LIBERATE MICHIGAN!', former Attorney General William Barr equating stay-at-home mandates with slavery, or conservative protesters repurposing the reproductive rights motto 'My Body, My Choice' by putting it next to crossed-out face mask pictograms.

The ideological inconsistency of this line of argument becomes particularly obvious when put in relation to the public security measures following 9/11. In the wake of the terrorist attacks, US society has seen a restrictive reorganisation of public life on an unprecedented scale. To this day, Americans of all ages are regularly subjected to intrusive controls and searches in quotidian situations such as taking public transportation or entering their workplace. Yet at no point in the past twenty years has visible conservative resistance formed under the banner of protecting individual liberties. A key reason for this may lie in the differently gendered paradigms. Unlike anti-terrorist legislation, which has been conceived within the 'masculine' militarist template of fighting an enemy, government efforts to stop the spread of the virus are understood mainly in terms of 'feminine' attributes such as sacrifice, passivity, mindfulness and caring. Put in colloquial terms, this behavioural package is simply 'uncool' within the value system of muscular US conservatism.

From freedom to responsibility: a shift in the national discourse

There have been targeted efforts to overcome this image problem. To evade the subtext of femininity, particularly male politicians have been prone to using mercenary metaphors, 'speak[ing] of their response as one of being at "war" with the COVID-19 "enemy", drawing upon discourses of militarism to emphasize supposedly "male" values of power, domination, and violence – and the rejection of "female" weakness and vulnerability'.[38] Most notably, in June 2020 anti-Trump Republican Liz Cheney launched the hashtag #RealMenWearMasks by posting a photograph of her father, former vice president and conservative icon Dick Cheney, donning a face mask and a cowboy hat. Aimed primarily at conservative men, the campaign essentially sponsored the message that 'wearing a mask is the testosteroney thing to do' by framing it as a manly act of protecting the weak and helpless. Alas, the crusade failed to gain much traction, with the sexist stigma remaining firmly attached to masks, social distancing, quarantining and vaccinations.[39] At the time of writing in July 2022, male Americans still lagged behind female Americans by approximately 10 million when it came to full vaccinations.[40]

A rationale commonly invoked by men for forgoing precautionary measures is that they are 'tough enough to beat the virus'. The problem with this mantra of assertive virility is that, apart from being medically illiterate, it fosters an inhumane survival-of-the-fittest mentality. Notions of being vigorous enough to brush off the infection 'risk implicitly writing off more vulnerable members of the community, when in reality, people have less control over their ability to survive the virus than they might like to believe'.[41] The sexist undercurrent in the COVID-19 debate is also reflected in the fact that vaccinations have graduated from being considered a mere sign of an unmanly character to being warned against as the actual cause of physical sterility or impotence, with notions of 'unvaccinated sperm' soon becoming a rare and valuable commodity proliferating on social media.[42] All this is evidence of how counterintuitive the conceptual shift from combat to caring, from competition to cooperation is for many men, especially if they subscribe to conservative notions of masculinity.

In this light, it is not surprising that, particularly in Republican strongholds like Florida, Texas, Alabama and Mississippi, surges in COVID-19 cases were accompanied by an intensification of conservative resistance to mask-wearing and vaccination mandates. The governors of these states not only refused to make mask-wearing mandatory in public spaces like schools and retail stores, but even went so far as to legally ban such mandates. It has often been suggested that Republican politicians' stalwart refusals to acknowledge the dangers of the virus were motivated by their fear of Trump and his supporters. While this may well be accurate, this conservative impasse was more fundamental in nature, going well beyond Trump's personal influence. What made it so hard for Republican leaders to change their stance on the pandemic is that acknowledging the need for broad government-mandated restrictions would have meant going against the very grain of a conservative ideology that combines libertarian freedom-from-government sentiments with masculinist ideals of robust individuality.

But in a remarkable recent development, conservative resistance has been met with a momentous shift in the national discourse over COVID-19. Whereas during the Trump presidency the main trope had been the clash of fact versus fiction, with Trumpian disinformation as the rival of scientific facts, the new leitmotif is balancing personal freedoms against public interest. This change in paradigm has come in the wake of the Biden administration's effort in the summer of 2021 to push the stagnating vaccine campaign by means of rules and incentives. 'I know people talk about freedom,' the president said in a press conference on 29 July 2021. 'But . . . with freedom comes responsibility.'[43] Echoing this view, Dr Anthony Fauci, Director of the National Institute of Allergy and Infectious Diseases, stated with uncharacteristic bluntness that in the face of the most devastating infectious disease in a century, 'you gotta say, liberties aside'.[44] Other public voices have censored 'this individualism garbage' and 'hyper-individualism' of the still-unvaccinated, which, in the words of news anchor Joe Scarborough, amounts to the notion that 'I have a right to infect my house, to infect my community, to kill everybody.'[45] One of the most memorable comments came from former California governor and ultimate Hollywood macho figure Arnold Schwarzenegger. 'Screw your freedom', was his unceremonious message to COVID deniers, 'because with freedom comes obligations.'[46]

What makes this discursive switch from individual suasion to civic duty so significant is that it moved the discussion out of the narrow context of Trumpism into the broader field of the long-standing American conflict between personal freedom and the common good. This amounts to the acknowledgement that US shortfalls in handling the pandemic are not exclusively a short-term product of the Trump administration's mismanagement and politicisation but also a long-term effect of ingrained cultural predispositions.

Conclusion

The COVID-19 pandemic has shaken America's status as global hegemon and leader in the fight against infectious disease. Even as the United States remains a powerhouse of medical research, its capacity to mount a robust response to the virus has been undermined by the instability of its domestic politics. This triggered a surge in narratives of American decline revolving primarily around the impact of the Trump presidency with its hyper-partisanship, anti-institutionalism, isolationism and hostility towards science. What has received far less attention is the embeddedness of the health crisis in a decades-long national debate about the meaning of American manhood. Supercharged by an individualistic cultural climate, the gendered symbolism that has been fuelling this partisan conflict is of a piece with an established conservative strategy of appealing to alienated White men by reframing economic and cultural anxieties in terms of gender identity. At the same time, it speaks to a liberal failure to adequately address the profound crisis of American masculinity that has been unfolding at the complex intersections of race, class, region and religion. Considering how much this ideological divide has been driven by affective reflexes as opposed to rational weighing of medical facts, it seems evident that mediating it will require a deeper acknowledgement of the mental disruptions experienced by men as a result of collective dislocations. Especially with a view to long-term solutions, this also entails a critical engagement with culturally imprinted individualistic assumptions concerning the relationship of self and society.

The aforementioned Missouri patient Daryl Baker is a quintessential example of how the pandemic challenged traditional notions of what it means to be a man. In an interview he gave from his ICU bed in summer 2021, he assured his family that he 'wasn't going to give up', especially for the sake of his young son. 'I'm that little boy's hero,' Barker said as he was struggling to breathe through oxygen tubes. 'I'm supposed to be the strongest person he knows.'[47] Barker's personal plight is a grim testimony to the fact that simplistic ideas of masculinity as physical dominance have become as glaringly dysfunctional as a political mindset that casts individual independence in opposition to social interdependence.

Notes

1. Ryan Bort, 'Take it From Them: Americans Hospitalized With Covid Regret Not Getting the Vaccine', *Rolling Stone*, 5 August 2021, available

at: https://www.rollingstone.com/politics/politics-features/covid-hospital-izations-unvaccinated-regret-1206032.

2. Carolina A. Miranda, 'US Individualism Isn't Rugged, It's Toxic – and It's Killing Us', *Los Angeles Times*, 30 October 2020, available at: https://www.latimes.com/entertainment-arts/story/2020-10-30/how-toxic-individuality-is-tearing-the-u-s-apart.

3. John Fabian Witt, *American Contagions: Epidemics and the Law from Smallpox to COVID-19* (New Haven, CT: Yale University Press, 2020), 13.

4. Kathryn Olivarius, *Necropolis: Disease, Power, and Capitalism in the Cotton Kingdom* (Cambridge, MA: Harvard University Press, 2022), 9; Nancy Tomes. '"Destroyer and Teacher": Managing the Masses During the 1918–1919 Influenza Pandemic', *Public Health Reports* (2010), available at: https://www.ncbi.nlm.nih.gov/pmc/articles/PMC2862334.

5. Wade Davis, 'The Unraveling of America', *Rolling Stone*, 6 August 2020, available at: https://www.rollingstone.com/politics/political-commentary/covid-19-end-of-american-era-wade-davis-1038206.

6. Amy Mackinnon and Robbie Gramer, 'Russia Scores Pandemic Propaganda Triumph with Medical Delivery to US', *Foreign Policy*, 1 April 2020, available at: https://foreignpolicy.com/2020/04/01/russia-scores-pandemic-propaganda-triumph-with-medical-delivery-to-u-s-trump-disinformation-china-moscow-kremlin-coronavirus.

7. Richard Wike et al., 'US Image Plummets Internationally as Most Say Country Has Handled Coronavirus Badly', Pew Research Center, 15 September 2020, available at: https://www.pewresearch.org/global/2020/09/15/us-image-plummets-internationally-as-most-say-country-has-handled-coronavirus-badly.

8. Sandy Ruxton and Stephen Burrell, *Masculinities and COVID-19: Making the Connections* (Washington, DC: Promundo, 2020), 17.

9. Ronald F. Levant et al., 'Masculinity and Compliance with Centers for Disease Control and Prevention Recommended Health Practices During the COVID-19 Pandemic', *Health Psychology* 41:2 (2022), 94–103.

10. Global Heath 5050, 'The Sex, Gender and COVID-19 Project', available at: https://globalhealth5050.org/the-sex-gender-and-covid-19-project/the-data-tracker/?explore=country&country=USA#search.

11. World Health Organization, 'WHO Coronavirus (COVID-19) Dashboard', available at: https://covid19.who.int.

12. Anton Golwitzer et al., 'Partisan Differences in Physical Distancing are Linked to Health Outcomes During the COVID-19 Pandemic', *Nature Human Behaviour* 4 (2020), 1186–97.

13. Jeffrey M. Jones, 'COVID-19 Vaccine-Reluctant in US Likely to Stay That Way', *Gallup*, 7 June 2021, available at: https://news.gallup.com/poll/350720/covid-vaccine-reluctant-likely-stay.aspx.

14. Joseph Biden, 'Inaugural Address by President Joseph R. Biden, Jr', *The White House*, 20 January 2021.

15. Sara Burnett, 'Whitmer Plot Underlines Growing Abuse of Women Officials', *Associated Press News*, 5 March 2022, available at: https://apnews.com/article/coronavirus-pandemic-health-business-michigan-gretchen-whitmer-afefc541df8d47d33c8032caf147e066.

16. Malachi Barrett, 'Sexist Attacks Cast Michigan Gov. Whitmer as Mothering Tyrant of Coronavirus Dystopia', *Michigan Live*, 22 May 2020, available at: https://www.mlive.com/public-interest/2020/05/sexist-attacks-cast-whitmer-as-mothering-tyrant-of-coronavirus-dystopia.html.

17. Nathan Layne and Gabriella Borter, 'Militia Members, Others Charged in Plot to Kidnap Michigan Governor; She Says Trump Complicit', *Reuters*, 8 October 2020, available at: https://www.reuters.com/article/uk-michigan-whitmer-idUKKBN26T37C.

18. Alicia Parlapiano, 'National Exit Polls: How Different Groups Voted', *New York Times*, 3 November 2020, available at: https://www.nytimes.com/interactive/2020/11/03/us/elections/exit-polls-president.html.

19. CNN, 'Exit Polls', availaable at: https://edition.cnn.com/election/2020/exit-polls/president/national-results.

20. Pew Research Center, 'An Examination of the 2016 Electorate, Based on Validated Voters', 9 August 2018, available at: https://www.pewresearch.org/politics/2018/08/09/an-examination-of-the-2016-electorate-based-on-validated-voters.

21. A historical overview of the polarisation of US politics over the question of masculinity is provided in *The Man Card: White Male Identity Politics from Nixon to Trump*, created by Jackson Katz, directed by Peter Hutchison and Lucas Sabean, Media Education Foundation, 2020.

22. Chris Megerian, 'Even Sick with COVID-19, Trump Refuses to Change Tune on Pandemic', *Los Angeles Times*, 5 October 2020, available at: https://www.latimes.com/politics/story/2020-10-05/even-sick-with-covid-19-trump-refuses-to-change-tune-on-pandemic.

23. Andrea Tantaros, 'Andrea Tantaros: Men Can Vote for Trump to "Get Their Masculinity Back"', *YouTube*, uploaded by Raw Story, 22 December 2015.

24. Kelefa Sanneh, 'Jordan Peterson's Gospel of Masculinity', *The New Yorker*, 5 March 2018, available at: https://www.newyorker.com/magazine/2018/03/05/jordan-petersons-gospel-of-masculinity.

25. Cf. Ruxton and Burrell, *Masculinities and COVID-19*, 20.

26. Kurt Andersen, *Evil Geniuses* (New York: Random House, 2020), 305–6.

27. For an in-depth discussion on how race and ethnicity impact mask-wearing adherence in connection with gender, see Brittany N. Hearne and Michael D. Niño, 'Understanding How Race, Ethnicity, and Gender Shape Mask-Wearing Adherence during the COVID-19 Pandemic: Evidence from the COVID Impact Survey', *Journal of Racial and Ethnic Health Disparities* 9:1 (2022), 176–83.

28. United States Census Bureau, 'Measuring Household Experiences during the Coronavirus Pandemic', 22 December 2021, available at:

https://www.census.gov/data/experimental-data-products/household-pulse-survey.html.

29. Yue Sun and Shannon M. Monnat, 'Rural–Urban and Within-Rural Differences in COVID-19 Vaccination Rates', *Journal of Rural Health*, 23 September 2021, available at: https://pubmed.ncbi.nlm.nih.gov/34555222.

30. James Chu, Sophia L. Pink and Robb Willer, 'Religious Identity Cues Increase Vaccination Intentions and Trust in Medical Experts among American Christians', *Proceedings of the National Academy of Sciences* December 2021, available at: https://pubmed.ncbi.nlm.nih.gov/34795017.

31. Annie Kibongani Volet et al., 'Vaccine Hesitancy among Religious Groups: Reasons Underlying this Phenomenon and Communications Strategies to Rebuild Trust', *Frontiers in Public Health*, 7 February 2022, available at: https://www.frontiersin.org/articles/10.3389/fpubh.2022.824560/full.

32. Tom Gjelten, 'For Evangelicals, a Year of Reckoning on Sexual Sin and Support for Donald Trump', *NPR*, 24 December 2018, available at: https://www.npr.org/2018/12/24/678390550/for-evangelicals-a-year-of-reckoning-on-sexual-sin-and-support-for-donald-trump?t=1661638511659; Samuel L. Perry, *Addicted to Lust: Pornography in the Lives of Conservative Protestants* (New York: Oxford University Press, 2019), 14.

33 Miranda, 'US Individualism Isn't Rugged, It's Toxic – and It's Killing Us'.

34. Robert N. Bellah et al., *Habits of the Heart: Individualism and Commitment in American Life* (Berkeley: University of California Press, 1985), 250.

35. Nina Eliasoph, *Avoiding Politics: How Americans Produce Apathy in Everyday Life* (Cambridge: Cambridge University Press, 1998), 128.

36. Kurt Andersen, *Fantasyland: How America Went Haywire* (London: Ebury Press, 2017), 174.

37. Robert Wuthnow, *American Mythos: Why Our Best Efforts to Be a Better Nation Fall Short* (Princeton, NJ: Princeton University Press, 2006), 160.

38. Ruxton and Burrell, *Masculinities and COVID-19*, 43.

39. Monica Hesse, 'Making Men Feel Manly in Masks is, Unfortunately, a Public-Health Challenge of Our Time', *Washington Post*, 27 June 2020, available at: https://www.washingtonpost.com/lifestyle/style/realmenwearmasks-may-be-helpful-but-the-fact-that-we-need-it-is-a-shame/2020/06/27/8f372340-b7eb-11ea-aca5-ebb63d27e1ff_story.html.

40. Centers for Disease Control and Prevention, 'Demographic Characteristics of People Receiving COVID-19 Vaccinations in the United States', available at: https://covid.cdc.gov/covid-data-tracker/#vaccination-demographic.

41. Ruxton and Burrell, *Masculinities and COVID-19*, 43.

42. Samantha Cole, 'Antivaxers Think Their "Pure" Semen Will Skyrocket in Value', *Vice*, 13 August 2021, available at: https://www.vice.com/en/article/epn8j4/antivax-semen-fertility-covid-vaccine-safe.
43. Joseph Biden, 'Remarks by President Biden Laying Out the Next Steps in Our Effort to Get More Americans Vaccinated and Combat the Spread of the Delta Variant', *The White House,* 29 July 2021.
44. Anthony Fauci, 'Slander: Dr Fauci Rebukes Rand Paul's Falsehoods | The Beat | MSNBC', *YouTube*, uploaded by MSNBC, 22 July 2021.
45. Tim O'Brian, 'Republicans Choose Cries of Freedom Over Science and Mandates', *YouTube*, uploaded by MSNBC, 9 August 2021; Joe Scarborough, 'President Biden Hopes to Revive Vaccine Effort With Rules, Incentives', *YouTube*, uploaded by MSNBC, 30 July 2021.
46. Arnold Schwarzenegger, 'With Freedom Comes Responsibility', *YouTube*, uploaded by Arnold Schwarzenegger, 11 August 2021.
47. Bort. 'Take it From Them'.

Conclusion

Gaetano Di Tommaso, Dario Fazzi and Giles Scott-Smith

This volume offers a complex and multifaceted image of US public health and how the challenge to improve people's welfare became interwoven with the building of modern America. The development of the public health system in the United States has overlapped with many crucial changes in the country's governance that have taken place since the early twentieth century. The expansion of citizenship and civil rights, the tremendous growth in economic productivity, and the emergence of an overpowering and all-encompassing concept of national security, among others, have profoundly modified the federal state's functions, operations and power projection. At the same time, the implementation of specific public health policies and reforms – regarding immunisation, sanitation and occupational safety, for example – has been at the core of the self-assigned, global mission that the country pursued during the American Century, and the liberal order Washington built around it.[1]

The contrast between these ambitions and the actual practices of American public health has been – and to a large extent still is – one of the most significant tests to American conceptions of democracy.[2] As the authors of the chapters presented in this volume recognise, the story of the public health system in America is one of expansion and progressive reform, as well as long-standing constraints and discriminations linked to cultural, economic, social and political determinants.

To better identify and explain such tensions, the contributors of this volume focus mainly on two inter-related issues. On the one hand, they explored the dynamic relationship between public health and the American state, looking at how the country's public institutions have coped with the growing need for care of people in the United States and, given Washington's increasingly global outreach, also abroad. On the other hand, they have problematised the role that public health has played in the shaping and evolution of American democracy. In doing so, they not only offered different case studies assessing how public health has further complicated the idea of US citizenship, but have also collectively contributed to critically examining public health as a crucial variable in the trajectory taken over the last century by American power.[3]

On the relationship between public health and the American state, one of the most straightforward takeaways from the analyses presented here is that the recurring appearance of public health threats favoured a progressive, albeit non-linear, expansion of the role and functions of the federal government. When confronted with public health crises, Washington has consistently stretched its authority and taken responsibility for coordinating and supervising national responses. The US government has, in other words, demonstrated a reactive stance in its management of public health crises, like many other healthcare systems worldwide.[4]

From this perspective, public health crises have been a booster for the transformation of American institutions at home. However, since such a process occurred while the United States was rising as a global power, this approach also allows us to see public health as a proving ground for America's ascendancy abroad. Indeed, rather than reading the evolution of public health in the United States simply as a story of piecemeal domestic reforms, this volume's essays confirm the idea that the growth of federal interventionism in public health, especially post-1945, was one of the many instruments through which the federal government tried to promote and project American power and ideology globally.[5] Public health became therefore one of the many battlegrounds of the Cold War – one in which citizens' well-being was instrumental to consolidating America's worldwide ambitions.[6]

However, these processes of simultaneous domestic expansion and outward promotion of Washington's public health management have been widely contested and constrained. At home, federal authority in the field of public health has been far from complete or independent during the last century, as most of this volume's chapters show. On the contrary, the US government has offered its responses to public health crises mainly through constant cooperation with both local institutions and private actors. As a result, the functioning of the federal healthcare system has been largely reliant on and intertwined with state regulations and private initiatives. The peculiar interdependence between the federal and state levels of governance in public health has been one of the central features of the US cooperative federalism during the American Century: social security programmes, Medicare and several other healthcare services have all historically depended on the interaction between federal and state agencies, which shared powers and assisted each other to safeguard local and national constituencies. As many of the case studies presented here show, such an interaction has at times evolved into a dialectical, if not often openly competitive and conflictual, relationship. The problem, in those cases, does not revolve around conflicts of attribution as much as the increasing polarisation affecting the United States, which undermines the legitimacy of the public health system and inter-institutional cooperation.[7]

Similarly, and in line with a consolidated historiographical trend, the chapters in this volume highlight the historical reliance of the US public health system on private organisations at home and abroad.[8] The combination of public and private healthcare initiatives, according to some of the previous chapters, has not only contributed to the blurring of the lines between public and private interests, but has also led to the progressive consolidation of a neoliberal, consumer-based model that, spearheaded by the United States, constitutes one of the most recent trends in global public health. To Naomi Rogers (Chapter 3) the historical origins of the increased role of private initiatives' in the US definition and execution of public health policies lay in America's own political identity. As Rogers explains, forms of opposition to the government's health plans and infrastructure have always been present in the American socio-political debate. Such forces, grounded on long-standing mistrust of public institutions as potentially disruptive of individual freedom, have limited the US government's room for manoeuvre in public health. In fact, once simple counterweights to the state in such a policy field, private entities are now becoming the main actors in the US healthcare system, raising numerous concerns directly connected to the second issue at the centre of this volume, namely, the role that public health plays in the definition and functioning of American democracy.[9]

The chapters presented in this volume have indicated that public health emergencies have simultaneously symbolised and deepened the crisis of American democracy insofar as they have mirrored and further aggravated socio-economic inequality. Indeed, while some of the most important US allies in Europe have adopted universalist models that could provide equitable and affordable access to healthcare resources, the American public health system has grown substantially as individualist and exclusionary.[10] The main reason for such a difference has been what Margaret Humphrey's book about malaria eradication in the United States defines as the 'peculiar nexus' between race and public health.[11] In that respect, most of this book's contributions confirm the country's difficulties in overcoming racial inequality when dealing with diseases.[12] Public healthcare in the United States has been historically pervaded and affected by institutional racism, which has conditioned how US citizens perceive their medical rights, from reproduction to access to treatment and disease prevention.

However, the discriminations of the American public health system, which per se are a manifestation of the many shortcomings of US democracy, have been deeply intersectional. As many chapters in this volume show, gender and class have been essential factors, in addition to race, in formulating official public health responses. In addition, the progressive and steady privatisation of healthcare services and the consolidation of neoliberal practices and policies have further corroborated the inherent uneven characteristics of a private-based model.[13] As a result, during the American Century we saw a reconceptualisation of the idea of the 'public', while formulating policy decisions has gone hand in hand with constantly renegotiating the notion of citizenship. Public health, thus, has come to represent a field in which American individualism, free-market ideology, capitalism and racial-based democracy have found some of its most profound embodiments.

Finally, the progressive securitisation of public health – a development characterising many public policy fields throughout the American Century – has further undermined the democratic features of public health in the United States since it has led to the subjugation of health policies and practices to security and political imperatives.[14] However, rather than looking at it only as the result of contemporary trends, this volume frames such a process in a broader historical context, one in which especially Cold War relations and goals become central to understanding the connections between disease, public health policy and America's global aspirations.[15] The trope of national security had a forceful comeback through President Donald Trump's polarising rhetoric characterising the COVID pandemic as the result of the global spread of a 'Chinese' virus, virtually equating public health threats to the actions of a supposedly hostile country. Unfortunately, this opportunistic political move has done nothing but exacerbate the difficulties in setting up an efficient and widely shared response to the ensuing crisis.

The chapters in this volume emphasise the contradictions and paradoxes of American public health policies: the country has been able to mobilise its almost unrestrained resources not only to the advantage of US citizens but actually to improve health worldwide. Scientific progress and medical developments have characterised the beginning and consolidation of the American Century, with a legacy still relevant today in terms of absolute standards of care and international institutionalisation of public health. At the same time, however, public health management's historical trajectory in the United States has shown how racial discrimination, social inequality, privatisation and market-oriented strategies can undermine public health objectives, social cohesion, institutional legitimacy and the country's leadership and authority in the global arena.

Notes

1. Elena Conis, *Vaccine Nation: America's Changing Relationship with Immunization* (Chicago: University of Chicago Press, 2015); Martin V. Melosi, *The Sanitary City: Urban Infrastructure in America from Colonial Times to the Present* (Baltimore, MD: Johns Hopkins University Press, 2010); David Cutler and Grant Miller, 'The Role of Public Health Improvements in Health Advances: The Twentieth-Century United States', *Demography* 42 (2005), 1–22.
2. Tara Templin, Joseph L. Dieleman, Simon Wigley, John Everett Mumford, Molly Miller-Petrie, Samantha Kiernan and Thomas J. Bollyky, 'Democracies Linked to Greater Universal Health Coverage Compared With Autocracies, Even in an Economic Recession', *Health Affairs* 40:8 (2021), 1234–42.
3. Natalia Molina, *Fit to Be Citizens? Public Health and Race in Los Angeles, 1879–1939* (Berkeley: University of California Press, 2006)
4. Christopher Hamlin, 'The History and Development of Public Health in Developed Countries', in Roger Detels, Martin Gulliford, Quarraisha Abdool Karim and Chorh Chuan Tan (eds), *Oxford Textbook of Global Public Health* (New York: Oxford University Press, 2015), 19–36.
5. Theodore M. Brown, Marcos Cueto and Elizabeth Fee, 'The World Health Organization and the Transition From "International" to "Global" Public Health', *American Journal of Public Health* 96:1 (2006), 62–72; Nicole Pacino, 'Stimulating a Cooperative Spirit? Public Health and US–Bolivia Relations in the 1950s', *Diplomatic History* 41:2 (2017), 305–35; Aiko Takeuchi-Demirci, *Contraceptive Diplomacy: Reproductive Politics and Imperial Ambitions in the United States and Japan* (Stanford: Stanford University Press, 2018); Deborah Kowal, *The China–US Partnership to Prevent Spina Bifida: The Evolution of a Landmark Epidemiological Study* (Nashville, TN: Vanderbilt University Press, 2015).
6. Bob H. Reinhardt, *The End of a Global Pox: America and the Eradication of Smallpox in the Cold War Era* (Chapel Hill: University of North Carolina Press, 2015); Erez Manela, 'A Pox on Your Narrative: Writing Disease Control into Cold War History', *Diplomatic History* 34:2 (2010), 299–323.
7. Anne Daguerre and Tim Conlan, 'Federalism in a Time of Coronavirus: The Trump Administration, Intergovernmental Relations, and the Fraying Social Compact', *State and Local Government Review* 52:4 (2020), 287–97.

8. Julia F. Irwin, *Making the World Safe: The American Red Cross and a Nation's Humanitarian Awakening* (New York, Oxford University Press, 2013); Josep L. Barona, *The Rockefeller Foundation, Public Health and International Diplomacy, 1920–1945* (London: Routledge, 2015); Benjamin B. Page and David A. Valone (eds), *Philanthropic Foundations and the Globalization of Scientific Medicine and Public Health* (Lanham, MD: Rowman & Littlefield, 2007).

9. Mariateresa Torchia, Andrea Calabrò and Michèle Morner, 'Public–Private Partnerships in the Health Care Sector: A Systematic Review of the Literature', *Public Management Review* 17:2 (2015), 236–61.

10. Jan E. Blanpain, 'Health Care Reform: The European Experience', in Institute of Medicine (US), *Changing the Health Care System: Models from Here and Abroad* (Washington, DC: National Academies Press, 1994).

11. Margaret Humphreys, *Malaria: Poverty, Race, and Public Health in the United States* (Baltimore, MD: Johns Hopkins University Press, 2001); W. Michael Byrd and Linda A. Clayton, *An American Health Dilemma: Race, Medicine, and Health Care in the United States, 1900–2000* (London: Routledge, 2001).

12. David Chanoff and Louis W. Sullivan, *We'll Fight It Out Here: A History of the Ongoing Struggle for Health Equity* (Baltimore, MD: Johns Hopkins University Press, 2022).

13. Sachin Silva and Juergen Braunstein, 'Opinion: How the Invisible Hand of the Free Market Screwed Up Coronavirus Testing in the US—And How To Fix It', *Project Syndicate*, 30 April 2020, available at: https://www.marketwatch.com/story/how-the-invisible-hand-of-the-free-market-screwed-up-coronavirus-testing-in-the-us-and-how-to-fix-it-2020-04-30, last accessed 7 November 2022.

14. Stefan Elbe, *Virus Alert: Security, Governmentality and the AIDS Pandemic* (New York: Columbia University Press, 2009).

15. Debra L. DeLaet, 'Whose Interests is the Securitization of Health Serving?' in Simon Rushton and Jeremy Youde (eds), *Routledge Handbook of Global Security* (London: Routledge, 2014), 339–48.

Index